HUMAN CANCER

ENCYCLOPAEDIA OF CANCER

Vol. IV

HUMAN CANCER

By

Dr. Amita Sarkar

Dept. of Zoology

Agra College

Agra (U.P.)

(India)

DISCOVERY PUBLISHING HOUSE PVT. LTD.

NEW DELHI-110 002

First Published-2008

ISBN 978-81-8356-356-7 (Set)

Published by:

DISCOVERY PUBLISHING HOUSE PVT. LTD.

4831/24, Ansari Road, Prahlad Street,
Darya Ganj, New Delhi-110002 (India)
Phone: 23279245 • Fax: 91-11-23253475
E-mail: dphbooks@rediffmail.com
dphtemp@indiatimes.com
Website: www.discoverypublishinghouse.com

Printed at:

Sachin Printers, Delhi-

Preface

Over the past 20 years, technological advances in molecular biology have proven invaluable to the understanding of the pathogenesis of cancer. The application of molecular technology to the study of cancer has not only led to advances in tumor diagnosis, but has also provided markers for the assessment of prognosis and disease progression. The aim of *Encyclopaedia of Cancer* is to provide a comprehensive collection of the most up-to-date techniques for the detection of molecular changes in cancer.

This book is intended to provide a relatively short overview of important concepts and notions on the molecular biology of human cancers, including many facts essential to find one's way in this field. It is, however, not meant to be compreshensive and probably cannot be, as our knowledge is rapidly growing.

The salient feature of this book is that it covers a wide range of molecular techniques and provides a source of information to readers at all levels. Although several books on cancer have been published in the last decade, most of either very shallow or cover few areas in depth. Rarely do they cover the broad spectrum of topics which would provide enough information for understanding the subject or provide simple protocols for execution of molecular change. In my opinion, this book can help the reader to easily understand the subject and also excecute the experiments very efficiently.

There can be no claim to originality except in the manner of treatment and much of the information has been obtained from the books and scientific journals available in the different libraries.

The author expresses his thanks to his friends and colleagues whose continue inspirations have initiated him to bring out this book.

The author is painfully aware of the shortcomings, errors and misprints that have crept in, and shall be greateful to receive suggestion for improvement of the next edition from all the readers.

The author expresses his gratitude to Mr. Wasan and staff of M/s Discovery Publishing House for their whole hearted co-operation in the publication of this book.

Author

CONTENTS

1

INTRODUCTION

Cancer is a complex disease occurring as a result of a progressive accumulation of genetic aberrations and epigenetic changes that enable escape from normal cellular and environmental controls. Neoplastic cells may have numerous acquired genetic abnormalities including aneuploidy, chromosomal rearrangements, amplifications, deletions, gene rearrangements, and loss-of-function or gain-of-function mutations. Recent studies have also highlighted the importance of epigenetic alterations of certain genes that result in the inactivation of their functions in some human cancers. These aberrations lead to the abnormal behavior common to all neoplastic cells: dysregulated growth, lack of contact inhibition, genomic instability, and propensity for metastasis.

The genes affected by mutations in cancer may be divided into two main classes: genes that have gain-of-function (activating) mutations, which are known as oncogenes; and genes for which both alleles have loss-of-function (inactivating) mutations, which are known as tumor suppressor genes. Close to 100 genes have been shown to play a role in the development or progression of human cancers, some of which have been implicated in a broad spectrum of malignancies, whereas others are unique to a specific type. Cancers can arise via the aberration of different combinations of genes, which in turn may be mutated, overexpressed, or deleted. The order in which these events occur has also proved to be important. For example, in breast cancer it has been proposed that at least 10 distinct gene alterations may be involved in disease initiation and progression. The study of colon cancer has shown that carcinogenesis is a multistage process involving the activation of cellular oncogenes, the deletion of multiple chromosomal regions, and the loss of function of tumor suppressor genes.

Technologic advances in molecular biology over the past 20–25 yr have led to a dramatic increase in the identification of the molecular processes involved in tumorigenesis. Over this period, the molecular basis of cancer no longer holds the mystery that it once did. It is, however, also clear that the knowledge that has been accumulated is insufficient to claim a total understanding of the mechanism of cancer development. This volume has brought together a number of relevant techniques by which genetic abnormalities occurring in cancer can be detected and analyzed. This, in turn, will give rise to other avenues of study, such as: how mutations affect function, how these genes are regulated, and how they interact with each other.

The mutational analysis of oncogenes and tumor suppressor genes can provide evidence for a specific association between these genes and tumor type. These genes can be altered during carcinogenesis by different mechanisms such as point mutations, chromosomal translocations, gene amplification, or deletion. Furthermore, these genes may be analyzed at different levels—DNA, RNA, or expressed proteins.

DNA Analysis

Mutational analysis can be performed using a variety of techniques. The amplification of specific regions of DNA or RNA by the *polymerase chain reaction* (PCR) has opened endless possibilities that can be used for the rapid and efficient detection of alterations, even single nucleotide changes. These PCR-based techniques rely on changes in electrophoretic mobility induced by altered single-stranded secondary structure (single-strand conformation polymorphism), by altered dissociation rates of the DNA fragments (denaturing gradient gel electrophoresis), or by RNase cleavage assays. PCR can also be used for the rapid and quantitative detection of chromosomal rearrangements, such as commonly observed in leukemia. PCR is designed to specifically amplify genomic fragments that are not normally contiguous and are, therefore, unique to that type of gene rearrangement. Converting the RNA to DNA with *reverse transcriptase* (RT) prior to the PCR stage is usually required for this assay. However, in some cases, genomic DNA can be used for the direct amplification of translocation break points. A variation on the PCR theme involves the use of DNA fingerprints to detect genetic rearrangements in cancer. The primers are often arbitrary or repeat (e.g., ALU) sequences, which will give, after electrophoresis, a DNA fingerprint that can be used for the detection of genetic abnormalities. Microsatellite repeats occur throughout the genome and can be used as markers for genetic alterations, usually for the loss of heterozygosity, which will indicate that a deletion has occurred that overlaps that specific marker. For specific genes involved in certain cancers, the mutational analysis can be carried out using a protein truncation assay. This assay involves the identification of abnormal polypeptides synthesized in vitro from RT-PCR products, and the truncating mutations are usually confirmed by sequence analysis.

RNA Expression Analysis

DNA microarray technology, which makes use of high-density two-dimensional oligonucleotide probe arrays containing hundreds or thousands of oligonucleotide probes, represents a powerful new DNA sequence analysis tool to test for a variety of genetic mutations. Hybridization to cDNA microarrays allows the simultaneous parallel expression analysis of thousands of genes. High-throughput gene expression profiling increasingly is becoming a valuable method for identifying genes differentially expressed in tumor vs normal tissues. Gene expression microarrays hold great promise for studies of human tumorigenesis, and the large gene expression data sets produced have the potential to provide novel insights into fundamental cancer biology at the molecular level. Indeed, cDNA microarray technology has already begun to aid in the elucidation of the genetic events underlying the initiation and progression of some human cancers. Differentially expressed genes can also be detected by other techniques such as differential display, which involves a random primed RT-PCR display or fingerprint of subsets of expressed RNA, or subtractive hybridization, which involves the enrichment of genes preferentially expressed in one tissue compared with a second.

Chromosomal Analysis

Fluorescence *in situ* hybridization (FISH) is one of the techniques with an expanding role in the molecular analysis of cancer. It can be used for the simple detection of numerical and structural chromosomal abnormalities that may occur in cancer cells and is particularly useful as a tool for the diagnosis of nonrandom translocations in leukemia and numerous other cancers. To date, most FISH studies have involved the use of single whole-chromosome or gene probes. This has been taken to new levels by the development of spectral karyotyping, which involves the hybridization of 24 fluorescently labeled chromosome painting probes to metaphase spreads in such a manner that simultaneous visualization of each of the chromosomes in a different color is accomplished. Using this method, it is possible to define all chromosomal rearrangements and identify all of the marker chromosomes in tumor cells. Comparative genomic hybridization (CGH) is a FISH-based technique that can detect gains and losses of whole chromosomes and subchromosomal regions. CGH is based on a two-color, competitive FISH of differentially labeled tumor and reference DNA to normal metaphase chromosomes and can scan the whole genome without prior knowledge of specific chromosomal abnormalities.

Analysis of Methylation Status

Some molecular methods will analyze specific changes to the DNA structure or genomic modifications. Changes in the DNA methylation status are one of the most common detectable abnormalities in human cancer. Hypermethylation within the promoters of selected genes is especially common and is usually associated with inactivation of the involved gene or genes and may be an early event in the pathogenesis of some cancers, whereas other genes become methylated during disease progression.

Telomere and Telomerase Activity

Telomeres are repetitive DNA sequences at chromosome ends, which are necessary for maintaining chromosomal integrity. A reduction in telomere length has been described in a wide range of human cancers, including both solid tumors and leukemias. The enzyme telomerase synthesizes *de novo* telomeric repeats and incorporates them onto the DNA 3' ends of chromosomes. Telomere shortening in normal cells is a result of DNA replication events, and reduction beyond a critical length is a signal for cellular senescence. However, the maintenance of telomere length, by the activation of the enzyme telomerase, is thought to be essential for immortalization of human cancer cells to compensate for the loss of DNA from the ends of chromosomes. Therefore, the measurement of telomere length and telomerase enzyme activity levels are important in monitoring disease progression or response to therapy. Recently, the possible manipulation of telomerase has generated some excitement as an anticancer strategy.

Clonal Origin of Cancer

The methods we have described allow the investigator to study the myriad of genetic alterations that can occur during the initiation, development, and progression of cancer. However, it is also possible to provide insight into the transition from somatic cell mutation to neoplasia. The clonal origin of cells can be assessed in patients with X chromosome-linked polymorphisms, taking advantage of the random inactivation of the X chromosome. The inactivation is related to the differentially methylated patterns on the active and inactive X chromosomes.

Common Types of Cancer

In 2003 more than 2 million new cancer cases were diagnosed in the United States alone, and in that same year, more than half a million Americans died of cancer. Cancer can strike anyone, but the risk increases with age, certain lifestyles, and the quality of the environment. Nearly 80 percent of all cancers are diagnosed in patients age 55 and older, and smokers are 20 times more likely to develop lung cancer than nonsmokers. Cancers can appear in any of our tissues and organs, but there are some tissues that are more susceptible than others: Skin cells and the epithelial cells lining the lungs and digestive tract are prominent members in this group. All of these tissues and organs are at the interphase between the external environment and our internal organs, and like a sailor on the mast, take the full force of the storm when it hits.

The skin is exposed to daily doses of ultraviolet (UV) radiation and a variety of chemicals in the environment. The lungs, while providing us with the oxygen we need to breathe, are exposed to many other gases, such as smoke and pollutants that happen to be in the air.Our digestive tract is in direct contact with the food and water that we consume; and much of what we eat and drink contains chemicals that are often unhealthy, many of which are known carcinogens or mutagens.

Some cancers, such as those affecting the brain, breasts, or prostate gland, do not have clear connections to lifestyle or the environment, but appear to be a consequence of normal physiology and cellular biochemistry. Our bodies, complex machines that they are, simply start to break down after many years, and cancer is one of the regrettable consequences.

The deadliness of a cancer varies depending on the tissue that is affected. Prostate cancer struck more than 200,000 American men in 2003, but the mortality was only 13 percent (that is, 28,900 men died of prostate cancer in the same year). By contrast, brain tumors have a mortality of 72 percent, and lung cancer is even worse,with a mortality of 88 percent. But the deadliest of all cancers are those that appear in the pancreas, where the mortality is a numbing 98 percent.

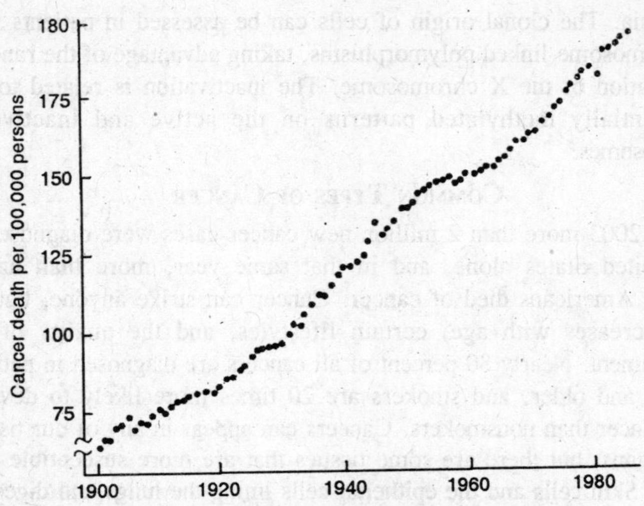

Fig. 1.1. Total deaths from cancer per 100,000 persons.

Table 1.1. New cancer cases and deaths

Cancer	*New Cases*	*Deaths*	*Mortality (%)*
Bladder	57,400	12,500	22
Brain	18,300	13,100	72
Breast	212,600	40,200	19
Digestive tract	204,400	89,200	44
Leukemia	30,600	21,900	72
Lymphoma	61,000	24,700	41
Liver	17,300	14,400	83
Lung	185,800	163,700	88
Mouth and throat	27,700	7,200	26
Pancreas	30,700	30,000	98
Prostate	220,900	28,900	13
Skin (melanoma)	54,200	7,600	14

The cancers shown in the table, and the seven covered in greater detail later in this chapter, kill millions of people worldwide every year. Brain tumors are described in this chapter; not because they are numerically common, but because of their notoriety, mortality, and the devastating effects they have on the patient's mental faculties.

TERMINOLOGY

Normal cells become cancerous through a process called *transformation*, leading to the uncontrolled growth of the cancer cells, which produces a *tumor* or *neoplasm*. As long as the tumor remains intact, and the cells do not try to invade other parts of the body, the tumor is called *benign*, and can easily be treated by surgical removal. Tumors become dangerous, and potentially deadly, when some of the cells develop the ability to leave the main tumor mass and migrate to other parts of the body, where they form new tumors; tumors like these are *malignant*, spreading the cancer by a process known as *metastasis*. Malignant cancers can be very difficult, if not impossible, to treat. The danger associated with all tumors is that they will switch from benign to malignant before being detected.

Cancers are classified according to the tissue and cell type from which they arise. Cancers that develop from epithelial cells are called *carcinomas*; those arising from connective tissue or muscles are called *sarcomas*; and those arising from blood-forming tissue, such as the bone marrow, are known as *leukemias*. More than 90 percent of all human cancers are carcinomas.

Cancer names are derived from their cell type, the specific tissue being affected, and whether the tumor is benign or malignant. An *adenoma*, for example, is a benign tumor originating in the adenoid gland, or other glandular tissue, that consists of epithelial cells. A malignant tumor from the same source is called an *adenocarcinoma*. A *chondroma* is a benign tumor of cartilage, whereas a *chondrosarcoma* is a malignant cartilage tumor. Some cancer names can be real tongue twisters: a type of leukemia that affects blood-forming cells is called *myelocytomatosis*.

Cancers generally retain characteristics that reflect their origin. One type of skin cancer called *basal-cell carcinoma* is derived from keratinocytes and will continue to synthesize keratin, the protein of hair and nails. Another form of skin cancer, called *melanoma*, is derived from pigment cells, and is associated with overproduction of the skin pigment melanin. It is for this reason that these tumors are usually very dark in color. Cancers of the pituitary gland, which produces growth hormone, can lead to production of excessive amounts of this hormone, the effects of which can be more damaging than the cancer itself.

Cancer progression is divided into five stages: *Stage 0* is noninvasive; that is, it has not begun to spread. *Stage I* and *stage II* mark the period when the cancer becomes malignant and begins to spread. At stage I, the tumor is no more than an inch across and the cancer cells have not spread beyond the organ or tissue in which it first appeared. Stage II tumors are still small (one inch or less) but have begun to spread to nearby tissues. A tumor that has increased in size to two inches, but has not begun to spread, is still at stage II. *Stage III* is a locally advanced cancer. In this stage, the tumor is large (more than 2 inches across) and the cancer has spread to nearby tissues. *Stage IV* is metastatic cancer. The cancer has spread to many other tissues and organs of the body. Correct staging is crucial for application of the appropriate therapy.

Bladder Cancer

This cancer is diagnosed in more than 50,000 people every year in the United States alone; it has a moderate mortality of 22 percent and appears to be especially sensitive to diet and the environment.

Anatomy

The bladder is a saclike organ that stores urine from the kidneys. Cancer cells appear in the epithelial cells that line the inside surface of the organ.

Risk factors

Bladder cancer is associated with several risk factors, or conditions that increases a person's chance of developing the disease: age, tobacco use, occupation, infections, race, and sex. The chance of getting bladder cancer increases dramatically with age. People under the age of 40 rarely get this disease. Cigarette smokers are six times more likely than nonsmokers to get bladder cancer. Pipe and cigar smokers are also at increased risk. Some workers have a higher risk of getting bladder cancer because of carcinogens in the workplace. Workers in the rubber, chemical, and leather industries are at risk. So are hairdressers, machinists, metalworkers, printers, painters, textile workers, and truck drivers. Being infected with certain tropical parasites increases the risk of developing bladder cancer. Caucasians are twice as likely as African Americans and Hispanics to get bladder cancer. (The lowest rates are among Asians.) Men are two to three times more likely than women to get bladder cancer.

Symptoms

Common symptoms of bladder cancer include blood in the urine, pain during urination, and frequent urination, or feeling the need to urinate without results. These are not sure signs of bladder cancer, since other problems, such as bladder stones, can produce similar symptoms.

Diagnosis

Bladder cancer is diagnosed with a simple physical exam, to check for obvious tumor growths; a urine test, to check for the presence of blood or cancer cells in the urine; X-ray photography of the bladder; and cystoscopy, whereby a lighted tube is inserted through the urethra to examine the lining of the bladder.

Staging

By stage 0, the cancer cells are found only on the surface of the inner lining of the bladder. This is called superficial cancer or carcinoma in situ. At stage I, the cancer cells are deep in the inner lining of the bladder, and by stage II they have spread to the underlying muscle tissue. By stage III, the cancer cells have spread through the muscular wall of the bladder to the layer of tissue surrounding the bladder. The cancer cells may have spread to the prostate gland (in men) or to the uterus or vagina (in women). By stage IV, the cancer extends to the wall of the abdomen or to the wall of the pelvis. The cancer cells may have spread to lymph nodes, the lungs, and many other parts of the body.

Brain Tumors

Although relatively rare, brain tumors are diagnosed in about 20,000 people in North America every year. Although the number of people affected is small compared with other forms of cancer, brain tumors are included here because they exact an especially heavy toll on those affected. Damage to virtually any area of the brain will leave its mark. Even if the tumor is removed or destroyed, the patient is often left with a lifelong disability.

Anatomy

The brain is divided into three major regions: the cerebrum, the cerebellum (a smaller area located at the lower-back of the brain), and the brain stem,which is continuous with the spinal cord. The brain, along with the spinal cord, is called the central nervous system and is constructed of three types of cells: the neurons, the astrocytes (star-shaped) and the oligodendrocytes, the latter two being supportive tissue to the neurons. The most common brain tumors are gliomas, which originate in the supportive glia tissue: Astrocytomas arise from astrocytes, and may grow anywhere in the brain or spinal cord. In adults, astrocytomas most often arise in the cerebrum. In children, they occur in the brain stem, the cerebrum, and the cerebellum. Brain stem gliomas occur in the lowest, stemlike part of the brain, where

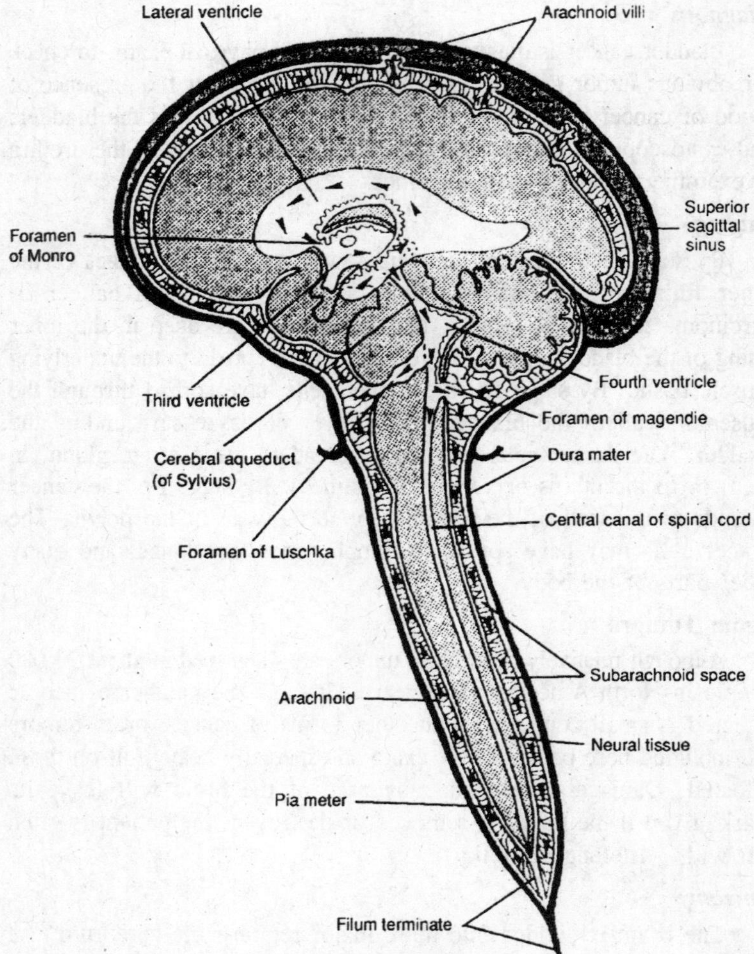

Fig. 1.2. Human nervous system.

they are difficult, if not impossible, to remove. Oligodendrogliomas arise in the glia cells that produce myelin, the fatty covering that protects nerves. These tumors usually arise in the cerebrum; they grow slowly and usually do not spread into surrounding brain tissue.

Brain tumors occur most often in middle-aged adults and are frequently secondary tumors; that is, tumors that originated in some other part of the body. Secondary tumors are named after the tissue of their origin. For example, a brain tumor that originated in the lung is called metastatic lung cancer, and the cells from such a tumor will resemble lung tissue, not neurons or glia cells.

Risk factors

The patient's age is the dominant risk factor. There is no clear link with lifestyle or environmental pollutants. Some people have suspected exposure to cell phone radiation, but this has not been proven, and several attempts to do so have met with failure.

Symptoms

The effect that tumors have upon the brain depends primarily on their size and location. Growing tumors may put pressure on surrounding tissue, damaging neurons and the many connections they make with other cells. Swelling and a buildup of fluid around the tumor also cause damage to the brain, a condition called edema. Tumors can also block the flow of cerebrospinal fluid, causing it to build up inside the brain, producing a condition known as *hydrocephalus*. Common symptoms of brain tumors include the following: headaches that tend to be worse in the morning and ease during the day; seizures; nausea or vomiting; weakness or loss of feeling in the arms or legs; stumbling or lack of coordination in walking; abnormal eye movements or changes in vision; persistent drowsiness; changes in personality, memory, or speech habits.

Diagnosis

Brain tumors are diagnosed primarily with a computed tomography (CT) scan or with magnetic resonance imaging (MRI). A CT scan is a series of detailed pictures of the brain that are created by a computer linked to an X-ray machine. In some cases, a special dye is injected into a vein before the scan, which increases tissue contrast. MRI produces computerized pictures of the brain that are based on the magnetic properties of the molecules in the tissue. A special dye may be used to enhance the likelihood of detecting a brain tumor.

Staging

Brain tumors rarely metastasize to other tissues or organs, but simply grow at their point of origin. Since damage to any part of the CNS is likely to have serious consequences, the main concern with a brain tumor is how fast it is growing. For these reasons, standard staging is not used. Instead, brain tumors are referred to as low, intermediate or high grade, with respect to their growth rate.

Breast Cancer

Other than lung and colon cancer, breast cancer is the most common type of cancer among women in North America, where more than 200,000 cases are diagnosed each year. Breast cancer also affects more than 2,000 men each year.

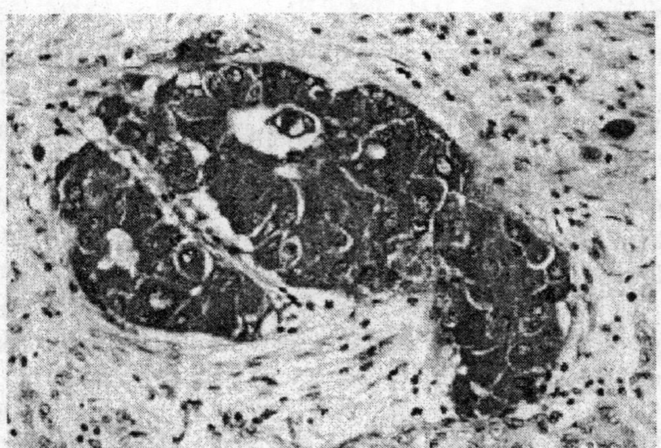

Fig. 1.3. Light micrograph of a carcinoma in human breast tissue

Anatomy

Each breast has 15 to 20 sections called *lobes*. Within each lobe are many smaller lobules. Lobules end in dozens of tiny bulbs that can produce milk. Thin tubes, called *ducts*, link all the lobes, lobules, and bulbs. These ducts lead to the nipple in the center of a dark area of skin called the *areola*. There are no muscles in the breast, but muscles lie under each breast and cover the ribs. The breasts also contain blood vessels and vessels for the lymphatic system, which consists of many lymph nodes found throughout the body. Many lymph nodes are found near the breast, under the arm, above the collarbone, and in the chest. The most common type of breast cancer is ductal carcinoma, which begins in the lining of the ducts. The second type occurs in the lobes and is called *lobular carcinoma*.

Risk factors

There are three major risk factors associated with both forms of breast cancer: mutations in two genes (BRCA1 and BRCA2), estrogen exposure, and late childbearing. The breast cancer genes 1 and 2 code for proteins that are needed to correct errors in DNA synthesis during the cell cycle. Estrogen is responsible for stimulating the breasts as part of normal reproductive physiology but over time may lead to the transformation of the duct cells. The connection between late childbearing and breast cancer is not clear.

Symptoms

There is no pain or discomfort associated with the early stages of breast cancer, which may produce a lump or thickening in or near the breast or in the underarm area; a change in the size or shape of the breast; nipple discharge or tenderness; or swelling, redness, or scaling of the skin of the breast, areola, or nipple.

Diagnosis

Breast cancers are diagnosed with a clinical breast exam, mammography, ultrasonography, and biopsy. The clinical exam is used to locate obvious lumps in the breast. It is often possible to tell if a lump is benign or malignant by the way it feels, how easily it moves, and its texture. Mammography uses X-rays to obtain a picture of the breast and any lumps that may be present. Ultrasonography uses high-frequency sound waves to determine whether a lump is a fluid-filled cyst (not cancer) or a solid mass (which may or may not be cancer). This exam may be used along with mammography. In some case, samples of a suspected tumor are obtained so the cells may be examined under a microscope. This procedure is referred to as a biopsy, and the tissue sample is usually collected with a hypodermic needle.

Staging

Stage 0 is noninvasive carcinoma. By stage I or II, the cancer has spread beyond the lobe or duct and invaded nearby tissue. At stage I the tumor is no more than an inch across, and the cancer cells are still inside the breast. Cancer cells begin to spread to underarm (axillary) lymph nodes by stage II. If the tumor increases in size to two inches but has not spread, it is still at stage II. Stage III is locally advanced cancer. The tumor is more than two inches across and the cancer has spread to the axillary lymph nodes and other nearby tissues. By stage IV, the cancer has spread beyond the breast to many other parts of the body.

Leukemia

Each year, nearly 32,000 adults and more than 2,000 children in the United States learn that they have leukemia, a cancer of the blood cells.

Anatomy

There are three different types of blood cells: red blood cells (RBC or *erythrocytes*), white blood cells (WBC, or *leukocytes*), and platelets (*thrombocytes*). Red blood cells contain hemoglobin and use it to carry oxygen from the lungs to the tissues. White blood cells do not carry oxygen but are part of the body's immune system. White blood cells are either lymphocytes (spend much of their time in the lymphatic system) or myeloid cells (spend much of their time in the

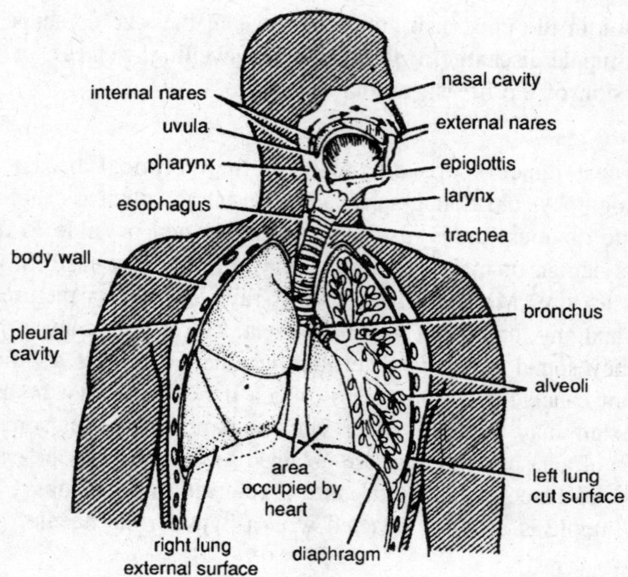

Fig. 1.4. The lungs are part of the respiratory system and fill most of the thoracic cavity. The trachea divides into two bronchial tubes, each of which branch out like a tree inside the lung. The branches are called bronchioles and terminate in grapelike clusters of alveoli, where gas exchange occurs between the air and the blood.

bone marrow or general circulation). Platelets are not complete cells but are fragments of certain kinds of leukocytes, and they are involved in blood clotting.

Leukemia affects white blood cells only and can arise in either lymphoid cells (lymphocytic leukemia) or myeloid cells (myelogenous leukemia). The disease has two forms: acute and chronic leukemia. Acute leukemia is a devastating disease that progresses very quickly, destroying the patient's immune system. Chronic leukemia progresses much more slowly, and even though the leukocytes are transforming, they retain some of their normal functions, so the immune system is not destroyed so quickly, or so completely.

Risk factors

The patient's age is the primary risk factor. Acute lymphocytic leukemia is the most common type of leukemia in young children and in adults who are 65 and older. Acute myeloid leukemia (also called *acute nonlymphocytic leukemia*) occurs in both adults and children. Chronic lymphocytic leukemia most often affects adults over the age of 55. It sometimes occurs in younger adults, but rarely affects children.

Chronic myeloid leukemia occurs mainly in adults. Very few children ever develop this form of leukemia.

Symptoms

Some symptoms of leukemia are fever, chills, and other flulike symptoms; weakness and fatigue; frequent infections; loss of appetite and/or weight; swollen or tender lymph nodes, liver, or spleen; easy bleeding or bruising; tiny red spots under the skin; swollen or bleeding gums; sweating, especially at night; and/or bone or joint pain. Leukemia metastasizing to the brain may cause headaches, vomiting, confusion, loss of muscle control, and seizures. Leukemia cells can also colonize the testicles, where they cause pain and swelling; the skin and eyes, where they produce sores; and many other organs and tissues of the body.

Diagnosis

The patient is examined for swelling in the liver, the spleen, and the lymph nodes under the arms, in the groin, and in the neck. A blood sample is examined under the microscope to check for abnormal white blood cells. The most definitive test is the microscopic examination of a bone marrow biopsy, which is obtained by inserting a needle into the hip and removing a small amount of bone marrow. If cancer cells are found, X-rays are obtained to evaluate the spread of the disease.

Staging

Staging is difficult to determine with this form of cancer, since the leukocytes normally travel throughout the body.Consequently, transformation and metastasis may occur simultaneously.

Lung Cancer

This cancer is very common and very deadly. More than 180,000 cases are diagnosed every year in the United States alone, and of these, nearly 90 percent die of the disease. Although it is one of the most deadly of all cancers, it is also the most preventable.

Anatomy

The lungs are a pair of cone-shaped organs that are part of the respiratory system. The right lung has three sections, called *lobes*, and is a little larger than the left lung, which has two lobes. When we breathe, the lungs take in oxygen, which our cells need to live and carry out their normal functions. When we exhale, the lungs get rid of carbon dioxide, a cellular waste product. Most lung cancers start in the epithelial lining of the bronchi, and occasionally in the trachea, bronchioles, or alveoli. All forms of lung cancer, being derived from epithelial cells, are carcinomas.

Risk factors

Scientists have discovered several causes of lung cancer, most due to atmospheric pollutants and the use of tobacco. The smoke from cigarettes, cigars, and pipes contains many compounds called *carcinogens* that can damage cells, leading to the formation of cancer. The likelihood that a smoker will develop lung cancer is affected by the age at which smoking began, how long the person has smoked, the number of cigarettes smoked per day, and how deeply the smoker inhales. Stopping smoking greatly reduces a person's risk for developing lung cancer. Environmental tobacco smoke, or second-hand smoke, is just as dangerous. Work-related exposure to radioactive gases, such as radon, and to asbestos dust is also known to cause cancer. Atmospheric pollutants, contributed by car and truck exhaust, are also believed to be risk factors, but the link is not proven.

Symptoms

Symptoms of lung cancer include a cough that doesn't go away and gets worse over time; constant chest pain; coughing up blood; shortness of breath, wheezing, or hoarseness; repeated problems with pneumonia or bronchitis; swelling of the neck and face; loss of appetite or weight loss and chronic fatigue.

Diagnosis

A chest X-ray to visualize possible tumors, and a lung biopsy are the most common methods used to diagnose lung cancer.

Staging

Lung cancer usually spreads to the brain and bones. CT scans and MRI are the most common methods for determining the stage of this form of cancer.

Prostate Cancer

Prostate cancer is the most common type of cancer in North American men. The number of men affected by prostate cancer is nearly equal to the number of women affected by breast cancer, but the mortality of prostate cancer is lower.

Anatomy

The prostate gland is part of the male reproductive system. It makes and stores portions of the seminal fluid, a fluid that is mixed with sperm to produce semen. The gland is about the size of a walnut and is located below the bladder near the base of the penis. It surrounds the upper part of the urethra, the tube that empties urine from the bladder. Because of its location, abnormal growth of the prostate can pinch the urethra, blocking the flow of urine. The prostate gland is regulated by the male sex hormone, testosterone.

Risk factors

Age, family history, and diet are the main risk factors. Prostate cancer usually occurs in men over the age of 55. The average age of patients at the time of diagnosis is 70. A man's risk of developing prostate cancer is higher if his father or brother has had the disease. This disease is much more common in African-American men than in white men. It is less common in Asian and American Indian men. Some evidence suggests that a diet high in animal fat may increase the risk of prostate cancer and a diet high in fruits and vegetables may decrease the risk. Studies are in progress to learn whether men can reduce their risk of prostate cancer by taking certain dietary supplements.

Symptoms

Common symptoms of prostate cancer are a need to urinate frequently, especially at night; difficulty starting urination or holding back urine; inability to urinate; weak or interrupted flow of urine; painful or burning urination; difficulty in having an erection; painful ejaculation; blood in urine or semen; or, in advanced stages, frequent pain or stiffness in the lower back, hips, or upper thighs.

Diagnosis

Digital rectal exam (DRE) and a blood test for prostate-specific antigen (PSA) are the methods used to diagnose prostate cancer. The patient's doctor inserts a lubricated, gloved finger into the rectum and feels the prostate through the rectal wall to check for hard or lumpy areas. The diagnosis, based on this simple procedure, is surprisingly accurate and informative. Confirmation of cancer, based on the DRE, is obtained by testing the patient's blood for the presence of PSA. PSA is a semen protein produced by the prostate, and under normal circumstances it should never appear in the blood. Blood that is positive for PSA is strong evidence of prostate cancer. This test is sometimes followed up with a biopsy and ultrasonography.

Staging

At stage I, the tumor cannot be felt during a rectal exam and there is no evidence that it has spread beyond the prostate. At stage

II, the tumor is large enough to be felt during a rectal exam, but is still noninvasive. By stage III, the cancer has spread outside the prostate to nearby tissues, and at stage IV, cancer cells have colonized the lymph nodes and many other parts of the body.

Skin Cancer

This is the most common type of cancer in North America,with 1 million cases being diagnosed each year. Nearly half of the North American population will develop some form of skin cancer by age 65. Although anyone can get skin cancer, the risk is greatest for people who have fair skin that freckles easily, often those with red or blond hair and blue or light-colored eyes.

Anatomy

The skin protects us against heat, light, injury, and infection. It helps regulate body temperature and stores water, fat, and vitamin D. The skin is made up of two main layers: the outer epidermis and the inner dermis. The epidermis is mostly made up of flat, scale-like cells called *squamous cells*. Under the squamous cells are round cells called *basal cells*. The deepest part of the epidermis also contains melanocytes, cells that produce melanin, which gives the skin its color. The dermis (just below the epidermis) contains blood and lymph vessels, hair follicles, and glands. These glands produce sweat to regulate body temperature and sebum, an oily substance that helps keep the skin from drying out. Sweat and sebum reach the skin's surface through tiny openings called *pores*.

The two most common kinds of skin cancer are basal cell carcinoma and squamous cell carcinoma. Basal cell carcinoma accounts for more than 90 percent of all skin cancers in North America. It is a slow-growing cancer that seldom spreads to other parts of the body. Squamous cell carcinoma also rarely spreads, but it does so more often than basal cell carcinoma. Another type of cancer that occurs in the skin is melanoma, which begins in the melanocytes. Melanomas are quick to metastasize and are often deadly. Basal cell carcinoma and squamous cell carcinoma are sometimes called nonmelanoma skin cancer.

Risk factors

The primary risk factor is excessive exposure to ultraviolet radiation. The use of sunscreens (particularly on children), hats, and protective clothing are strongly recommended for lengthy outdoor excursions.

Symptoms

The most common warning sign of skin cancer is a growth or a sore that does not heal. Skin cancers vary considerably in the way they look. Some begin as a pale waxy lump, whereas others first appear as a firm red lump. Sometimes, the lump bleeds or develops a crust. Skin cancer can also start as a flat, red spot that is rough, dry, or scaly. Both basal and squamous cell cancers are found on areas of the skin that are often exposed to the sun: the face, neck, hands, and arms. Actinic keratosis, which appears as rough red or brown scaly patches on the skin, is known as a precancerous condition because it sometimes develops into squamous cell cancer.

Diagnosis

Basal and squamous cell carcinomas are generally diagnosed and treated in the same way. When an area of skin does not look normal, all or part of the growth is removed and a portion of the biopsy will be examined under a microscope.

Staging

Basal and squamous cell carcinoma rarely spread beyond the skin. Melanoma, however, can metastasize to other tissues and organs. CT and MRI are commonly used to assess the invasiveness of malignant melanoma.

2

Cancer Around the World

Cancer has become one of the most devastating diseases worldwide. Every year, 10 million people are diagnosed with cancer, and of these, 6 million will die of this disease. Virtually every family, in every country of the world, has at least one member afflicted with this disease. The disease burden is immense, not only for the victims and their families, but for the medical establishments that struggle to meet the demand for care and treatment.

In 1948 the United Nations established the *World Health Organization* (WHO) to help people around the world attain the highest level of health. As part of the fight against cancer, WHO has collected data on the worldwide incidence of cancer to give governing bodies an estimate of the magnitude of the problem. This information has provided crucial insights into the causes of cancer and possibilities for treatment and prevention.

Magnitude of the Problem

Although there are more than 100 different forms of cancer, more than 80 percent of cases involve just 14 types of cancers. WHO has collected detailed information on each of these cancers for nearly every country in the world. Africa and South America are the only major regions of the world that record fewer than 1 million cases each year, while North America, Europe, and Asia have between 1 million and 3 million cases each year. When other regions of the world are included, such as the Philippines, Australia, and New Zealand, the combined total exceeds 10 million new cancer cases worldwide each year. The relatively low number of cases recorded in Africa and South America is partly due to inadequate diagnostic facilities, but it also reflects a real regional variation in cancer incidence.

The magnitude of the cancer epidemic defies the medical capabilities of most places in the world. Treatment in North America alone exceeds $1 billion each year, and for the millions of cancer patients who live in poorer countries, the treatments are unavailable or too expensive for the local population to afford. Wealthier countries can better afford cancer treatment; this is fortunate for them, since the highest incidence of nearly all cancers occurs in developed countries.

Developed Countries Have the Highest Cancer Rates

Of the 14 cancers, all but two occur with a higher incidence in developed countries (located in North America, Europe, and parts of Asia). The difference is often profound. Prostate cancer, is nearly six times more prevalent in developed companies than it is in undeveloped or less developed countries of the world (located in South America, Africa, and large parts of Asia). Skin cancer, specifically melanoma, is seven times more prevalent in developed countries, while the remaining cancers, are two to three times more prevalent in developed countries. There are two exceptions to this trend: stomach cancer, which occurs with about the same incidence in developed and undeveloped countries, and liver cancer, which is more common in undeveloped countries. The equalized incidence of stomach cancer may point to the ingestion of environmental carcinogens that are present throughout the world. The elevated incidence of liver cancer in less developed countries is likely due to the storage of grains in equatorial countries, which promotes the growth of a powerful fungal toxin that is known to cause liver cancer.

The data are averages, and thus they tend to obscure some of the more dramatic differences in cancer prevalence throughout the world. Individual comparisons between specific locations, show a striking trend for each type of cancer. Again, cancers tend to be more prevalent in developed countries, but in a specific comparison the magnitude of the difference is staggering. The incidence of prostate cancer in the United States is more than 60 times greater than it is in China. Liver cancer in Mongolia is almost 40 times more prevalent than is in Northern Europe, and stomach cancer in Japan is 12 times more common than it is in Africa. These differences are not due to genetic predispositions or resistance to cancers. Chinese people who move to the United States develop prostate cancer at a rate typical for the location. Similarly, West Africans develop colon cancer at a higher rate when they move to North America. Scientists interpret the worldwide variation in cancer rates as an indication that most cancers are caused by diet and lifestyle, and are therefore avoidable.

Cancer and the North American Diet

According to the U.S. Centers for Disease Control (CDC), 64 percent of Americans are overweight. The typical American diet is high in fat and calories, with insufficient quantities of whole grains, fresh fruits, and vegetables. Whole grain breads and cereals, along with fresh fruit and vegetables, are known to reduce the risk of cancer development, particularly colon cancer. The issue of high- versus low-fat diets has traditionally focused on improving an individual's resistance to cardiovascular disease and diabetes. But it has recently become clear that a high-fat diet is directly responsible for the high incidence of many cancers in the developed countries.

Fat has been thought of as a harmless substance, intended for the storage of energy, and historically, this has been the case. When human society was based on hunting and gathering there were periods of the year when individuals would deposit fat as a reserve for the winter months. During other periods of the year, when food was plentiful, the fat reserves were depleted and the individual's physique became slimmer. Women, during their reproductive years, store fat in preparation for childbirth, but again this deposit was transitory, so that men and women cycled between robust and lean physiques. However, in recent times, there has been a clear trend toward the deposition of permanent body fat, and research has shown a direct link between increased cancer rates and obesity.

Adipocytes, the cells that store fat, increase or decrease in number, depending on the amount of fat being consumed and used. The fat in high-fat diets cannot be metabolized at the rate that it is being ingested, and yet the digestive system is programmed to absorb as much as it can. Consequently, the unused portion is stored in adipocytes, which are capable of proliferating to meet the demand. In other words, development of obesity involves storage of fat and an increase in the number of fat-storing cells. Adipocytes were first identified around the turn of the 20th century, and for more than 90 years these cells were thought of as simple fat-storage depots. This perception changed dramatically in 1995, when several research groups in the United States and Europe discovered that adipocytes synthesize and secrete several growth factors, one of which is called *leptin*. Leptin has since been shown to be a potent growth factor, capable of stimulating the proliferation of many kinds of cells, including those of the pancreas, liver, lung, stomach, skin, and mammary glands. Even more remarkable is the observation that leptin stimulates the synthesis and secretion of estrogens by adipocytes and by other cells throughout the body, particularly in the ovaries and testes.

The realization that fat cells have an endocrine function came as a surprise to physiologists and endocrinologists. Normally, hormone production is regulated by an area in the brain called the hypothalamus, which in turn controls the pituitary gland, the so-called master gland of the body. Stimulation of the pituitary gland by the hypothalamus leads to the production and release of pituitary hormones that regulate the activity of secondary glands and tissues throughout the body. A specific example is the control of the ovaries and the reproductive cycle. In this case, the pituitary gland releases *follicle-stimulating hormone* (FSH), resulting in the growth and development of ovarian follicle cells. These cells, under the influence of FSH, begin to synthesize and secrete large amounts of the hormone estrogen. The physiological role of estrogen is to stimulate the growth and development of the mammary glands for eventual lactation, and of the uterine lining, in preparation for fertilization, implantation, and development of the fetus. The ovarian reproductive cycle is characterized by monthly fluctuations in the amount of estrogen released into the blood. After menopause, when the ovaries stop responding to FSH, the level of estrogen in the blood decreases and remains low thereafter. However, because of the endocrine function of adipocytes, obese women have chronically high levels of estrogen in their blood throughout their lives. The constant stimulation of cells in the breast, uterus, and other areas by estrogen and possibly leptin is believed to be the single most important cause of cancer development in these tissues.

Scientists have shown that obese women have much higher levels of estrogen (130 percent more) than do thinner women. A similar relationship is believed to influence the incidence of prostate cancer in men. In this case, the estrogen produced by the adipocytes overstimulates the cells in the prostate gland, thus increasing the risk of cancer development. The discovery of leptin and the endocrine function of fat cells provides a direct link between obesity and the high incidence of cancer in the developed world. Breast and prostate cancers are only two of the many cancers that are likely to be induced by a high-fat diet. Additional cancers, of the pancreas, liver, lung, stomach, and skin, may be attributable to both the elevated levels of sex steroids and to leptin.

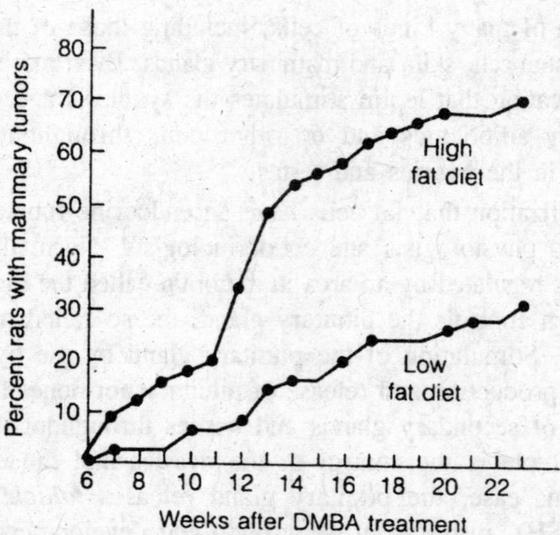

Fig. 2.1. Rate given the carcinogen dimethylbenzanthracene (DMBA) develop mammary tumours more often when given a high-fat-diet than when given a low-fat diet.

High fat content is only one element in the North American diet that predisposes people to cancer. A second, and very important, element is insufficient fiber in the diet. Dietary fiber is thought to protect against cancers in general, but most particularly colorectal cancer. Two epidemiological studies completed in 2003 examined the relationship between dietary fiber and colon cancer. These studies, involving 519,978 Europeans and 33,971 Americans, are unprecedented for their size and scope. Participants in the study completed a dietary questionnaire in 1992–98 and were followed up for cancer incidence. The results showed a clear inverse relationship between the incidence of colon cancer and intake of dietary fiber. In other words, high fiber intake is associated with a low incidence of cancer. No food source of fiber was more protective than others. That is, the fiber could come from bread, vegetables, or breakfast cereal. The authors of the studies concluded that in populations with low-fiber diets, an approximate doubling of total fiber intake from foods could reduce the risk of colorectal cancer by 40 percent. The American and European studies were both published in the May 3, 2003, issue of the medical journal *The Lancet*.

Cancer and Lifestyle

Although cancer risk increases with obesity and with lack of dietary fiber, many people who are not overweight and eat a healthy diet still develop cancer. A striking example is lung cancer induced by the smoke from cigarettes. This type of cancer is the product of a lifestyle

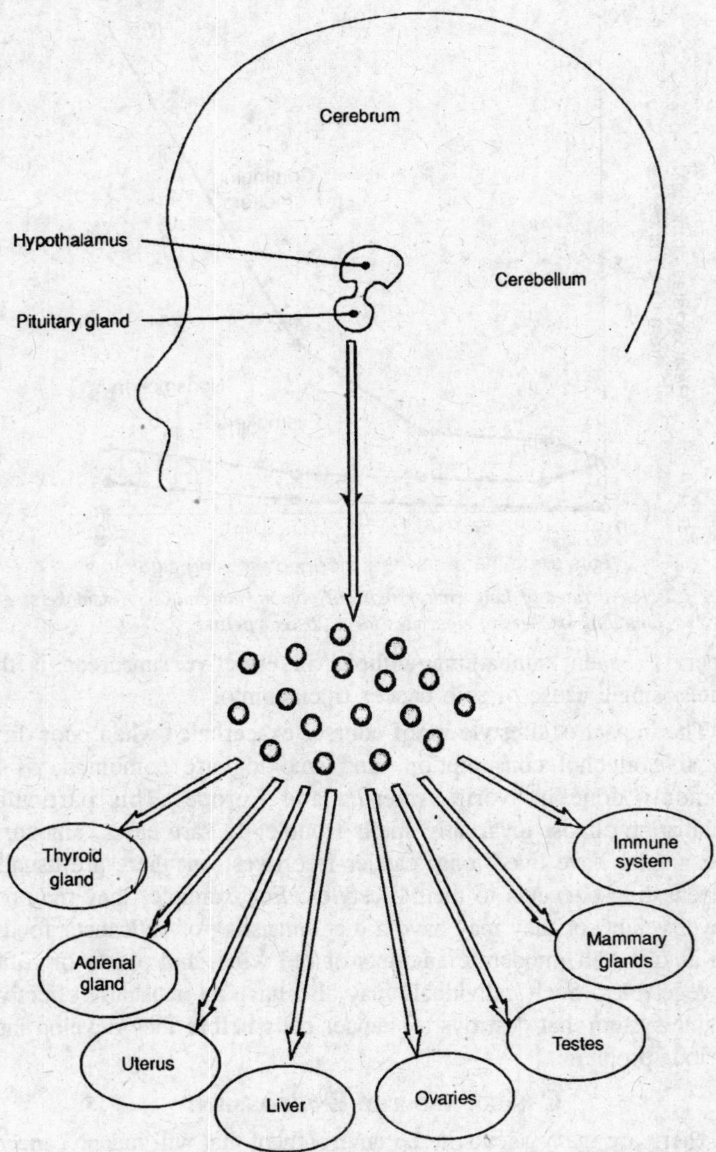

Fig. 2.2. The human endocrine system is controlled by the hypothalamus, which regulates the production and release of various hormones from the pituitary gland.

that counteracts the beneficial effects of a healthy diet and slim physique. Another lifestyle variable, excessive alcohol consumption, is associated with increased risk of various cancers, particularly liver

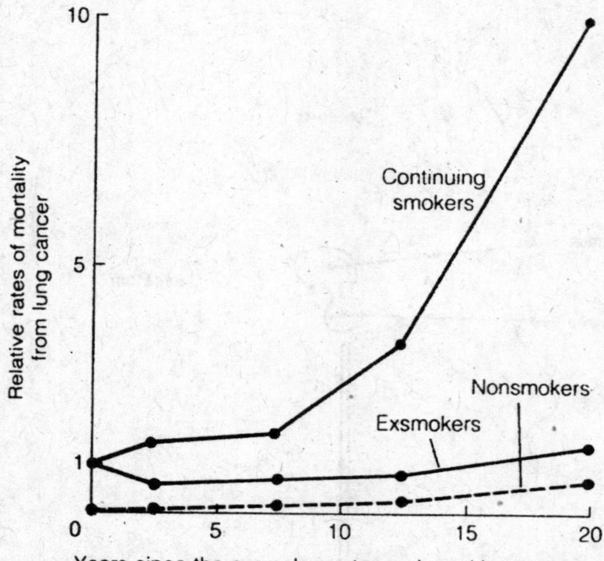

Fig. 2.3. Relative rates of lung cancer mortality among nonsmokers, exsmokers, and continuing smokers of cigarattes for a 20 year period.

cancer. Frequent sunbathing without an effective sunscreen is the greatest single cause of skin cancer (melanoma).

The impact of lifestyle is, of course, exacerbated when poor diet, excessive alcohol consumption, and smoking are combined, as is commonly done in North America and Europe. This particular combination almost invariably spells trouble. In rare cases, smokers, for example, have lived long, cancer-free lives, but there are usually compensating elements to their lifestyles. For example, they may not be overweight, or they may have a diet consisting of anticancer foods, such as olive oil, moderate amounts of red wine, and plenty of fruits and vegetables. Such individuals may also have an unusually effective immune system that destroys all cancer cells before they develop into a serious problem.

Cancer and the Environment

There are many agents in the environment that will induce cancers in people who are otherwise healthy and careful about what they eat and drink. The first involved a fungal carcinogen that causes liver cancer in people living in the tropics, and the second was asbestos, which damaged the lungs of British factory workers in the 1950s. The incidence of stomach cancer among the Japanese, shown in the table, may be due to the consumption of fish containing high pesticide or mercury residues.

Food additives, pesticides, and herbicides are believed to be responsible for causing cancers. While many of these compounds have been shown to be mutagens in vitro, there is very little evidence thus far to support their role as carcinogens. Much of the difficulty associated with confirming such a link stems from the problem of distinguishing the effects of a specific pesticide or herbicide from other factors, such as obesity or cigarette smoke. While food additives and pesticides may cause cancer, the number of cases resulting from these carcinogens is believed to be very small compared to the quantity arising from dietary practices (such as fat and fiber intake) and lifestyle.

Cancer is a disease of the genes, but the incidence of this disease is greatly influenced by what we eat and how we live. DNA, though a stable molecule, can be damaged by environmental compounds, radiation, and errors in replication that occur during the cell cycle. The cell has very efficient DNA repair systems, but they can only do so much.

A detailed comparison of cancer rates around the world has shown that most cancers are avoidable. DNA damage, at the heart of cancer induction, can be minimized with a careful attention to diet and lifestyle. A cancer-resistant diet is low in fat and high in fiber, fruits, and vegetables. A cancer-resistant lifestyle includes regular exercise, no smoking, regular use of a sunscreen, and moderate consumption of alcohol. Studies have shown that these simple measures can reduce the incidence of cancer by almost 40 percent, or 4 million cancer cases worldwide each year.

3

Skin Cancer

The skin is the largest organ and the most frequent site of cancers in humans. The life-time risk of skin cancer for fair-skinned individuals may now add up to 40%. Fortunately, the two most frequent subtypes, *basal cell carcinoma* (BCC) and *squamous cell carcinoma* (SCC), are rarely life-threatening. The rarer melanoma is and its incidence appears to increase alarmingly.

The most important carcinogen in the skin is UV radiation. It is incriminated by a clear correlation of incidence with exposure and by typical mutations found in skin cancers, i.e. point mutations at dipyrimidine sequences. This is a paradigmatic example for molecular epidemiology, which aims at determing the causes of cancer from the mutation patterns observed. In skin cancer, UV radiation acts not only as a mutagen, but also by altering gene expression in epidermal keratinocytes and mesenchymal dermal cells. It also modulates immune responses in skin.

The incidence of skin cancer is strongly influenced by inherited genetic variation. At the population level, skin pigmentation is the most obvious factor modulating risk. Individuals with inherited deficiences in the repair of UV-damaged DNA are at even greater risk, prominently xeroderma pigmentosum patients. In a different fashion, *PTCH1* in BCC, certainly, *ESS1* in SCC, perhaps, and *CDKN2A* in melanoma, in rare cases, behave as classical '*gatekeeper*' tumor suppressors predisposing to skin cancer.

Basal cell carcinoma consists of undifferentiated keratinocytes resembling basal cells of the epidermis. They often carry *TP53* mutations which show the diagnostic signature of being induced by UV radiation.

Other consistent mutations lead to constitutive activation of the hedgehog pathway. This pathway normally helps to maintain basal cells in a precursor state. Its activation explains the morphological appearance of BCC. BCC cells exhibit mutations in either an inhibitory or an activatory component of the hedgehog pathway. Most inactivating mutations affect PTCH1, which is a classical tumor suppressor. Germ-line mutations in *PTCH1* occur in the Gorlin syndrome which predisposes to BCC and selected other cancers. This syndrome encompasses developmental defects which occur without mutations in the second copy of *PTCH1*, i.e. by haploinsufficiency. Alternatively, hedgehog pathway overactivity in BCC is caused by mutations that activate the SMO membrane protein. So, *SMO1* as an oncogene.

In normal skin, the main reservoir of proliferating keratinocytes consists of basal cells from which the upper protective layers of the skin are formed by terminal differentiation. This '*transient amplifying*' fraction of cells can be replenished from stem cells. Normally, hedgehog activity is restricted to precursor cells. Its constitutive activation in BCC appears to confer a precursor cell phenotype to the tumor cells.

In SCC, keratinocyte differentiation is more advanced but proliferation does not cease. Regularly, UV-induced *TP53* mutations are found, with LOH on 17p. Additional LOH is found on chromosomes 9 and/or 13q, and may signify loss of cell cycle control by $p16^{INK4A}$ and RB1. Together, these changes could account for blocked cell cycle exit and immortalization in SCC.

Melanoma develops from melanocytes which synthesize protective pigments. They have a different developmental origin than keratinocytes, viz. neural crest cells which migrate to the epidermis during fetal development. Melanomas are often highly invasive and form metastases much more readily than BCC and SCC. Melanoma cells maintain the expression of differentiation antigens specific for melanocytes such as gp100 and tyrosinase. In addition, they express '*cancer testis antigens*' which occur otherwise only in male germ cells. These antigens may be targets of host anti-tumor immune responses and are exploited in (experimental) immunotherapy, for which melanoma seems a promising target.

Although epidemiology does not link the causation of melanoma as clearly to UV exposure as that of SCC and BCC, typical point mutations are found in many cases. They activate either the *NRAS* or the *S BRAF* gene, which likely stimulate *F* cell proliferation and cell migration. These mutations may be complemented by mutations in

TP53, *CDKN2A*, *CDK4*, and *PTEN* that may inactivate the mechanisms by which inappropriate proliferation induces apoptosis or replicative senescence. Altered responses to melanocyte-specific growth factors may also contribute to melanoma development.

Carcinogenesis in the Skin

The skin is the largest organ in humans. As it covers and protects our external surface, it is subject to mechanical damage and is exposed to a variety of potential carcinogens, chemicals, infectious agents, and radiation alike. Thus, a strong capacity for repair and regeneration is mandatory. This requirement is met by continuous turnover of the epidermis in a structural arrangement that minimizes the impact of carcinogenic agents and protects the body as a whole and the skin itself from cancer development.

The outmost layer of the epidermis ('*stratum corneum*') is composed of crosslinked dead keratinocytes filled with filamental proteins. This layer forms a barrier that rejects many infectious agents, reacts with chemicals and absorbs radiation. The underlying layers ('*stratum granulosum*' and '*stratum spinosum*') are formed by living cells which are irreversibly committed to terminal differentiation. Therefore, genetic changes afflicted upon these cells become rarely permanent, because the cells are destined to becoming incapable of proliferation, losing their nuclei, and being eventually eliminated by shedding. Even the basal layer of epithelial cells in the skin, to which proliferation activity is largely confined, consists mostly of cells with a limited replicative potential. They form the transient amplification compartment. The actual stem cells of the skin are rare and are thought to proliferate normally very slowly, except during wound repair. Nevertheless, even then, the brunt of expansion is borne by the transient amplifying fraction.

Another factor in the protection against infection and carcinogenesis is the immune system of the skin. Langerhans cells are dendritic cells which present antigens for recognition by T-cells to elicit immune response against infectious agents and cancer cells.

Melanocytes help to protect specifically against light by producing melanin pigments which are deposited in the keratinocytes. As they differentiate, they carry the pigments to the upper layers of the skin. The extent of pigmentation is the most obvious factor modulating skin cancer risk.

In spite of its intricate protective system, the skin is the most frequent site of cancers in humans. The combined life-time risk for all skin cancers is estimated as 30-40% for lightly pigmented (Northwestern) Europeans, albeit lower for others according to pigmentation. Three different types of skin cancer are prevalent, in decreasing order *basal cell carcinoma* (BCC), *squamous cell carcinoma* (SCC), and melanoma. Conversely, melanoma is by far the most lethal of these cancers, in ≈ 20% of all cases. SCC metastasizes only rarely, and BCC almost never.

The incidences of all three types of cancer have increased over the last decades, often steeply. This is particularly worrying in the case of the life-threatening melanoma. The presumed cause of the rise is an increased exposure to UV-rich sunlight. While the risk of skin cancers is modulated by a variety of genetic factors, short wavelength light is the most important exogenous carcinogen in the skin. Accordingly, most skin cancers, SCC and BCC, and to a lesser degree melanoma, develop in light-exposed areas of the skin.

UV light is categorized by wavelength into UVC (200-280 nm), UVB (280-320 nm), and UVA (320-400 nm). UVC cannot penetrate the upper layer of the skin, but ≈ 0.4% of UVB and a few percent of UVA reach the basal layer of the epidermis. Some UVA even penetrates into the dermis, as does most visible light. How much UVA and visible light reaches the deeper layers of the skin depends on the intensity of pigmentation.

Exposure to sunlight has a range of effects on the skin. At moderate doses, it is beneficial, while higher doses of UV-rich light are problematic. In DNA, UVC can induce single-strand and double-strand breaks and even ionization of bases by direct action. Like ionizing radiation, it also generates reactive oxygen species like hydroxyl radicals that damage DNA by reaction with bases and with the deoxyribose-phosphate backbone. The typical consequence of UVC exposure encountered by living cells is therefore death.

The effects of UVB are more subtle and therefore more dangerous. UVB can be absorbed by DNA, albeit weakly, and lead to photoproducts like thymine dimers and thymine-cytosine 6-4 adducts. These are normally removed by nucleotide excision repair. Hereditary defects in nucleotide excision repair cause xeroderma pigmentosum which is characterized by greatly enhanced photosensitivity and risk of skin cancers.

Extensive DNA damage by UV radiation elicits activation of cellular checkpoints, and activates TP53 which can initiate apoptosis. This happens at a large scale during '*sunburns*'. In many skin cancers, inactivation of *TP53* therefore appears to be a necessary initiating step, which has to take place before further mutations can be acquired. Indeed, *TP53* mutations can be detected in morphologically altered, but non-cancerous regions of the skin.

UVA is only weakly mutagenic, but induces cellular reactions in different skin cell types such as modulation of immune responses, altered cytokine production, and activation of stress responses and proliferative signaling pathways. It is now thought that alterations of cellular interactions also contribute to the carcinogenic effect of UV radiation and are elicited by UVA as well as UVB. Diminuation of immune surveillance by inhibition of dendritic Langerhans cells and cytotoxic T-cells may be particularly important. In fact, even manifest carcinomas of the skin often still respond to treatment with stimulators of T-cell responses such as '*imiquimod*'.

The complex mode of UV action illustrates that carcinogenesis requires more than mutations in DNA. Typically, it involves an altered tissue environment, in which tumor cells can more easily proliferate, escape from interactions with normal neighboring cells, and evade immune responses. Strong carcinogens, therefore, elicit such tissue reactions as well as a high rate of mutations. For instance, tobacco smoke inhalated in the lung also acts by several means including, of course, mutagenesis by polyaromates like benzopyrene, but also cell death with tissue repair, chronic inflammation induced by tar and particles, and a direct inhibitory effect of (nonmutagenic) nicotine on normal cells in the tissue.

Squamous Cell Carcinoma

Squamous cell carcinomas (SCC) are composed of differentiated epithelial cells, which show many typical markers of differentiated keratinocytes like keratins, involucrin, and other structural proteins. However, unlike normal keratinocytes SCC cells do neither cease to proliferate nor undergo cell death, and the tissue becomes severely disorganized. Squamous cell carcinomas develop from precursor lesions such as actinic keratoses. They sometimes progress to invasive and even metastatic tumors.

Almost invariably, SCC show mutations in the *TP53* gene and often LOH at 17p, where the gene is located. Such mutations are also highly prevalent in actinic keratoses. Activation of TP53 is responsible for the apoptotic death of epidermal cells during sunburns. The cells that survive may do so, because they have acquired mutation in the gene. This may set the stage for the eventual development of skin cancers.

Typically, *TP53* mutations in skin and skin carcinomas such as SCC are located at pyrimidine-pyrimidine dinucleotides identifying them as caused by UV radiation. Absorption of UVB by DNA causes Py-Py dimers, either cyclobutane or 6-4 photoproducts. These are usually removed by nucleotide excision repair, but in rare cases they are bypassed by error-prone DNA synthesis, e.g. using DNA polymerase . In this type of repair, if the damaged dipyrimidine cannot be read, the sequence AA is inserted by default. This makes sense in so far, as thymine-thymine dimers are most frequent. However, TC and CC dinucleotides are misrepaired in this strategy. Therefore UVB induces TC$\rightarrow$TT or CC$\rightarrow$TT mutations at pyrimidine dimer sites. These are exactly the mutations most frequently found in *TP53* in SCC and other skin carcinomas, implicating UVB as the responsible carcinogen.

This relationship is an example of molecular epidemiology. If a particular molecular alteration can be related to a specific carcinogen, it is possible to determine to which extent cancers are caused by that carcinogen. For instance, carcinogenic aflatoxins add to a specific guanine in the *TP53* gene, causing 249G$\rightarrow$T mutations. By following this particular change, it can be proven that aflatoxins contribute to a large proportion of hepatomas in Africa and Asia, but not in Europe or North America. This approach has its limits, however, because many carcinogens do not leave specific fingerprints or several carcinogens can leave the same one. For instance, it was thought for a while that C$\rightarrow$T mutations at CpG sites were mostly due to an increased rate of mutation of methylated cytosines following spontaneous deamination, which would exculpate exogenous carcinogens. More recently, however, methylated cytosines were shown to preferentially react with several activated carcinogens, re-opening this issue to debate.

Inactivation of TP53 in SCC is thought to lead to diminished apoptosis and to favor genomic instability. A second consistent change in this cancer is loss of chromosome 9, in particular of the short arm harboring the *CDKN2A* gene. Loss of $p16^{INK4A}$ is clearly involved in the progression of actinic keratosis to carcinoma. It may contribute to deregulation of the cell cycle leading to continuing proliferation and failure of terminal differentiation of the tumor cells. In some SCC, losses of 13q are found which would be suspected to lead to decreased or abolished RB1 function with basically the same biological outcome as $p16^{INK4A}$ loss. Loss of either $p16^{INK4A}$ or RB1 is found in many human carcinomas, particularly those with a more differentiated phenotype.

While *CDKN2A* is generally accepted to represent the critical target of 9p loss in SCC, the relevant gene affected by the likewise frequent loss of 9q is not known. In basal cell carcinoma of the skin and a limited range of other cancers, the loss contributes to a decreased function of *PTCH1*. This change is clearly not involved in the development of SCC. Instead, a locus tentatively named *ESS1* in the 9q22-31 region has been implicated through linkage analysis in a small number of families and seems to behave as a classical tumor suppressor.

Several further prevalent alterations in SCC are characteristic of a wider range of epithelial cancers.

1. Loss of 3p is not only frequent in SCC of the skin, but also in SCC of the head and neck, which has a different etiology, and in lung cancers. In these cancer types, it may be the frequent chromosomal change. Loss of 3p is even diagnostic for clear-cell carcinoma of the kidney where it contributes to lack of the *VHL* gene function that constitutes the gatekeeper event in this tumor type. *VHL* remains functional in other cancers, including skin SCC. Therefore, other potential tumor suppressor genes on 3p are thought to be more important in SCC. Good candidates are *RASSF1A* and *RARB2*. RARB2 is a receptor for retinoic acid which is known to regulate proliferation and differentiation particularly of the epidermis.
2. Either *KRAS* or *HRAS* are mutated in SCC, at moderate frequencies. Perhaps, *S* inactivation of RASSF1A which relays a signal limiting RAS action, occurs as a complementary change to these mutations. RAS activation by mutation is certainly pleiotropic and may yield a proliferative signal mainly through the MAPK pathway and/or an anti-apoptotic signal through the PI3K pathway. In either case, it may contribute to independence of external growth factors.
3. Overactivity of the EGFR as a consequence of gene amplification or autocrine stimulation by EGF-like factors would be expected to have similar consequences. Again, this is a widespread change in human carcinomas, occuring in some at an early stage of development, while being associated with progression and metastasis in others. SCC of the skin appears to belong to the latter group. As in general, it is not clear why this is so. One speculation goes as follows. Proliferation in normal epidermis is regulated by

paracrine interactions with mesenchymal cells in the underlying dermis. Increased EGFR activity may diminish the dependence of the cancer cells on paracrine stimulation and enable them to survive in a wider range of environments, thus creating one prerequisite for invasion and metastasis.

Table 3.1. Prevent genetic changes in different cancer of the skin

Squamous cell carcinoma	*Basal cell carcinoma*	*Melanoma*
TP53 mutation and LOH	TP53 mutation and LOH oncogenic SMO activation	TP53 mutation and LOH
Chromosome 9q loss	HRAS mutation	HRAS or BRAF mutation
Chromosome 13q loss		Chromosome 6q loss
Chromosome 3p loss		PTEN inactivation
EGFR overexpression		Loss of TGFβ response

In summary, thus, while skin SCC appears less malignant than most other carcinomas, it is prototypic, showing an assembly of alterations also found in these cancers. These alterations comprise inactivation of the TP53 and RB1 regulatory systems, activation of RAS-dependent pathways, EGFR overactivity, and 3p loss.

Basal Cell Carcinoma

Among those carcinomas that are very different from SCC of the skin is basal cell carcinoma of the skin. Whereas the tumor cells in SCC resemble differentiated keratinocytes, those in basal cell carcinoma look similar to those of the basal layer and indeed carry their typical markers such as basal cell cytokeratins (CK5 and CK14) and integrins ($\alpha_2\beta_1$). However, while they proliferate like basal cells, they do not differentiate. Furthermore, proliferation in the tumor is no longer restricted to cells in the basal layers.

The crucial genetic alterations in BCC lead to constitutive activation of the hedgehog (SHH) pathway. Normally, this pathway is activated in the skin by binding of SHH (sonic hedgehog) to the PTCH1 (patched) protein. This relieves the inhibition of SMO (smoothened) by PTCH, turning the SHH intracellular signal cascade on. The steps following SMO activation are not precisely known, but may involve an activating G-protein and be subject to some form of regulation by protein kinase A. The next components definitely known are Fused and SUFU (suppressor of fused) which are part of a protein complex located at microtubules. This complex binds GLI transcription factors maintaining them in an inactive state.

Three GLI proteins are known in humans. Of these, GLI1 and GLI2 are activated by SHH in basal cells of the skin. The factors migrate to the nucleus to activate target genes of the pathway. Among the proteins induced – directly or indirectly – are activators of cell growth and proliferation like Cyclin D1 and MYC, and the transcription factor gene FOXM1, but also PTCH1 and another membrane protein HIP1, which serves as a feedback inhibitor of the pathway together with PTCH1. GLI1 and GLI2 are also regulated by SHH signaling.

The activity of the SHH pathway is normally restricted to a subset of the basal cells in the epidermis and is thought to define these cells as keratinocyte precursor cells with stem cell character. It is not clear how the restriction to this subset is achieved. Perhaps, the NOTCH pathway, which is capable of repressing hedgehog signals, may be involved. If so, it would be plain why the NOTCH pathway tends to be inactive in BCC.

Constitutive activation of the SHH pathway in BCC can occur by one of several mechanisms. Most frequently, the function of *PTCH1* is lost by inactivation of both alleles. The *PTCH1* gene is located at 9q22. Many BCC show LOH in this region and inactivating mutations in the remaining allele. Not surpringly, as UVB is also implicated as a carcinogen in BCC, some mutations in *PTCH1* show the characteristic signature of this carcinogen.

Since PTCH1 inactivation leads to increased activity of the SHH pathway, of which it itself is a transcriptional target, BCC overexpress the mRNA of mutated *PTCH1*. In fact, a hallmark of SHH pathway activation is the overexpression of several target genes including those encoding GLI factors and HIP1.

PTCH1 is also the gene mutated in the germ-line of patients with nevoid basal cell carcinoma syndrome (NBCCS or Gorlin syndrome), a rare autosomal dominantly inherited disease. Patients develop multiple nevi and BCC at a relatively young age, even during childhood or more frequently around puberty. Like sporadic BCC, those in Gorlin syndrome also preferentially develop in light-exposed areas. Moreover, LOH at 9q22 is found in these tumors. Thus, *PTCH1* is a classical tumor suppressor gene in the Knudson definition and belongs to the 'gatekeeper' class. Gorlin syndrome patients are also at risk for a selected range of other cancers, including medulloblastoma. Indeed, many sporadic cases of this type of brain tumor, but not of others such as glioma, also contain mutations in SHH pathway genes. One pecularity sets Gorlin syndrome apart from other '*gatekeeper*' cancer syndromes. Patients often present with a characteristic range of developmental abnormalities, mostly of the skeleton. These do not seem to require inactivation of the second *PTCH1* allele or a dominant-negative function of the mutated gene product. Hedgehog signaling is crucially important during development. So, in some organs, expression of one intact *PTCH1* allele may not suffice to ensure proper regulation of the pathway. Thus, *PTCH1* may display haploinsufficiency with regard to its function in human development. Clearly, this begs the question whether haploinsufficieny of the gene may also occur in the context of tumor development.

The second most frequent alteration leading to constitutive SHH signaling in BCC – and actually in medulloblastomas as well – are point mutations in *SMO1*. These mutations occur in specific sites and lead to constitutive activity of the protein. In particular, they abolish regulation of SMO by PTCH1. For a while, it was thought that the mutations affected the interaction between the two proteins. Now, it is assumed that PTCH1 regulates SMO indirectly and in a non-stochiometric fashion by directing a low-molecular inhibitor towards it. So, the mutations may prevent binding of this – unknown – inhibitor. As *PTCH1* has to be regarded as a tumor suppressor, *SMO* is obviously a proto-oncogene which is activated by specific point mutations.

Inactivation of *PTCH1* and oncogenic activation of *SMO* are very likely not the only alterations which can lead to SHH overactivity in BCC. Mutations in *PTCH2* have already been observed, and others are expected, since the pathway is not yet fully elucidated. Moreover, distinct modes of activation may take place in other cancers. For instance, amplification of a region at 12q where *GLI1* is located close to *HDM2* may not only lead to overexpression of HDM2, but also of GLI1.

An entirely different mechanism appears to be at work in *small-cell lung cancer* (SCLC). SCLC could be regarded also as sort of a stem-cell cancer, in so far as it is composed of neuroendocrine cells who are thought to be produced by activation of tissue stem cells. In this case, however, an autocrine SHH loop may be responsible for over-activity of the pathway. This mechanism has also been observed in some pancreatic carcinomas.

Of course, activation of the SHH pathway is not the only alteration in BCC. Other genetic changes do occur and are probably required for development as well as progression of this cancer. As in SCC, RAS mutations are observed and TP53 is very frequently inactivated. It may be significant, however, that alterations in the RB1 pathway do not seem to be as essential in BCC as they are in SCC.

In addition to BCC and SCC, there are further cancers derived from the wider keratinocyte lineage. Keratinocytes share precursor cells with the cells of the hair bulges and the sebaceous glands from which rarer tumors can arise. These are again characterized by different patterns of genetic alterations, such as activation of the WNT pathway in hair follicle tumors.

This suggests two alternative possibilities how the diverse tumors may arise. One possibility is that each type of cancer is formed by different mutations in the common tissue precursor cell: Mutations impeding the RB1 regulatory system might lead to SCC because keratinocytes can differentiate, but not exit from the cell cycle, whereas mutations activating the SHH pathway would arrest the development of keratinocytes at the basal cell stage, etc. The second possibility is that cells at a more advanced stage of commitment and differentiation might require different types of genetic alterations to turn them into tumor cells. For instance, activation of the SHH pathway would not be possible or would not be able to induce tumor formation once a certain stage of keratinocyte differentiation has been reached. Whichever of these alternatives holds, the elucidation of the molecular basis of skin cancers has made very clear that specific molecular therapies need to be directed at different targets in BCC, SCC, and other skin cancers.

Melanoma

The third most frequent cancer of the skin, melanoma, is derived from melanocytes. These cells belong to a distinct cell lineage as keratinocytes. During development, melanocyte precursors migrate from the neural crest to the basal layer of the skin. Melanocytes specialize in synthesizing the pigment melanin from tyrosine. The enzymes of melanin biosynthesis, such as tyrosinase, are only expressed in this cell type. The insoluble pigment is transported by dendritic processes to surrounding epidermal keratinocytes and deposited in them. Differentiating keratinocytes transport melanin to the upper layers of the skin where it absorbs visible and UV light, protecting the living cells of the skin.

Skin pigmentation in man is highly variable. It ranges from a complete lack due to mutations in tyrosinase ('*albino*') to very intense, e.g. in populations from equatorial Africa. In most humans, pigmentation is inducible in response to sun exposure. It is regulated by interaction of melanocytes with the neighboring keratinocytes and by the hormone αMSH (*melanocyte stimulating hormone*).

The hormone acts specifically on melanocytes because they express the MC1R receptor. This is a classical '*serpentine*' receptor coupled to trimeric G_s proteins that activate adenylate cyclase. As in all cell types, increased cAMP activates protein kinase A which induces transcription through the CREB transcription factor. Specifically in melanocytes, CREB induces another transcriptional activator, MTF, which is actually responsible for the induction of melanocyte-specific genes and increased production of melanin. In normal melanocytes proliferation is also dependent on MSH.

The differences in pigmentation and its inducibility are categorized as '*skin types*' by dermatologists. For instance, persons with skin type I have low pigmentation and very little inducibility, whereas persons with skin type II have also relatively pale skins, but develop some pigmentation in response to sun-light. Skin type I is prevalent in Northern and Northwestern European populations, presumably as an evolutionary adaptation to less intense sun exposure. Therefore, travel and migration of Northern European to areas with intense sun exposure is a major factor in the alarming rise of skin cancer incidence in these countries and in states like Australia with a high proportion of immigrants from Northern Europe. Skin types are mostly caused by polymorphisms in the MSH receptor MC1R. *MC1R* is thus a cancer predisposition gene.

Melanoma is a much more lethal cancer than BCC and SCC, because of its stronger invasive and metastatic potential. However, many genetic alterations in this cancer are not too different from those in SCC, in particular. Frequent chromosomal losses affect chromosomes 9p and 17p and contribute to inactivation of *CDKN2A* and *TP53*. The second alleles of these genes are subject to point mutations. These carry occasionally the signature of UVB carcinogenesis, but not as regularly as in BCC and SCC. In many cases, *CDKN2A* is inactivated by homozygous deletions which obliterate expression of $p14^{ARF1}$ in addition to that of $p16^{INK4A}$ and in many cases $p15I^{NK4B}$ as well. The overall effect of these changes would be loss of function of the TP53 and RB1 regulatory systems contributing to immortalization, loss of cell cycle control, and genomic instability.

In melanoma, loss of $p16^{INK4A}$ function may be particularly important. In some of the families prone to melanoma development, germ-line mutations in *CDKN2A* were found which inactivate p16[INK4A] or at least diminish its function as an inhibitor of CDK4 in biochemical assays. In fact, in a few families with predisposition to melanoma, mutations were detected in *CDK4*, always affecting the part of the kinase to which the p16[INK4A] inhibitor binds. Of note, in melanoma-prone families, an association between UV exposure and cancer development is maintained. So, this may be regarded as a border-line case between high-risk gene mutations and mutations modulating the sensitivity to exogenous agents.

Germ-line mutations in *CDKN2A* have also been observed in patients with pancreatic cancers, and melanomas, too, have occurred in these families. However, germ-line mutations in *CDKN2A* do not lead to a severe generalized cancer syndrome such as the Li-Fraumeni-syndrome caused by TP53 mutations. This is certainly unexpected in view of the frequent inactivation of the locus in a wide range of human cancers.

Further chromosomal losses in melanoma affect chromosomes 3p, 6q, and 10q. At 10q, the *PTEN* gene is likely involved, and as in many other human cancers, this may an important step during progression.

A further set of alterations in melanoma activate the canonical MAPK pathway. Activating mutations in the *NRAS* gene occur in a subset of melanomas. In a complementary fashion, the *BRAF* gene harbors mutations that lead to an increased *F* activity of the protein kinase. There are multiple pathways emerging from RAS and three different RAF genes and proteins in humans. The complementarity of these mutations indicates that the MAPK pathway is particularly important in tumor formation by activated RAS and that BRAF, among the three protein kinases, is the one transducing the most relevant signals. However, since this constellation has, so far, been found in a restricted number of cancers, it could reflect a cell-type specific '*wiring*' of the MAPK signaling network.

There is also some evidence for altered responses to melanocyte-specific growth factors like αMSH in melanoma.

Finally, the most pressing question is of course, what makes melanoma so much more invasive than SCC and BCC? Several points are discussed in this regard. (1) Melanocytes are ontogenetically derived from a highly mobile and migratory cell type. So, they may easily fall back into a '*fetal*' pattern of behavior. (2) Melanocytes are very peculiarly located. They sit as single cells at the basis of the epithelium and while they maintain cell-cell-contacts with keratinocytes, these are flexible and certainly not comparable to the multiple junctions between proper epithelial cells. So, it may be less complicated for them to dissociate from the epithelium and grow or migrate into the dermis. (3) There are more molecular changes in melanoma typically associated with invasion and metastasis. Melanoma appear to express higher levels of certain metalloproteinases, they exhibit more consistently down-regulation of responsiveness to TGF, and they express chemokine and cytokine receptors that may allow '*homing*' to certain metastatic sites.

Tumor Antigens

Diminished immune responses to tumor cells are thought to constitute one component in the initial carcinogenic action of UV radiation. Immune responses remain important, however, during tumor progression. In the case of melanoma, the tumor cells may be particularly immunogenic, although this does obviously not present an insurmountable obstacle to tumor progression. However, immune cells directed against tumor cell antigens can be detected in melanoma patients. Several different types of tumor cell antigens can be recognized.

Cell-type Specific Antigens

Melanocytes express specific proteins which are not found in any other cell-type. These comprise, of course, the enzymes and proteins involved in melanin production such as tyrosinase, but also surface proteins like gp100.

Viral Antigens

Some tumor cells harbor viral genomes. SCC of the skin, e.g., often contain HPV genomes and consequently present viral antigens on their surface. While the role of HPV in SCC etiology is debated, the expression of viral proteins may aid in containment of these cancers.

Oncofetal Gene Expression

Many cancers express ectopic proteins. Some of these are normally expressed only in the respective fetal tissues and are therefore called oncofetal antigens. *Carcinoembryonic antigen* (CEA) in gastrointestinal tumors and α-fetoprotein (AFP) in liver cancers belong to this category.

Cancer-testis Antigens

Melanoma cells strongly express a somewhat different type of ectopic markers, called '*cancer testis antigens*'. These proteins, comprising several MAGEs, GAGEs, etc. each, are otherwise only expressed in testicular tissue in adult humans. It is not clear, why these genes are also activated in melanoma, or in some other cancers. Reactivation is often associated with promoter hypomethylation, but this is probably not sufficient.

In the majority of cases, obviously, immune cells directed against such antigens cannot eliminate the cancer completely. It is thought, however, that they limit its progression and it is hoped that the immune response towards cancer antigens can be harnessed for the purpose of '*immune therapy*'.

4

Stomach Cancer

Stomach cancer (or *gastric cancer*) is the second most frequent cause of cancer death worldwide with almost 1 million new cases per year. It poses a serious health problem because of its low cure rate and its severe impact on the quality of life. Fortunately, its incidence has plummeted in many industrialized countries for several decades. The causes of this unique decrease are presumed in improved hygiene, altered diet, and widespread use of antibiotics reducing the prevalence of *Helicobacter pylori* infection.

Helicobacter pylori infection is associated with most cases of stomach cancer. About 50% of the world population carry strains of the bacterium, but <10% develop inflammatory disease and ulcers, and even fewer stomach cancer. The outcome of the infection is determined by genetic variability of the germ and of the host which act in a strongly synergistic fashion. In the bacterium, variations in babA2, cagA, and vacA genes and in the host, polymorphisms in cytokine genes, particularly *IL1B*, influence the risk of chronic inflammation, ulcers, and cancer. Furthermore, carcinogenesis is dependent on cofactors, such as dietary carcinogens and protective ingredients.

Most stomach cancers arise in the antrum and corpus. The predominant histological subtypes are the intestinal type and the diffuse type. The intestinal type develops from gastric atrophy in areas of intestinal metaplasia. The highly invasive diffuse type consists of small groups of easily scattering undifferentiated cells. Both histological types share some alterations such as the TP53 inactivation. Intestinal metaplasia is associated with altered expression of transcription factors that regulate the segmentation of the gut tube during fetal development. From benign metaplasia, intestinal-type gastric cancer develops in a fashion resembling colon carcinoma in some respects.

The most distinctive alterations in diffuse-type stomach cancers are mutations of the *CDH1* gene encoding E-Cadherin. Rare familial cases of this cancer type are caused by germ-line mutations in E-Cadherin. So, *CDH1* behaves as a classical tumor suppressor gene in this specific cancer type.

The decreased incidence of '*classical*' gastric cancer in industrialized countries is partly offset by a rising incidence of cancers of the esophagus and the upper parts of the stomach. These cancers are associated with alcohol consumption and smoking, and they may be promoted by enhanced acidity of the stomach juice as a consequence of *H. pylori* eradication. They are also typically associated with metaplasia.

Etiology of Stomach Cancer

Worldwide, about 900,000 persons are diagnosed with stomach cancer (or '*gastric cancer*') each year, making it the second most frequent cancer. Since the 5 year survival rate is 3 – 20%, it is also one of the most lethal malignancies. Survival most strongly depends on the tumor stage at diagnosis. Cures can be achieved by complete or partial surgical removal of the stomach. As with many other metastatic carcinomas, chemotherapy is only marginally successful.

While stomach cancer thus clearly remains a major health problem worldwide, the situation is at least improving in many developed countries. For almost 50 years now, the incidence rates have steadily declined in Western Europe and North America. This fortunate decline would be admirable, if it had been achieved by conscious human intervention. It was, however, not and only to a small degree caused by improvements in diagnosis and therapy. Instead, the decline in stomach cancer incidence appears to be associated with an altered life-style, in particular with improvements in food quality and with the use of antibiotics. It is important to understand the causes underlying this decrease as thoroughly as possible, not only to further reduce the incidence of stomach cancer in the industrialized countries, but even more to address the problem in those developing countries where high incidence rates persist.

Like liver cancer, gastric cancer most often develops in the context of chronic inflammation, named '*chronic gastritis*' in the stomach.

However, chronic inflammation in this organ is not caused by viruses like HBV and HCV and less strongly by alcoholic drinks. Rather, the crucial agent is a bacterium, *Helicobacter pylori*.

Again as in the liver, complex interactions between the host and the pathogen determine whether chronic inflammation ensues at all and whether it develops further towards cancer. Moreover, some of the co-carcinogens and protective factors are the same, as alcohol abuse and diets low in fresh fruit and vegetables increase the risk of cancers in both organs. Even the role of aflatoxins in the liver may have its complement in the stomach, where dietary nitrosamines are thought to act as mutagens. These factors appear to act in a synergistic fashion, although bacterial infection may be the most crucial prerequisite.

Table 4.1. Causes of stomach cancer cancer

Individual factors causing stomach cancer in humans
Helicobacter pylori
Nitrosamines
Low consumption of fresh fruits and vegetables
Alcohol
Tobacco smoking
Genetic predisposition by high risk gene mutations (*CDH1*)
Genetic predisposition by polymorphisms (*IL1B*)

Accordingly, the geographical differences in the incidence of gastric cancer can be ascribed to a combination of factors. They appear to result from a synergistic effect of eridication of *Helicobacter pylori* by antibiotic treatment (intentional or incidental) and improvements in food quality. Importantly, stomach cancer is the only clear-cut example of a human cancer caused by bacterial infection. It may not be the only one, though, since bacterial infections causing chronic infections may also lead to an increased risk of cancers in other organs. Another well-documented case of infections causing cancer involves a trematode parasite, *Schistosoma mansoni*, which induces chronic inflammation, metaplasia and a metaplastic cancer, squamous cell carcinoma, in the urinary bladder. With the change in gastric cancer incidence in industrialized countries, the localization of the cancers within the stomach and the relative frequencies of the histological subtypes have also changed. Whereas formerly the vast majority of stomach cancers originated in the lower parts of the stomach, i.e. the corpus (body) and antrum, an increased proportion of cases now originates in the upper sections, the fundus and cardia. In fact, this shift may continue further upwards within the gastrointestinal tract, since the decreased incidence of stomach cancer appears to be accompanied by an increased incidence of carcinoma in the esophagus. The shift between the histological subtypes takes place, because the decrease in incidence is stronger for the '*intestinal*' than the '*diffuse*' subtype, which are the major histological subtypes of stomach cancer.

The intestinal subtype develops in metaplastic areas. Normally, the surface of the stomach is lined by a simple columnar epithelium in which several different cell types reside. Chief cells produce the protease precursor pepsinogen and enteroendocrine cells secrete peptides and transmitters regulating the function, but also the growth of intestinal and gastric cells. Parietal cells secrete hydrochloric acid to generate the low pH in the stomach. These cells are located in pits, which are protected by mucus produced by epithelial surface cells.

During intestinal metaplasia, this well-organized structure is replaced by a glandular epithelium which resembles the villous structure of the intestine. Metaplasia of the stomach epithelium precedes the development of cancer. It is one of several clearly defined '*preneoplastic*' stages in the development of intestinal type stomach cancer. As in the liver, most cancers in the stomach arise in a context of chronic inflammation, i.e. gastritis. Chronic gastritis in some cases progresses to an atrophic stage from which intestinal metaplasia develops. Initially, well-differentiated glandular structures are formed, which can develop into benign and increasingly dysplastic adenomas progressing towards invasive carcinomas.

The histological progression of diffuse-type stomach cancer is less well documented. This carcinoma is named for its its characteristic histology. It presents as small groups of loosely attached, highly invasive and undifferentiated tumor cells proliferating into the tissues underlying the gastric mucosa and metastasizing through the peritoneum.

Both types of stomach cancer are linked to *Helicobacter pylori* infection, although the relationship to the intestinal subtype is stricter. Patients with the diffuse type cancer are on average younger, whereas intestinal-type stomach cancer usually develops through several preneoplastic stages in older people after decades of gastritis.

Molecular Mechanisms in Gastric Cancer

The two major histological subtypes of stomach cancer share many genetic alterations, e.g. *TP53* mutations. Other alterations differ significantly between them and account for typical characteristics of each subtype.

The crucial molecule in the diffuse type is E-cadherin. This 882 amino acid membrane glycoprotein mediates homotypic adhesion between epithelial cells. It connects to the cytoskeleton by way of the catenins, of which β-Catenin doubles as a signaling molecule in the WNT pathway and a transcriptional co-activator. In many different types of carcinomas, E-Cadherin is frequently down-regulated during tumor progression. However, it is infrequently mutated. To name just one example from the gastrointestinal tract, down-regulation of E-cadherin and LOH of its gene (*CDH1*) at 16q are frequent in hepatocellular carcinoma.

In >50% of all diffuse-type gastric cancers, *CDH1* is mutated, and in almost all others, E-cadherin is strongly down-regulated. Many mutations in the gene are small in-frame deletions or splice site mutations affecting the adhesion domain. They lead to a shortened protein that has lost the ability for homotypic interactions. It may, instead, interfere with the function of intact E-cadherin and of related proteins such as N-cadherin. The consistent dysfunction of E-Cadherin provides an obvious explanation for the decreased adhesiveness and the '*diffuse*' growth pattern of the tumor cells of this cancer. Moreover, loss of E-Cadherin may contribute to WNT-pathway deregulation.

The importance of E-Cadherin mutations in sporadic diffuse-type gastric cancer is underlined by the genetic defect in its – very rare – familial form. In a small number of families in which young people succumb to diffuse-type gastric cancer, the disease co-segregates with mutations in *CDH1*. In the cancers that develop, the second, wild-type allele is lost. So, *CDH1* is a classical '*gatekeeper-type*' tumor suppressor gene for diffuse-type gastric cancer, with germ-line mutations in familial cancers and biallelic inactivation in sporadic cases. Remarkably, no other cancers appear at elevated rates in the affected families. Thus, there must be something particular about E-Cadherin in the stomach epithelium. Another consistent genetic alteration in diffuse-type gastric cancer are *TP53* mutations, as one might expect in a tumor exhibiting aneuploidy and high invasiveness.

There is no similarly evident genetic predisposition for intestinal-type cancer of the stomach. An increased risk of gastric cancer is observed in HNPCC families. A significant proportion of sporadic cases, overall >10%, also exhibit microsatellite instabilities. Some mutations in genes found in these cases are similar to those in colon cancers arising by the microsatellite instability pathway, e.g. in the *APC*, *CTNNB1*, and *TGFBRII* genes. This suggests that *I* intestinal type gastric cancer is a sort of colon cancer arising in the wrong organ. Indeed, constitutive activation of the WNT pathway can also be detected in some gastric cancers without an MSI phenotype. It is most often caused by inactivation of *APC*, but other changes like oncogenic mutations of β-Catenin are also found. The changes in the WNT pathway may be compounded through loss of E-Cadherin by LOH and down-regulation (rather than mutation), and by mutations of TP53.

Compared to colon cancer, the TGFβ response may be a more important and probably earlier target of mutations in the stomach. Inactivation of components of the actual pathway does occur, but in gastric cancer a more widespread target may be a '*downstream*' transcription factor, RUNX3, which regulates gene expression in gastric cells in response to TGFβ signaling. This factor is inactivated in many gastric cancers by deletion of one *RUNX3* gene copy and promoter hypermethylation of the second, remaining allele.

Metaplasia as such is not a malignancy, although metaplastic tissue is functionally disturbed. Metaplastic intestinal tissue in the stomach is not suited for an environment with a pH as low as 1 and, of course, cannot secrete proteases and peptides like normal gastric pit cells. Similarly, metaplastic squamous epithelium in the urinary tract is not as impermeable to urine components as normal urothelium. In both organs, therefore, the presence of metaplastic tissue tends to aggravate ongoing tissue damage and inflammation.

A straightforward explanation for the development of metaplasia in the context of chronic inflammation is that damage to the tissue over a long period cannot be compensated simply by division and expansion of existing differentiated cells. Rather, chronic tissue damage may necessitate the recruitment of tissue precursor cells. While some of these may differentiate correctly and replenish the damaged tissue, others may be deviated by the adverse conditions in the inflammated organ towards a different cell fate. Conceivably, direct influences from a pathogen like *H. pylori* might also disturb the direction of differentiation.

In a sense, intestinal differentiation in the stomach is not exotic, because the stomach and intestine develop from consecutive segments of the embryonal gut tube. During development, a network of transcriptional regulators determines whether segments of the gut assume an anterior, i.e. gastric, or a posterior, i.e. intestinal, identity.

There is indeed evidence that intestinal metaplasia in the stomach is associated with and maybe caused by a shift in the pattern of these regulators. The factors involved belong to the HOX and SRY box (SOX) family. The most clearly identified components are the caudal homeobox proteins CDX2 and CDX1 and SOX2. In addition, specific (canonical) HOX proteins are implicated. Expression of CDX2 is normally restricted to the intestine and the protein is not detectable in gastric epithelial cells, whereas SOX2 shows the reverse pattern, being present in cells in the stomach, but not in the intestine. As one might expect, in metaplastic intestinal epithelium in the stomach CDX2 is expressed and SOX2 is down-regulated.

Although they both act as determinants of an intestinal phenotype, CDX2 and CDX1 are actually antagonists. CDX2 promotes the terminal differentiation of intestinal cells, e.g. by inducing $p21^{CIP1}$, whereas CDX1 maintains intestinal cells in a proliferative state. Accordingly, in well-differentiated metaplastic intestinal tissue in the stomach, CDX2 is expressed, but CDX1 only weakly. When dysplastic adenomas and carcinomas develop from metaplastic precursor tissue, expression of CDX1 increases and CDX2 becomes down-regulated, in some cases bolstered by hypermethylation of its gene promoter.

Helicobacter pylori and Stomach Cancer

Since *Helicobacter pylori* was discovered in 1983 (!) and soon after suggested as a cause of gastritis, '*peptic ulcers*', and stomach cancer, a large body of evidence has been assembled that supports its classification as a human carcinogen. Unusual in cancer epidemiology, even controlled prospective longitudinal studies have been performed. These demonstrate that infected persons, as indicated by the presence of antibodies against proteins of the bacterium (*seropositivity*), have a higher risk of developing chronic gastritis as well as stomach cancer and that the risk for stomach cancer increases the longer the bacterium persists in the stomach. The converse approach, intervention, has also been attempted and shown to be successful. Antibiotic treatment that eradicates *Helicobacter* prevents gastritis and cancer. In particular, it appears to prevent in many cases the progression from gastric atrophy to metaplasia and cancer.

Helicobacter pylori is one of several related bacteria which live in the human gastrointestinal system. Usually they do not cause severe disease, but only an initial gastroenteritis, which can even pass without symptoms. Most people become infected by *Helicobacter pylori* as children and remain so for life, unless the germ is eliminated by antibiotic treatment (usually prescribed for a different infection). The stomach environment is designed to kill or damage bacteria and other infectious agents through its low pH and through the action of the protease pepsin.

Helicobacter pylori manages to survive in this environment by a variety of mechanisms developed during the >10,000 years in which it has co-evolved with its host. For instance, it buffers gastric hydrochloric acid by hydrolysing urea to bicarbonate and ammonia through the enzymatic action of urease produced by all *H. pylori* strains. Some strains cling closely to the epithelial surface which is relatively protected by buffering mucins.

Several bacterial proteins mediate the interaction between the bacteria and the epithelial cells of the stomach mucosa.

The *babA2* protein, e.g., attaches to the Lewis^b (blood group) antigen on the surface of gastric epithelial cells.

The bacterial '*cag island*' encompasses 31 genes within 40 kb. This '*pathogenicity island*', which may move as a unit between bacterial species and strains, encodes a secretion and translocation system that transports the cagA protein into stomach epithelial cells. Within the host cell, the cagA protein becomes tyrosine phosphorylated by SRC tyrosine kinases. This phosphorylation elicits changes in cellular cytoskeletal proteins, cell shape and adhesion. The tyrosine phosphate in the bacterial protein is recognized by the adaptor proteins SHP2 and GRB2 that activate MAPK and other signaling pathways. The resulting change in the epithelial cells may facilitate adhesion of the bacteria and allow them to take cover between and behind the mucosal cells. Introduction of cagA into epithelial cells also induces the expression and secretion of the interleukin IL8. This is a pro-inflammatory cytokine which induces a cellular immune response to the infection. This response is accompanied by increased expression of further cytokines, prominently IL1β and TNFα (tumor necrosis factor α). On one hand, these cytokines further promote inflammation, on the other hand they decrease the secretion of hydrochloric acid by the parietal cells of the gastric epithelium. This constitutes a second important mechanism by which *Helicobacter pylori* increases the pH in the stomach fluid and can survive in this hostile environment.

The effect of the bacterium on the gastric epithelium is compounded by its *vacA* protein which induces vacuolization (hence its name) and apoptosis of host cells. This leads to the release of nutrients and further facilitates penetration of *H. pylori* through the mucosal barrier.

The vacA protein is also immunosuppressive, diminishing responses by macrophages and T-cells.

In summary, as the bacterium changes its environment to fit its needs, it induces regenerative proliferation of the gastric epithelium which is stimulated by the peptide gastrin and by cytokines that also contribute to an immune reaction which can lead to tissue reorganization and to chronic inflammation.

The outcome of an *H. pylori* infection can vary substantially. Most infected humans do not experience any symptoms over decades. So, one potential, frequent outcome appears to be a stable equilibrium between tissue damage by the bacterium and immune response by the host. In other cases, fulminant inflammation and permanent tissue damage lead to the symptoms of a peptic ulcer and in some individuals, cancer develops. Overall, while between 10% and 65% of individuals in different populations worldwide are infected, only a few percent of them develop chronic gastritis and again a fraction of these eventually come down with stomach cancer. Nevertheless, worldwide, one million cases per year result, with huge differences between different populations. These differences in the relative incidences are caused by an interaction of several factors.

H. pylori Strain Differences

There are substantial differences between strains of *Helicobacter pylori* in each of the three pathogenetic determinants discussed above, babA2, cagA, and vacA. Strains without functional babA2 genes are much less apt at inducing intestinal-type stomach cancer, probably because fewer bacteria adhere to epithelial cells. The babA2$^+$ strains also tend to induce autoimmune reactions much more strongly than others. The cagA island, likewise, is present in most, but not in all strains. Strains lacking cagA induce less inflammation and do not appear to promote cancer development. The presence of actively secreted vacA is also statistically correlated with an increased cancer risk. However, the interpretation of vacA associations is complicated by the peculiar distribution of the vacA genotypes. There are several major polymorphic forms of the gene, designated s_1a, s_1b, s_1c and s_2 (with further subtypes). Each is associated with a particular human population to such an extent that they can be used to follow human migrations. While this association gives good reason to believe that vacA polymorphisms may account for geographic differences in stomach cancer incidence, it complicates studies in those mixed human populations, where people of different origins live under different socioeconomic conditions, and prevents studies of the influence of vacA in homogeneous human populations. Moreover, cagA and vacA genotypes are not completely independent of each other.

Host Reaction

There are also substantial differences in the host reaction towards *H. pylori* infection. Some are caused by genetic polymorphisms, while others may be determined by co-infections, e.g. worm parasites. Most of the genetic polymorphisms concern co-determinants of the immune response such as the MHC type or genes encoding cytokines and cytokine receptors. Since stomach cancer is a multifactorial disease, it is not surprising that not all studies agree on the importance of every polymorphism implicated. However, the case for polymorphisms affecting the expression of the cytokine IL1β has been confirmed by several independent studies. This suggests that the effect is large and relevant in different populations.

The *IL1B* gene is polymorphic in man. Functional polymorphisms in its promoter influence the expression level of the cytokine, most strongly a C/T polymorphism at –31 in the TATA box of the gene. In T-alleles, transcription factors bind more strongly than in C-alleles, and expression of IL1B is more strongly inducible. The presence of T-alleles is associated with an ≈10-fold increased risk of gastric ulcers and cancer. Of note, the genes encoding IL1β, IL1α, and their receptor IL1R are all located close to the *ILB* gene. Polymorphisms in these genes, including the *IL1B* -31C/T polymorphisms are often in linkage disequilibrium with others in the gene cluster. This means that a particular form (allele) of the *IL1B* gene is as a rule found together with a particular form (allele) of the *IL1R* gene. Indeed, other studies have found associations of cancer risk with the *IL1R* genotype. As one might suspect, the effect of the *IL1B* polymorphism is synergistic with that of the *Helicobacter pylori* genotype. Across all human populations, the risk of stomach cancer is estimated to be ≈2-3-fold elevated by becoming infected with any strain of *Helicobacter pylori*. By comparison, the risk of *IL1B* –31T carriers infected with cagA$^+$, vacA s1m1 strains is almost 100-fold enhanced.

Dietary Carcinogens and Irritants

A third important factor in the development of gastric cancer appears to be the presence of co-carcinogens in the diet, specifically alcohol, excessive salt and nitrosamines. Alcohol and salt may act primarily as irritants, aggravating tissue destruction and inflammation. Nitrosamines are implicated as direct mutagens. They are alkylating reagents that react, in particular, with DNA bases and as a rule cause point mutations. They are therefore thought to be responsible for many of the point mutations found in gastric cancers, e.g. in *TP53*, *CDH1* (E-Cadherin), and *CTNNB1* (β-Catenin). They are present in the diet, e.g. in pickled foods, or are contained in cigarette smoke. Some may be generated in the acidic milieu of the stomach by reaction of nitric acid with amines contained in food. Nitric acid is produced by reduction of dietary nitrates in the oral cavity and during passage through the esophagus. Its concentration is particularly high in spoiling salted or pickled food. Improvements in food quality over the last decades, specifically the replacement of pickling by refrigeration, may have made an equally important contribution to the decline of stomach cancer as the eradication of *Helicobacter pylori* by antibiotics in many individuals.

Fruit and Vegetables

Conversely, several other components of the diet appear to protect against stomach cancer. Particularly important may be antioxidants like vitamin C and the methyl group carrier folate, which are present in fresh fruit and vegetables. The increasing availability of fresh fruit and vegetables in the Western industrialized countries throughout the year, as opposed to use of pickled, salted and dried food before the advent of global transport and refrigeration, may also have contributed to the decline in stomach cancer.

These compounds may exert their protective effect partly by extracellular and partly by intracellular mechanisms. In the stomach fluid, vitamin C reduces and inactivates nitrosamines. In the inflammated stomach epithelium, antioxidants diminish the effect of reactive oxygen species. They may therefore protect against cell damage and decrease the rate of mutations. A sufficient supply of the methyl group carrier folate ensures that thymidine pools are adequate, preventing uridine misincorporation and DNA strand breaks, and ensures an adequate supply of S-adenosylmethionine needed to maintain proper DNA methylation patterns.

In summary, therefore, the development of stomach cancer as a consequence of infection by *Helicobacter pylori* is not only a multistep, but also a multifactorial process. As in the development of liver cancer following HBV infection, chronic inflammation is a crucial prerequisite and is contingent on the genotypes of both pathogen and host. Chronic inflammation as such is likely mutagenic, but most of all it creates an environment in which cells with an altered phenotype are selected for and expand. It may therefore be significant that *TP53* mutations are found already at some frequency in chronic gastritis. Again as in liver cancer, both the creation of altered cells and their progression towards cancer cells are accelerated by the presence of mutagens and a lack of protective compounds. In stomach cancer, the part of mutagenic aflatoxins in the liver is apparently performed by nitrosamines.

It is likely that each of the above factors may be needed for this cancer to arise at the excessive rate still seen in several parts of the world. The epidemiological data clearly shows that stomach cancer can be largely prevented. Conceivably, each factor involved in gastric carcinogenesis can be addressed for this purpose.

5

Hepatic Cancer

Liver cancer is one of the major lethal malignancies worldwide. The main histological subtype is hepatocellular carcinoma, which is derived from hepatocytes, the predominant epithelial cell type in the liver, and often retains biochemical and morphological markers of hepatocyte differentiation.

Hepatocellular carcinoma develops as a rule in the context of chronic inflammation and liver cirrhosis caused by the hepatitis viruses HBV or HCV, by chronic alcohol abuse, or more rarely by hereditary diseases such as hemochromatosis. Chemical carcinogens such as aflatoxin B1 from the mold Aspergillus flavus act synergistically with the causes of inflammation, in particular with chronic HBV infection. Aflatoxins cause a diagnostic G→T mutation at codon 249 of TP53.

In addition to disrupting the TP53 network, genetic and epigenetic alterations in hepatocellular carcinoma inactivate cell cycle regulation by RB1 and cause constitutive activity of the WNT signaling pathway, most often by mutations of β-Catenin and more rarely by inactivation of Axin1 and APC. WNT pathway activation may be exacerbated by loss of E-cadherin.

Several growth factors and their receptors controlling normal hepatocyte proliferation and regeneration are also implicated in the growth and survival of hepatocellular carcinoma, by autocrine and paracrine mechanisms. In addition to activation of HGF/MET and TGFα/ERBB1 circuits, a particular important change may consist in increased stimulation by the insulin-like factor IGF2 through the IGFIR receptor tyrosine kinase, while the scavenger receptor IGFRII may become inactivated.

The pivotal role of HBV in liver carcinogenesis appears mainly to be due to a continuous hepatocyte destruction by T-cells which attempt to eliminate the infection and their repletion from differentiated cells and eventually liver stem cells. This process may select for genetically altered cells with diminished response to the virus and to apoptotic signals. Increased oxidative stress in the inflammated tissue may contribute to mutagenesis and at the same time increase the selective pressure. Inhibition of TP53 function by the viral HBX protein may aid in down-regulation of apoptosis during early stages carcinogenesis and permit the accumulation of cells with aberrant genomes. Furthermore, integration of viral genomes may promote genomic instability.

Importantly, while therapeutic options are limited once HCC is established, vaccination against HBV and anti-viral treatment against HCV appear to be efficacious in preventing this cancer.

Etiology of Liver Cancer

Although the liver is a frequent site of metastases from other organs, primary liver cancer is nowadays one of the rarer malignancies in Western industrialized countries. The main histological subtype is *hepatocellular carcinoma* (HCC), derived from the major cell type in the liver, the epithelial hepatocyte.

A long way into their development, HCC cells remain similar to normal hepatocytes to the extent that early stage cancers can be difficult to distinguish morphologically from normal parenchyma or benign adenomas. Some secrete the oncofetal albumin homolog α-fetoprotein, which is a useful marker in such cases. Molecular histological techniques such as fluorescence-in-situ-hybridization can be used to detect chromosomal abnormalities and support a diagnosis of cancer.

Notwithstanding their morphologically differentiated appearance, hepatocellular carcinomas are highly lethal cancers. In spite of progress in surgery, including even the use of liver transplantation, overall survival is <20% two years after diagnosis. As a rule, only small cancers with diameters <2 cm can be cured by surgery. Currently available chemotherapy is unsuccessful.

In many developing countries, the situation is worse. Primary hepatocellular carcinoma is a major health problem in East and Southeast Asia as well as Central and Southern Africa, the more so, as patients tend to be much younger than in the Western world, and even include children. In many countries, the possibilities for treatment are even more limited than in the Western world. As a result, HCC remains the (approximately) fifth-most frequent cause of cancer deaths worldwide.

Independent of geography and socioeconomic factors, HCC arises typically in the context of chronic liver inflammation and liver cirrhosis. For instance, some patients suffering from hereditary hemochromatosis develop chronic liver inflammation leading to cirrhosis, and eventually to HCC in some cases.

Hemochromatosis is an iron storage disease caused by missense mutations in the *HFE* gene. Its product is a membrane protein similar to MHC proteins which regulates iron uptake and transport. Inadequate function of HFE leads to iron overload in the liver. Normally, iron is stored in the liver bound to proteins such as ferritin. In hemochromatosis the protein storage capacity is exceeded and free iron ions cause damage to the tissue. Protein-bound ferrous iron ions (Fe^{2+}) are relatively innocuous, while Fe^{2+} free in solution or associated with low molecular ligands can be more easily oxidized to the ferrous state (Fe^{3+}) in the Fenton reaction, which yields highly reactive hydroxyl radicals. Hydroxyl radicals damage macromolecules and lipids, causing necrotic cell death and chronic inflammation. They also react with DNA bases and with deoxyribose, causing strand-breaks and base mutations.

HFE mutations are highly prevalent in Europeans. In this population, 10% may be heterozygous for the 282Cys>Tyr mutation, and up to 20% for the 63His>Asp mutation. Only homozygotes or compound homozygotes (i.e. persons carrying two different mutations in the *HFE* alleles) develop hemochromatosis. In fact, not all do, and only a fraction of these progress towards cirrhosis and hepatocellular cancer. This demonstrates that further factors modulate the risk of inflammation and cancer. Nowadays, patients with early signs of hemochromatosis disease can be treated with iron chelators to prevent organ damage, cirrhosis, and cancer.

Hemochromatosis is a comparatively rare disease, but its pathophysiology is well understood. It provides an example for other, more prevalent, but less well understood factors that cause liver cancer by a basically similar pathway through chronic inflammation and cirrhosis. The most important ones are the hepatitis viruses HBV and HCV, and alcohol abuse. In a typical Central European population, ≈3% of all HCC cases might be associated with hemochromatosis, and 30% each with HBV, HCV, and alcohol, the remainder with other known or unknown causes. A rising incidence of HCC in industrialized countries over the last decades is mainly caused by an according increased prevalence of HCV infections. Tellingly, the rise in cancer incidence is delayed by ≈15 years compared to that of the viral hepatitis. So, this is the period required for development of cirrhosis and cancer.

Table 5.1. Causes of human hepatocellular cancer

Individual factors causing hepatocellular cancer in humans
Alcohol
Hepatitis virus B
Hepatitis virus C
Steatosis (fatty liver)
Inherited diseases leading to chronic liver damage
Hemochromatosis and other diseases leading to iron or copper overload
Other causes of liver cirrhosis
Aflatoxins

HBV persists as a chronic infection in ≈10% and HCV in >50% of infected persons. In chronic viral hepatitis, hepatocytes are continuously destroyed by cytotoxic T-cells attempting to eliminate the virus and need to be replaced. Replacement of hepatocytes is partly achieved by proliferation of differentiated hepatocytes and partly, especially during continuous damage, by recruitment of liver stem cells. These are thought to reside in the ducts of Herring at the origin of the bile duct. Their activation can be recognized by spreading of undifferentiated small epithelial-like cells with oval nuclei ('*oval cells*') into the hepatic parenchymal structure. During chronic alcohol abuse, hepatocyte destruction is initiated by the substance and its metabolites.

During chronic tissue damage and inflammation, nonepithelial cells in the liver become activated and proliferate. While their activation and proliferation initially serves to support the immune response and the regeneration of the tissue, during chronic liver damage and with increasing inflammation their expansion predominates and they gradually replace epithelial structures in the organ. This process eventually manifests as cirrhosis, in which the well-organized parenchymal tissue is displaced by more disorganized and dysfunctional fibrotic tissue.

In this disturbed tissue, hepatocellular cancer may develop from liver stem cells or from more differentiated hepatocytes that are more resistant to the adverse conditions in the organ. Hepatic cancer cells are typically more resistant to viral infection, store less iron, or are less easily triggered to apoptosis by cytotoxic immune cells. So, they may be selected for their ability to survive in the cirrhotic tissue environment. Specifically, their increased resistance to apoptosis, e.g. by the CD95 pathway, may be one reason for the primary resistance of HCC to chemotherapy.

Hepatocellular carcinoma is preceded by several morphological alterations in the parenchymal epithelium. These were initially identified in experimental animals, and later confirmed in humans. In some cases, the proliferation of liver stem cells can actually be observed. Otherwise, the first morphological stage are small dysplastic foci, which increase in size to form nodules with progressively aberrant cells.

While these precursor stages remain restricted to the epithelial parenchyma, actual HCC invades interstitia and vessels and may form metastases in distant parts of the liver or in other organs. A critical stage, both biologically and clinically, appears to be reached at a tumor volume of $\approx 1\ cm^3$. Here, angiogenesis by branches of the hepatic artery and capillaries appears to become activated and the tumor cells become more invasive. This transition is quickly followed by spreading of the cancer cells through the liver, and later to other organs.

Genetic Changes in Hepatocellular Carcinoma

Hepatocellular carcinoma cells are aneuploid with a number of consistent chromosomal changes. In short, gains of 1q, 6p, 8q, 11q, 17q and the entire chromosome 7 are prevalent, while losses concern predominantly 4q, 6q, 8p, 13q, 17p and both arms of chromosome 16. The 'cancer pathways' targeted by these alterations and further genetic and epigenetic changes are the RB1 network regulating the cell cycle, the WNT pathway, the STAT pathway and the TP53 network. In addition, autocrine or paracrine growth factors loops appear to be set up. While these may promote proliferation, they may also contribute to decreased apoptosis together with altered responses to death receptor ligands and overexpression of anti-apoptotic proteins.

Regulation of the cell cycle through RB1 is disrupted in most HCC by loss and mutation of *RB1* itself, by hypermethylation, mutation or deletion of *CDKN2A*, and - perhaps more often than in other carcinomas - by overexpression of Cyclin D1 as a consequence of amplification of its gene, *CCND1*, at 11q13. The *MYC* gene at 8q24.1 is also quite often amplified, promoting cell cycle progression and cell growth. These alterations leading to deregulation of the cell cycle resemble those in many other carcinomas, e.g. squamous cell carcinoma of the skin and bladder cancers.

The WNT pathway is also activated in many hepatocellular carcinomas, although not as regularly as in colorectal cancer. In fact, the mode of activation is usually different. In colorectal cancer, constitutive activation of the pathway is most often caused by inactivation of both alleles of the *APC* tumor suppressor gene, and in a smaller fraction of cases by point mutations in *CTNNB1* that turn β-Catenin into an oncogenic protein. These mutations occur in the part of the protein that is recognized by GSK3β and prohibit the phosphorylation that allows the recognition of β-Catenin by the βTRCP ubiquitin ligase complex.

This type of *CTNNB1* mutation is also prevalent in HCC, at a frequency of 25-30%, whereas inactivation of APC is the exception rather than the rule. Instead, two other alterations promote overactivity of the pathway in some cases. Mutations of Axin1, a protein that helps to assemble the APC/GSK3β/β-Catenin complex, are found in ≈5% of HCC. Accordingly, LOH at 16p13, where the *AXIN1* gene is located, is relatively common. In many HCC, loss of the long arm of this chromosome, i.e. 16q, together with mutation and promoter hypermethylation lead to decreased activity of E-Cadherin. Loss of this protein from the cell membrane causes decreased adhesiveness between neighboring epithelial cells and thereby favors invasion and metastasis. Moreover, on the cytoplasmic side of the cell membrane, E-Cadherin anchors a network of fibers through the α-Catenin and β-Catenin proteins. In this fashion, in some cell types, E-Cadherin seems to act as a kind of '*buffer*' for β-Catenin and to modulate the activity of the intracellular WNT signaling pathway dependent on this protein. In HCC, specifically, the loss of E-Cadherin appears to contribute to enhanced β-Catenin concentrations in the nucleus.

HCC is one of those solid tumors in which enhanced STAT activity has been observed. Among the defects leading to STAT overactivity in these cases is hypermethylation of the *SOCS1* promoter combined with LOH at 16p13 (the same region containing *AXIN1*). SOCS1 is a feedback inhibitor of JAK2 that relays growth and survival signals from cytokines such as IL6. In the absence of SOCS1, signals through the STAT pathway may be prolonged and more strongly promote resistance to apoptosis, in particular. It is important to remember in this context, that although IL6 is labeled a '*cytokine*', because it influences the proliferation and function of many cell types of the immune system, it also affects the growth and modulates the function of several epithelial cell types, especially of hepatocytes.

TP53 function is disturbed in most HCC, usually by the mechanism most prevalent across all cancers, i.e. point mutations in one allele and loss of the second allele by deletion or recombination. In HCC from Europe, the USA, as well as in Japan and Taiwan, these mutations are spread across the central DNA binding domain of the TP53 protein. In HCC from Africa and other Asian countries, a mutational 'hotspot' is observed at codon 249. A transversion in its third base changes AGG to AGT and thus Arg to Ser in the TP53 protein. This particular mutation can be experimentally induced by aflatoxin B_1. Food contaminated with the fungus *Aspergillus flavus*, which produces this carcinogen, is mostly consumed in the hot and humid regions of the world where this mutation is prevalent. So, like the mutations at pyrimidine dimers that are diagnostic for DNA damage by UVB, the G→T mutation at codon 249 reveals the influence of a particular carcinogen. Moreover, this mutation is predominantly found in HCC patients with chronic HBV infection, so there is clearly some selection for the mutation from this side.

Throughout all HCC, mutations of TP53 tend to occur together with altered β-Catenin signaling. The mechanism underlying this association is not entirely clear, but it is notable that these changes also concur in colon carcinoma. A plausible explanation is that constitutive WNT/β-Catenin signaling activates wildtype TP53 because it induces MYC and Cyclin D1 which increase (directly and indirectly) the transcription of $p14^{ARF1}$. In this fashion, a selective pressure for mutations in TP53 could be exerted. As in many other cancers, loss of TP53 function may contribute in HCC to decreased apoptosis and increased angiogenesis. Both may favor cell survival in the environment of a cirrhotic liver.

Among the growth factors and receptors particularly important in HCC are those which also direct normal liver growth and regeneration: TGFα acting through the EGFR (ERBB1), hepatocyte growth factor (HGF) acting through MET and – perhaps more critical than in other cancers – insulin-like growth factor 2 (IGF2) and its receptors.

TGFα may be produced by hepatoma cells themselves. If these also express the EGFR, autocrine stimulation of growth and survival may result. In contrast, HGF is produced by nonepithelial cells in the liver. During cirrhosis and development of HCC, mesenchymal cells become activated. In particular, Ito cells which are normally located in the space of Disse (between endothelial and epithelial cells), change to myoepithelial cells that proliferate themselves, but also secrete growth factors and cytokines acting on other stromal and epithelial cells. They are the likely source of HGF in hepatocellular carcinoma, whose action is enhanced by overexpression of the MET receptor on the hepatoma cells. Production, secretion and maturation of HGF may all be stimulated by factors from the tumor. The genes encoding the EGFR and MET are both located on chromosome 7 which is typically gained in HCC, as in many other carcinomas.

Overexpression of IGF2 is a central event in some cases of the childhood nephroblastoma, Wilms tumor, but it is not at all uncommon in carcinomas afflicting older people. Insulin and/or insulin-like growth factors are necessary for the proliferation and function of normal hepatocytes. In HCC, IGF2 can be overproduced as a consequence of various mechanisms. In some cases 'loss of imprinting' is responsible. More complex mechanisms include altered usage of the four promoters of the *IGF2* gene.

IGF2 acts through the receptor tyrosine kinase IGFRI or an alternatively spliced form of the insulin receptor IR1 to promote cell survival and proliferation via the MAPK pathway, but perhaps more importantly via the PI3K pathway. In principle, insulin exerts the same effects as IGF2, but it is a relatively weak growth factor, whereas IGF2 affects metabolic functions not as strongly as insulin.

The growth-promoting activity of IGF2 is normally limited by IGFRII. This protein is rightly named a '*receptor*', in that it binds IGF2. However, ligand binding does not elicit a proliferation or survival signal. Instead, IGF2 is directed towards the lysosomes for degradation. Therefore, IGFRII is a '*scavenger receptor*' that limits the action of insulin-like growth factors. Another limitation to their action is provided by binding proteins like IGFBP3, which is induced by TP53.

So, the cellular reaction to IGF2 is not only dependent on its concentration and expression level of its gene, but also regulated by several other factors. Specifically, the cellular reaction towards IGF2 is dependent on the relative expression levels of the IGFRI and IGFRII receptors. The *IGFR2* gene is located at chromosome 6q27, where LOH is frequent in HCC. Therefore, it is considered as the most likely candidate for a tumor suppressor in this region. There are, however, conflicting findings on this issue. One source of confusion is that Igfr2 is an imprinted gene in mice, and was initially reported to be imprinted in some human tissues as well. Although this idea has now been largely refuted, the notion tends to persist. The importance of insulin-like growth factors in liver cancer, however, is a fact and underlined by occasional point mutations that activate the IGFRI.

Viruses in HCC

The genetic and epigenetic changes that cause HCC develop in a context of chronic tissue inflammation, with infiltration of cytotoxic cells, activation of stromal cells, continuous damage to hepatocytes and according need for regeneration in a tissue that becomes more and more disorganized. Hereditary diseases like hemochromatosis, chronic alcohol abuse, or chronic infection by the hepatitis viruses HBV and HCV can elicit this state each by themselves or together. Chronic inflammation in the liver provides an environment that is per se mutagenic, relieves some of the growth controls in a normal tissue, promotes proliferation of hepatocytic cells and selects for expansion of cells that are resistant to the adverse conditions. Thus, chronic infection by hepatitis viruses by itself would be thought to be sufficient to increase the risk of developing liver cancer. In fact, the risk of HCC in men chronically infected with HBV is increased ≈200-fold, which suggests that the virus may contribute to cancer development by additional mechanisms.

In humans, DNA viruses rather than retroviruses are implicated in carcinogenesis, with few exceptions. The best understood human tumor virus is human papilloma virus. Oncogenic strains like HPV16 and HPV18 contain E6 and E7 proteins which bind and inactivate TP53 and RB1, respectively, thereby interfering with two of the most crucial networks that control cell growth, differentiation, and genomic integrity. A causative role of HPV in cervical cancer is established beyond doubt and it is very likely in squamous carcinoma of the head and neck. The evidence is weaker for other cancers. The papovaviruses SV40, JCV, and BKV might act in a similar fashion by impeding the function of TP53 and RB1 through their multifunctional large T proteins. However, there is no conclusive evidence for their active involvement in human cancers, with the arguable exception of mesothelioma and SV40. A large part of the human population carries JC or BK viruses without obvious adverse effects.

The same is almost true for the herpes virus EBV, although the normally relatively innocuous virus is quite clearly a cofactor in specific lymphatic cancers such as Burkitt lymphoma. As far as known, EBV does not act via TP53 or RB1. Instead, it appears to expand the population of cells amenable to transformation by specific translocations that activate oncogenes like MYC and complements their action by diminishing apoptosis.

HBV is also a DNA virus. However, its life cycle can best be characterized as that of a reverse retrovirus. The virus contains a ≈3.3 kb DNA genome in an icosahedrical capsid formed by 240 hepatitis B virus core antigen (HBcAg) proteins. This core is surrounded by a membrane, derived from the host endoplasmatic reticulum, into which several isoforms of the HBV surface antigen (HBsAg) are embedded.

In infectious viruses, the genome is a circular incomplete double-stranded DNA. One strand is complete, but the circle is not closed, because it is covalently linked at its 5'-end to a tyrosine residue in the terminal protein (TP) encoded by the virus. This complete strand is called the minus-strand, because it is used exclusively as the template for transcription of the viral genome. The plus-strand in the virus is incomplete and of variable length, but always overlaps the gap in the minus-strand. At its 5'-end, it contains a conserved short, capped RNA primer and the viral polymerase is bound to its 3' variable end. After infection, the synthesis of this partly double-stranded genome is completed, with removal of the RNA primer. Three different RNAs can be transcribed from the viral genome. They encode the HBcAg, the HBsAg and a shorter secreted isoform of the same protein named HBeAg, the TP protein, and the regulatory HBx protein.

Following uptake into endosomes, the viral capsid escapes into the nucleus, where it is unpacked for replication and transcription to begin. As a rule, the DNA genome remains episomal, although it occasionally integrates into the host DNA, usually by recombination involving the single-strand segment of the genome. Replication proceeds through an RNA intermediate. This RNA intermediate, like all other viral RNAs, is synthesized by host RNA polymerases. It is then used by the own polymerase of HBV, a combined reverse transcriptase/ DNA polymerase with RNase H activity to generate the minus and plus DNA strands of the genome. The covalently linked polymerase molecule at the 5'-end serves to prime the first strand, and a capped RNA primer is used for the second strand. The genome contains two short direct repeats, which are used for template switching, similar as in retroviruses.

Replication and transcription of HBV take place concurrently. Transcription is stimulated by a liver-specific enhancer in the viral genome, which is responsive to glucocorticoids and – to a lesser extent – to androgens. Once sufficient amounts of viral proteins have become synthesized, the genome is packed into the capsid and the virus assembles in the endoplasmatic reticulum. Complete and incomplete virus particles appear to be secreted via a Golgi pathway.

HBV does not usually lyse cells. Hepatocyte death during infection is mainly caused by cytotoxic lymphocytes (CD8+ T-cells) which appear to act by the FAS/FAS-ligand route. During chronic infection, NK cells become as well involved. Acute infections last several weeks and end, when the patient develops a sufficient titer of IgG antibodies against the viral surface and core antigens. Development of immunity is impeded by the secretion of the HBeAg and incomplete viral particles. Young children and other not fully immunocompetent individuals cannot mount an efficient IgG response, if any immune response at all, and the infection becomes chronic, sometimes without symptoms, but often with development of liver cirrhosis and eventually of HCC. Transmission from mother to child is an important route in areas where HBV is endemic.

Cures of HBV infections can sometimes be achieved by interferons α and β which activate intracellular responses that prohibit virus replication. However, the best protection against HBV is vaccination using an HBsAg produced in yeast. This vaccine prevents both acute and chronic disease. Importantly, although a few related animal viruses are known, the only known host of HBV are humans and, experimentally, chimpanzees. There is thus a chance to eradicate the virus. So, what is there in HBV that might specifically promote hepatocarcinogenesis? Obviously, not really much beyond the factors already mentioned, i.e. an increased rate of hepatocyte cell death and regeneration and inflammation with tissue remodeling. Two further factors are debated.

1. Many HCC arising in HBV-infected patients carry integrated HBV DNA in their genome. These copies are usually incomplete and not replication-competent (even if they could be excised from the genome back into an episomal form). In rare cases, they are integrated into an proto-oncogene such as a Cyclin gene, and may lead to its over-expression through the action of the viral enhancer. In other rare cases, viral integrates may disrupt tumor suppressor genes. There is also evidence that integrates are unstable and favor chromosomal rearrangements, creating a sort of extra 'fragile site'. This effect may pertain to integrates of many different viruses, beyond HBV.
2. Other than episomal genomes, HBV integrates tend to express substantial amounts of HBx. This is a regulator protein which can

transactivate cellular promoters by interaction with cellular transcription factors, even though it does not bind to DNA itself. It is thought that HBx in this manner increases the expression of anti-apoptotic proteins during acute and chronic infection. HBx may also activate cell proliferation by interacting with PKC enzymes. Certainly, HBx binds TP53 and promotes its degradation, like the HPV E6 protein. However, its effect is much weaker than that of E6. In fact, the geographical regions where both HBV and HCC are endemic are those in which co-carcinogens are common. In tropical Africa and Asia, the main co-carcinogen is likely aflatoxin B_1 which often causes the very specific G→T mutation at codon 249 of TP53. It is possible that this specific mutation is not only selected for by the action of the mutagen, but also because it optimally complements the effect of HBx.

Mechanisms of Human Hepatocarcinogenesis

The primary hepatocellular neoplasms include hepatocellular adenoma, *hepatocellular carcinoma* (HCC), and hepatoblastoma. Together, these neoplasms constitute a clinically important group of human cancers that are diagnostically and therapeutically challenging. Of these primary liver neoplasms, HCC is the most common. Early detection and diagnosis of HCC is inefficient in the absence of well-known risk factors and appropriate surveillance, and most currently available treatments for this tumor are ineffective. Consequently, HCC is nearly uniformly fatal. Clinical and basic research on mechanisms of hepatocarcinogenesis has produced a tremendous amount of information about the pathologic settings in which HCC develops and the major etiologic factors that are responsible. Recent progress has begun to unravel the molecular pathogenesis of HCC in response to specific etiologic factors. The accumulated evidence suggests that HCC emerges through a multistep process (with well-characterized histopathologic manifestations), in which HCC develops in the context of the pathologic liver (chronic hepatitis and/or cirrhosis), from aberrant cells contained in dysplastic hepatocyte nodules or adenomatous hyperplasia. However, in the absence of an obvious genetic predisposition for HCC development, the identification of critical genes and genetic pathways has been difficult, precluding the elucidation of the rate-limiting steps in multistage hepatocarcinogenesis.

Epidemiology of Hepatocellular Carcinoma

Cancers of the liver and intrahepatic bile ducts are relatively rare in the United States, with 18,920 new diagnoses and 14,270 deaths in 2004. This represents ~1.3% of all new cancer diagnoses and 2.5% of cancer-related deaths in the United States. In contrast, liver cancer occurs at high incidence when the world population is considered. In 1990 there were 437,000 new cases of liver cancer worldwide, representing 5.4% of all cancers and making it the fifth leading cause of cancer incidence. Deaths attributed to liver cancer for the same year totaled 427,000, which represents 8.2% of all cancer deaths and makes it the fourth leading site for cancer mortality. In 2000 the worldwide incidence of liver cancer increased, with 564,000 new cases and 549,000 deaths, representing 5.5% (fifth leading site) of new cases and 8.8% of all cancer deaths (third leading cause of cancerrelated deaths).

The prevalence of primary liver cancer varies greatly among world regions. The highest incidence of liver cancer worldwide is found in China, where men exhibit an incidence rate of ~36 cases per 100,000 population. High rates of liver cancer incidence are found throughout large portions of Asia and Africa, with much lower incidence rates for this tumor found in Europe and the Americas. Early studies called attention to the extremely high incidence of hepatocellular carcinoma among black males in Mozambique, which demonstrates the highest incidence worldwide at 113 cases per 100,000 population. In fact, the incidence of this tumor among black Mozambican males aged 25–34 years is more than 500-fold higher than the incidence for comparably aged white males in the United States and United Kingdom. These statistics strongly suggest that factors related to genetic background and/or environmental exposure contribute significantly to the incidence of this tumor among world populations.

There has been a dramatic increase in HCC incidence among Japanese men during the last 30 years. Likewise, significant increases in HCC have been reported in the United States, the United Kingdom, and France. These increases in the incidence of HCC may reflect significant changes in risk factors or environmental exposures in affected populations. It has been suggested that the increased incidence of HCC in Japan, Europe, and the United States is related to increased incidence of HCV infection. Migration of individuals from one world region to another can affect their relative risk for development of HCC. Indians who migrate to Singapore or parts of China acquire incidence rates of HCC that are similar to those of the native population and significantly increased from that of their home country. In contrast, migrants from world regions with high risk for HCC development to regions of low risk for HCC demonstrate a decline in HCC incidence with successive generations. These observations suggest that exposure to environmental factors are more important contributors to HCC risk than population-based genetic factors or susceptibilities.

Liver cancer affects men more often than women. The ratio of male to female incidence in the United States is ~2:1, and worldwide it is ~2.4:1. However, in high-incidence countries or world regions, the male to female incidence ratio can be as high as 8:1. This consistent observation suggests that sex hormones and/or their receptors may play a significant role in the development of primary liver tumors. Some investigators have suggested that HCCs overexpress androgen receptors, and that androgens are important in the promotion of abnormal liver cell proliferation. In fact, anecdotal evidence suggests that therapeutic exposure of patients to androgenic–anabolic steroids increases the chances of HCC development. Conversely, some investigators suggest that female hormones (or their metabolites) are protective against development of HCC. In addition to the strong linkage between gender and development of HCC, there is evidence that the progression of the disease is less severe in women and that their longterm survival is much better than that of affected men. Others have suggested that the male predominance of liver cancer is related to the tendency for men to drink and smoke more heavily than women and the fact that men are more likely to develop cirrhosis.

Natural History of Hepatocellular Carcinoma

Hepatocarcinogenesis is a continuous and slowly unfolding process that leads from the initial genetic and epigenetic alterations in one or a few hepatocytes to the acquisition of a neoplastic phenotype by one or a few cells with the capacity to grow autonomously and to metastasize to distant sites outside the liver. The descriptive natural history of HCC, including the pathologic tissue patterns and clinical course, provides a framework for attempting to trace the sequence of molecular genetic alterations that drive its development. Hepatocellular carcinoma is strongly associated with chronic liver diseases, including chronic hepatitis and cirrhosis. In fact, the majority of cases of primary hepatocellular carcinoma worldwide develop in cirrhotic livers, most commonly nonalcoholic posthepatitic cirrhosis.

Chronic hepatitis

Chronic hepatitis is a prolonged inflammatory condition of the liver that is characterized by the presence of an inflammatory cell infiltrate, hepatocyte necrosis and death, and accelerated proliferation of residual hepatocytes to replace cells lost to injury and death. The inflammatory cells of chronic hepatitis consists of a mixture of B and T lymphocytes, dendritic cells, plasma cells, and macrophages. These cells infiltrate the connective tissue of the portal tracts and may also invade the adjacent lobular parenchyma. Lymphocytes and macrophages accumulate in the chronically inflamed liver as a result of increased expression of chemotactic cytokines by endothelial cells of the portal vessels and interlobular sinusoids. The inflammatory cell infiltrate of chronic hepatitis express numerous cytokines, including chemotactic cytokines of the CC and CXC types, and immunomodulatory cytokines, including tumor necrosis factor alpha (TNFα), various interleukins, and various interferons. The chemotactic cytokines recruit additional inflammatory cells and induce higher levels of expression by endothelial cells of adhesion molecules and receptors for inflammatory cell ligands.

The immunomodulatory cytokines stimulate both inflammatory cells and resident liver cells, including hepatocytes, to secrete cytokines, growth factors, and proteases, which stimulates destruction and repair of liver tissue. Where the inflammatory cells (infiltrate) touch the lobular parenchyma, cytotoxic T lymphocytes surround individual hepatocytes or small groups of hepatocytes; many of these hepatocytes die as a result of activation of death-signaling pathways mediated by Fas receptor or TNF1 receptor. The resulting persistent hepatocyte cell death produces a pathologic pattern in the liver that is characterized by zone 1 (periportal) necrosis.. Residual hepatocytes are stimulated to proliferate by the loss of cells and as a result of direct stimulation by cytokines and growth factors produced by inflammatory cells.

Cirrhosis

Cirrhosis is a diffuse form of hepatic fibrosis resulting from severe, long-standing hepatitis with extensive necrosis. In the cirrhotic liver, the normal hepatic architecture is destroyed by fibrous septa that encompass regenerative nodules of hepatocytes. Thus, the normally continuous liver parenchyma is dissected and subdivided into nodular aggregates of varying size, each of which is segregated by encircling bands (septa) of collagenous connective tissue. Several general pathologic features characterize cirrhosis: (i) the hepatic parenchyma is separated into nodular aggregates of regenerative hepatocytes that vary in size; (ii) the entire liver is involved and normal parenchymal structure is destroyed by septa of connective tissue; and (iii) both afferent and efferent arms of the liver vasculature are consumed by connective tissue septa.

Two major morphologic types of cirrhosis are recognized, termed micronodular cirrhosis and macronodular cirrhosis. In micronodular cirrhosis, regenerative hepatocyte nodules are scarcely larger than the size of a normal lobular unit of parenchyma, and are separated by thin connective tissue septa. However, the nodules show none of the landmarks observed in the normal liver, such as portal tracts or central veins. Macronodular cirrhosis is characterized by the presence of large irregular nodules that may contain portal tracts and efferent vessels. This form of cirrhosis may result from multilobular necrosis and formation of scars surrounding an area of parenchyma larger than a single lobule. In addition, micronodular cirrhosis can progress to the macronodular form through persistent regeneration and expansion of existing nodules.

The functional consequences of cirrhosis reflect the obstruction of normal blood flow through the liver. In the cirrhotic liver, the connective tissue septa preclude the normal passage of blood via the sinusoids through the formation of shunts from the portal triads to the central vein. The decreased hepatic function observed in with cirrhosis patients is the direct result of the rerouting of blood around the parenchyma. In addition to decreased liver function, portal hypertension results from the obstruction of liver blood flow secondary to regenerative nodules impinging on the hepatic veins. Complications from portal hypertension include bleeding from gastroesophageal varices, formation of ascites, and development of splenomegaly.

Cirrhosis is a result of chronic hepatitis, and most hepatocellular carcinoma occurs in the setting of cirrhosis in humans. Despite the observation that cirrhosis is not an obligate precursor lesion for HCC development, cirrhosis of any morphologic type or etiology is associated with increased risk for development of the disease. However, the magnitude of excess risk for development of HCC reflects the specific etiology of cirrhosis, suggesting that the nature of the causative agent may be determinant.

Hepatocellular carcinoma develops annually in 5–8% of the population affected by cirrhosis related to chronic hepatitis C virus (HCV) infection (IARC). A similar level of risk is associated with cirrhosis resulting from hemochromatosis. In contrast, risk for development of HCC is less for patients with hepatitis B virus (HBV)-related cirrhosis (IARC). Likewise, alcoholic cirrhosis and cirrhosis associated with certain genetic diseases (e.g., Wilson's disease and α1-antitrypsin deficiency) are accompanied by an even smaller risk for HCC. Nonalcoholic fatty liver disease (or nonalcoholic steatohepatitis) can result in development of cirrhosis, and in these patients there is an increased risk for HCC as well.

Phenotypic alterations and dysplasia

In the setting of simultaneous hepatocellular necrosis and proliferation, nodular aggregates of hepatocytes may develop in either cirrhotic or noncirrhotic livers that are affected by chronic hepatitis. These nodular aggregates of hyperplastic hepatocytes may express a variety of aberrant metabolic phenotypes before obvious genomic abnormalities occur. Alterations in the metabolic phenotype of a few hepatocytes, evidenced by the occurrence of foci of phenotypically altered hepatocytes, are one of the earliest morphologic changes detected in hepatocytes during the process of hepatocarcinogenesis. Phenotypically altered hepatocytes express and store various metabolic products, such as glycogen, lipid, and iron. Three major types of phenotypically altered hepatocytes have been identified: (i) glycogen-storing, (ii) mixed-cell type, and (iii) basophilic. Phenotypically altered hepatocytes occur in 76% (84/111) of cirrhotic livers, in 91% (29/32) of cirrhotic livers containing HCC, and in 70% (55/79) of cirrhotic livers without HCC.

Glycogen-storing (clear-cell) foci were found to be smaller than mixed-cell foci, which were often associated with larger hepatocyte nodules and the development of small-cell (dysplastic) change. Glycogen-storing foci contain hepatocytes with the earliest preneoplastic alterations, whereas mixedcell foci (containing both glycogen-storing and basophilic hepatocytes) represent more advanced lesions. Hyperplastic hepatocyte foci composed of cells with small-cell change appear to be the direct precursors of dysplastic nodules, which exhibit a higher probability of undergoing malignant transformation. Numerous studies of preneoplastic alterations in human livers have reported morphologic changes associated with hepatocyte dysplasia and suggested that dysplastic lesions are important in the evolution of HCC. Further, prospective studies have shown that the presence of dysplastic hepatocytes in cirrhotic livers is correlated with increased risk for HCC.

Emergence and progression of hepatocellular carcinoma

Development of HCC occurs in or near (and presumably from) dysplastic hepatocytes contained within either small foci or larger nodules. Liver cell dysplasia refers to morphologic alterations of hepatocytes, including cellular enlargement with a normal nuclear to cytoplasmic ratio, nuclear pleomorphism with hyperchromasia, and multinucleation. Regenerative hepatocyte nodules containing dysplastic cells in cirrhotic livers have been referred to as atypical adenomatous hyperplasia, macroregenerative nodules, or dysplastic nodules. Nodular aggregates of hepatocytes in cirrhotic livers range in size from less than 3 mm to greater than 5 cm in diameter, with size primarily reflecting the cause and chronicity of the cirrhotic process. Similar nodules (with or without dysplastic hepatocytes) can also occur in noncirrhotic livers that are the affected by chronic hepatitis. HCC can also occur in the setting of chronic hepatitis in the absence of cirrhosis but is always accompanied by hyperplastic nodules and foci of dysplastic hepatocytes. In Alaskan natives chronically infected with HBV (who are often infected with HBV at young ages), HCC usually occurs in livers affected by chronic inflammation and mild fibrosis but lacking frank cirrhosis. Furthermore, dysplastic hepatocytes can also develop as a focal lesion that is not contained in a regenerative hepatocyte nodule.

Etiology of Hepatocellular Carcinoma in Humans

The etiology of human HCC is clearly multifactorial. Numerous causative factors have been identified that are suggested to contribute to the development of HCC in humans, including exposure to naturally occurring carcinogens, industrial chemicals, pharmacologic agents, and various pollutants. Furthermore, viral infection, genetic disease, and lifestyle factors (e.g., alcohol consumption) contribute to the risk for development of HCC. The major human hepatocarcinogens that have been identified are the hepatotropic viruses HBV and HCV. Another major hepatocarcinogenic risk for humans is the dietary consumption of aflatoxins in food grains contaminated with *Aspergillus flavus* and related fungi. Consumption of alcoholic beverages (ethanol exposure) poses a carcinogenic risk to humans, with liver as the major target organ. In addition, several chemicals, complex chemical mixtures, industrial processes, and therapeutic drugs are recognized as potentially hepatocarcinogenic in humans. Some genetically determined liver disorders are associated with elevated risk for development of HCC. In common among all of these etiologic factors is the risk for development of chronic hepatitis and cirrhosis.

Hepatitis viruses

Numerous studies have shown a strong correlation between HBV infection and increased incidence of HCC. More recently, an association between chronic HCV infection and HCC has been recognized. Chronic infection with either HBV or HCV results in greatly increased risk for development of HCC in humans (100-fold to 200-fold) compared to individuals who are not infected. These associations led to the suggestion that these viruses might contain transforming oncogenes. However, the evidence suggests that this is not necessarily the case. Rather, the pathologic consequences of infection by HBV and/or HCV frequently include development of chronic hepatitis and cirrhosis, and these pathologic states are the settings in which HCC occurs most often in humans. Thus, infection by HBV and/or HCV may contribute to the risk of development of HCC by setting up a predisposing condition in the chronically injured liver.

Aflatoxins

The most well-studied hepatocarcinogen is a natural chemical carcinogen known as aflatoxin B_1, which is produced by the *Aspergillus flavus* mold. This mold grows on rice or other grains (including corn) that are stored without refrigeration in hot and humid parts of the world. Ingestion of food that is contaminated with *Aspergillus flavus* mold results in exposure to potentially high levels of aflatoxin B_1. Aflatoxins are toxic to the liver in humans and numerous animal species. The effects of these compounds are dose-related and demonstrate some dependency on age and sex. Aflatoxin B_1 is a potent, direct-acting liver carcinogen in humans, and chronic exposure leads inevitably to development of HCC.

Methods for accurately measuring human exposures to aflatoxins have been difficult to develop. Nonetheless, epidemiologic evidence suggests that rates of HCC are highest in populations that are exposed to the greatest levels of aflatoxin. Aflatoxin-DNA adducts have been exploited as a molecular biomarker of aflatoxin exposure. Using this biomarker in a prospective study of 18,000 men in Shanghai, a significant increase in risk for development of HCC was noted in individuals who demonstrated urinary excretion of aflatoxin–DNA adducts. The acute and chronic effects of aflatoxin exposure have not been well documented in humans, but in animal studies these exposures resulted in hepatocyte necrosis and steatohepatitis with acute exposure and fibrosis and cirrhosis with chronic exposure.

Ethanol consumption and smoking

Chronic alcohol (ethanol) consumption is associated with an elevated risk for HCC. However, alcohol is not directly carcinogenic to the liver; rather, it is thought that the chronic liver damage produced by sustained alcohol consumption (hepatitis and cirrhosis) may contribute secondarily to liver tumor formation. In fact, $>80\%$ of hepatocellular carcinoma in alcoholics occurs in cirrhotic livers. Furthermore, ethanol appears to potentiate the hepatocarcinogenicity of chronic HBV and chronic HCV infection. Other lifestyle factors may also contribute to risk for development of HCC, including tobacco smoking. However, some epidemiologic studies find no association between cigarette smoking and risk for development of HCC.

Hepatotoxic drugs and chemicals

Several chemicals, complex chemical mixtures, industrial processes, and/or therapeutic agents have been associated with development of HCC in exposed human populations. These include therapeutic exposure to the radioactive compound thorium dioxide (Thoratrast) for the radiologic imaging of blood vessels and exposures to high levels of certain industrial chemicals, such as vinyl chloride monomer, in the workplace. Furthermore, specific occupations are associated with slightly elevated risk for HCC, including asphalt workers and farmers exposed to pesticides. Pharmacologic exposure to anabolic steroids and estrogens can lead to development of liver cancer. Other agents are occasionally associated with development of HCC in humans, including ingestion of inorganic arsenic compounds.

Genetic diseases of the liver

Several genetic diseases that result in liver pathology can increase the risk of development of HCC. These genetic conditions include hemochromatosis, hereditary tyrosinemia, glycogen storage diseases, Wilson's disease, α1-antitrypsin deficiency, and others. Most of these genetic liver diseases are related to inborn errors of metabolism that result in the accumulation of metabolic products in hepatocytes. Liver damage resulting from this abnormal accumulation of metabolic products leads to chronic hepatitis and cirrhosis. Hereditary predisposition to HCC (in the absence of genetic liver disease) has been suggested based on the observation of tumor clusters in families. However, such familial clustering of HCC could reflect common exposures of family members to environmental risks factors such as HBV infection or aflatoxin exposure.

Cellular Pathogenesis of Hepatocellular Carcinoma

Development of HCC is typically in the pathologic setting of chronic hepatitis or cirrhosis. As such, chronic hepatitis and cirrhosis represent significant preneoplastic conditions of the liver. A number of cellular alterations characterize the hepatocytes of the regenerative nodules that are found in these livers. These changes, including increased cellular proliferation and development of monoclonal cell populations, have been documented in preneoplastic liver, and they persist in HCC.

Development of monoclonal hepatocyte populations in preneoplastic and neoplastic liver

A monoclonal cell population is defined as one that develops through multiple cycles of cell proliferation from a single progenitor cell. The importance of monoclonality in carcinogenesis relates to the accumulation of genetic changes in an emerging population of cells. Genetic alterations affecting the original progenitor cell will be passed to its progeny, and development of additional genetic alterations can result in the outgrowth of new clonal subpopulations. The clonality of regenerative hepatocyte nodules in cirrhotic livers has been addressed in several studies using various molecular techniques. Of the methods used, analysis of the chromosomal integration of HBV deoxyribonucleic acid (DNA) into the genomic DNA of infected hepatocytes appears to be the most sensitive and specific but depends on integration of the viral genome. In the livers of patients chronically infected with HBV, the integration of viral DNA in nonneoplastic hepatocytes suggests clonal expansion in regenerative hepatocyte nodules. Furthermore, molecular analysis of regenerative hepatocyte nodules in HBV-related cirrhosis determined that subsets (6–31%) of these nodules are monoclonal. Likewise, using molecular techniques, a significant fraction (43%) of hepatocyte nodules in HCV-related cirrhosis has been shown to be monoclonal. The monoclonality of hepatocyte nodules in the preneoplastic liver extends from regenerative hepatocyte nodules to more progressive lesions, including dysplastic nodules. Dysplastic hepatocytes in HBV-infected livers have been shown to be monoclonal using various molecular techniques. These observations demonstrate that monoclonal populations of hepatocytes (often phenotypically altered or dysplastic) occur in preneoplastic liver before the involved hepatocytes display characteristics of neoplastic transformation. Repetitive clonal proliferation from one progenitor (parent) cell facilitates the accumulation of genetic alterations in a large population of progeny cells.

Monoclonal populations of hepatocytes (regenerative and/or dysplastic) have been shown in preneoplastic livers (chronic hepatitis and cirrhosis). In a few studies, neoplastic lesions have been shown to reflect clonal outgrowths from a monoclonal population of nonneoplastic hepatocytes. Identical HBV DNA integration patterns were observed between HCC and adjacent nontumorous liver in one study. Similarly, the HBV integration pattern of hepatocytes contained in a dysplastic nodule was shown to be identical to that of a small HCC arising within the dysplastic nodule. These observations suggest that monoclonal hepatocyte populations represent preneoplastic lesions with potential to undergo neoplastic transformation to give rise to HCC and that dysplastic lesions may represent the direct precursor for HCC.

A number of studies have evaluated the monoclonality of HCC. Nearly all (105/109, 95%) small HCCs examined (using HBV integration or other molecular techniques) have been shown to be monoclonal. However, with increasing size of the HCC resulting from continued cell proliferation, new genetically distinct subpopulations of tumor cells emerge. The clonal divergence that accompanies increasing size of HCC has been demonstrated through DNA fingerprint analysis. HCCs less than 6 mm in diameter (mean = 4.7 mm) were found to be monoclonal, whereas HCCs greater than 6 mm in diameter (mean = 15.4 mm) were composed of multiple genetically divergent cell populations (clones).

Increased hepatocyte proliferation in preneoplastic and neoplastic liver

In the normal liver, the rates of cell proliferation and cell death are negligible and in near balance, reflecting the facts that hepatocytes are long lived and that there is very little cellular turnover in the adult. However, cell death and cell proliferation are both significantly increased in chronic hepatitis and cirrhosis. In the normal liver, less than 0.5% of hepatocytes are proliferative as evidenced by bromodeoxyuridine (BrdU) labeling index, whereas regenerative hepatocytes in cirrhotic livers exhibit BrdU labeling indices that are more than 8-fold that of normal liver. The increased cell proliferation that occurs in pathologic livers reflects increases in the proliferation of regenerative hepatocytes as well as foci of phenotypically altered hepatocytes.

In nodular lesions that also contained dysplastic hepatocytes, further increases in cell proliferation were noted. Corresponding increases in cell density accompany the increased rates of cell proliferation in preneoplastic liver lesions. High rates of hepatocyte proliferation correlate with increased risk for HCC. In preneoplastic liver (involving chronic hepatitis or cirrhosis), greatly increased rates of hepatocyte proliferation are accompanied by increased rates of cell death (apoptosis). However, rates of proliferation always exceed rates of apoptosis, resulting in expansion of aberrant cell populations.

Compared to normal liver and to preneoplastic liver lesions, HCC demonstrates high rates of cellular proliferation. BrdU labeling indices of HCC have been shown to be 28-fold higher than for normal livers. However, HCCs do not exhibit uniformly high rates of cell proliferation. Rather, there appears to be an inverse correlation between cell proliferation rate and the histologic differentiation of the tumor. Well-differentiated tumors exhibit BrdU labeling indices that are 18-fold higher than those of normal livers and 2.5-fold higher than those of cirrhotic livers. Moderately differentiated HCCs display BrdU labeling indices that are 24-fold higher than those of normal livers and 3-fold higher than those of cirrhotic livers. In contrast, poorly differentiated HCC exhibit BrdU labeling indices that are 42-fold higher than those of normal livers and 5-fold higher than those of cirrhotic livers. Increasing tumor grade has also been shown to be associated with higher rates of cellular proliferation in HCC. Furthermore, several studies suggest that larger (more advanced) tumors have dramatically increased rates of cellular proliferation compared with early tumors.

Mechanisms governing increased hepatocyte proliferation in preneoplastic and neoplastic liver

Usually HCC develops in the pathologic liver (involving either chronic hepatitis or cirrhosis), in which hepatocytes proliferate continuously and at higher rates than in nondiseased liver. The proliferative tissue microenvironment of the preneoplastic liver is characterized by elevated expression of several mitogenic factors for hepatocytes, including growth factors and their receptors, proinflammatory cytokines, and hormones. A comprehensive review of these mitogenic signaling molecules in HCC has recently appeared.

The major growth factors in HCC include transforming growth factor α (TGFα), insulin-like growth factor-2 (IGF-2), and hepatocyte growth factor (HGF). Normal hepatocytes do not express TGFα, but TGFα is expressed by hepatocytes in chronic hepatitis and cirrhosis, with the greatest expression in nodular lesions containing dysplastic hepatocytes. TGFα expression is immunohistochemically detectable in a significant fraction of HCCs, and expression levels do not correlate with tumor differentiation.

The cognate receptor for TGFα is the epidermal growth factor receptor (EGFR), which is expressed at similar levels in HCC and hepatocytes of nontumorous liver. Furthermore, coordinate expression of EGFR and TGFα in HCC has been shown, suggesting the establishment of an autocrine mechanisms for self-sustaining cellular growth stimulation. The concentration of IGF-2 increases significantly in cirrhotic livers (>threefold) and HCC (>ninefold) compared to normal livers. Similarly, immunohistochemical staining of pathologic livers has identified overexpression of IGF-2 in chronic hepatitis, cirrhosis, and HCC.

The IGF-2 protein generally co-localizes with proliferative cells of HCC, suggesting a correlation between autocrine expression of IGF-2 and cellular proliferation in those tumors. IGF-2 signaling is mediated by the IGF-1 receptor and the insulin receptor. Both of these receptors are ubiquitously expressed in normal cells and tissues, but no studies have been reported that describe their expression in HCC. Hepatocyte growth factor is not expressed by normal hepatocytes but is expressed by the neoplastic hepatocytes of many HCCs. However, the elevated levels of HGF in neoplastic hepatocytes of HCC is thought to reflect uptake and accumulation of the growth factor, rather than autocrine synthesis.

The HGF receptor c-met is expressed by normal hepatocytes and the neoplastic cells of HCC. Elevated c-met expression has been correlated with both increased cell proliferation in HCC and with poorer differentiation of tumors in some studies. Expression or overexpression of c-met in neoplastic hepatocytes in the presence of HGF (autocrine or paracrine) might drive tumor cell proliferation as a result of increased mitogenic stimulation. In the case of each of these major growth factor/receptor pathways (TGFα/EGFR, IGF-2/IGFIR, HGF/c-met) in HCC, the cognate receptors are expressed (or thought to be) by the neoplastic hepatocytes, and the growth factor is produced in autocrine fashion or is available through paracrine signaling pathways.

The inflammatory cells that infiltrate the liver in chronic hepatitis and cirrhosis represent a rich source for production of proinflammatory cytokines. In addition, the expression of certain cytokines and cytokine receptors can be induced in cells of the liver, including hepatocytes. Cytokines exert various effects in the liver, including mediating inflammation and immune responses. In addition, specific cytokines are required for activation of hepatocyte proliferation, especially TNFα and interleukin 6 (IL6). It has been suggested that these cytokines may play a role in the regulation of cellular proliferation leading to and following the development of HCC. However, the significance and specific role of these cytokines in human hepatocarcinogenesis has not yet been elucidated.

Molecular Pathogenesis of Hepatocellular Carcinoma

The molecular mechanisms that govern neoplastic transformation of hepatocytes leading to HCC have been extensively studied in humans and rodent models. The major molecular features of HCC include aneuploidy and chromosomal aberrations, activation of positive mediators of cellular proliferation (including classic cellular protooncogenes), and inactivation of negative mediators of cellular proliferation (including classic tumor-suppressor genes). Both genetic and epigenetic mechanisms play significant roles in the molecular pathogenesis of HCC.

Genomic alterations in hepatocellular carcinoma

The genomic alterations documented in human HCC include aberrations in chromosome structure, aneuploidy and abnormal chromosome numbers, allelic losses, and microsatellite instability. Approximately 40% of HCCs exhibit an aneuploid DNA content and numeric chromosomal abnormalities. Aneuploidy has also been documented in dysplastic lesions, suggesting that the genetic abnormalities may represent a significant determinant of neoplastic transformation in the liver. Further, aneuploidy has been shown in some studies to increase with decreasing differentiation of HCC, suggesting that continued genomic instability accompanies tumor progression. Karyotype analysis has been performed on a limited number of HCCs using cells taken directly from the neoplasm and cultured for short periods. Most HCC-derived cells were aneuploid with increased numbers of chromosomes and contained numerous structurally altered abnormal chromosomes as well. Approximately half of the HCCs examined contained a subtetraploid chromosome number (64–99 chromosomes per cell), whereas the remainder were near diploid. Among these studies of HCC, structural alteration of chromosome 1 was most frequently reported. Chromosomal regions most frequently involved in structural rearrangements included 1p11, 1p22, 1p32, 1p34, 1p36, 1q10, 1ql2, 1q25, 6q13-q15, 6q22-q25, 8q10, 16q24, and 17p11.

Comparative genomic hybridization has been used in a number of studies to examine gains and losses of chromosome arms in HCC. Chromosomal gains have been described in HCC involving 1p, 4q, 5p, 6q, 8p, 9p, 10q, 11q, 12q, 16q, 17p, and 19p. In some cases, significant gains were observed, suggestive of gene amplification. Chromosomal losses involving 1q, 6p, 8q, 11q, 17q, and 20q also occur in HCC. Some studies have addressed the possibility that specific genetic aberrations occur in HCC related to a specific etiologic agent. In one study, chromosomes 4q, 8p, and 16q were affected in HBV-related HCC, whereas 11q was affected in HCV-related HCC, suggesting that specific genetic abnormalities can be attributed to specific etiologic agents or mechanisms. However, other investigators conclude that no such association exists. Furthermore, it appears that the most commonly affected chromosome across all studies is 1q, which is affected in HCC of all etiologies at high frequency.

More recent studies have used spectral karyotyping to examine chromosomal rearrangements in primary HCC and derived cell lines. These analyses identified aberrant chromosomes involving 1p13-q21, 8p12-q21, 17p11-q12, 17q22, and 19p10-q13.1. These studies also noted that HCC of larger size contained increasing numbers of chromosomal abnormalities, suggesting continued genomic evolution as tumors progress. Spectral karyotyping also identified novel chromosomal breakpoints involving numerous pericentromeric chromosomal regions. These breakpoints could be important for large-scale chromosomal deletions (involving chromosome arms) that are recognized through allelotyping studies.

The development of HCC involves numerous chromosomal alterations. Comprehensive allelotyping of HCC has been performed by several groups of investigators using large numbers of polymorphic microsatellite markers spanning the entire genome with an average spacing of markers of ~20 cM. Additional allelotyping studies have appeared, but many examined only a few chromosomal arms or used very few markers per chromosomal arm. When the most comprehensive of these studies are considered, there is very good agreement on the fraction of allelic loss in HCC and the identification of specific chromosomal arms that demonstrate significant allelic losses during hepatocarcinogenesis and tumor progression. The mean fractional allelic loss per HCC was 13–24%, and ranged from 0–43%. Recurring allelic losses affecting more than 30% of all HCCs examined have been documented on a number of chromosome arms, including 1p, 1q, 4q, 5q, 6q, 8p, 8q, 9p, 13q, 14q, 16p, 16q, and 17p, but the frequency of loss of heterozygosity (LOH) involving loci on these chromosome arms is rarely more than 60%. Nonetheless, allelic imbalance of 60–85% involving 4q, 8p, 9p, and 16q has been identified in some studies.

In theory, the chromosomal regions affected by deletion (LOH) may harbor genes with tumor-suppressor activity. In fact, several well-known tumor-suppressor genes reside on chromosome arms that are frequently affected by regional chromosomal deletions, such as *p53* at

17p and *Rb1* at 13q. These observations suggest that chromosomal losses can be exploited to infer the location of important tumor-suppressor genes that are subject to inactivation through this mechanism. Furthermore, the diversity of chromosomal aberrations supports the suggestion that multiple genes and molecular pathways contribute to the development of HCC. Studies of gene expression in HCC support this suggestion.

Microsatellite instability is a specific form of genomic instability that is characterized by mutational alteration of simple repetitive sequences, including both expansions (insertional mutagenesis) and contractions (deletional mutagenesis), usually resulting in frameshift mutations. The molecular defects responsible for microsatellite instability in human tumors involve the genes that encode the proteins required for normal mismatch repair. A limited number of studies have examined microsatellite instability in HCC. When all studies are combined, 25/218 (11%) HCCs demonstrated microsatellite alterations involving at least one locus. However, with application of more stringent criteria (microsatellite alterations involving at least two loci), 25/88 (28%) of hepatocellular carcinomas exhibit microsatellite instability. Microsatellite instability involving a small number of loci was noted in two comprehensive allelotyping studies of a large number of HCCs. More recent studies have suggested that microsatellite instability affects only ~7% of loci investigated. Other studies have failed to identify microsatellite instability in HCC.

Comprehensive studies of the mutation status of mismatch repair genes have not been performed for HCC. However, there is evidence that mismatch repair genes (including *hMSH2* and *hMLH1*) are affected by loss of heterozygosity in HCC that exhibits microsatellite instability. In addition, *hMSH2* has been shown to be mutated in some HCCs that display microsatellite instability. These studies suggest that microsatellite instability may be mechanistically involved with the molecular pathogenesis of a subset of HCC. In fact, in some cases microsatellite instability may precede the development of HCC, as has been documented in preneoplastic cirrhotic livers and in nontumorous liver adjacent to HCC. Microsatellite instability could contribute to the pathogenesis of HCC through the inactivation of critical genes for growth control, regulation of apoptosis, or some other pathway. In support of this suggestion, microsatellite alterations involving the *TGFβRII, M6P/IGFIIR,* and *BAX* genes have been documented in one case study of HCC.

Cellular protooncogenes and hepatocarcinogenesis

The setting for HCC is the hyperproliferative liver associated with chronic hepatitis and cirrhosis. The repetitive proliferation of regenerative hepatocytes (and progressive lesions) is promoted by the presence of numerous mitogenic growth factors and cytokines. However, neoplastic transformation of hepatocytes is accompanied by perturbation of the numerous intracellular signaling pathways leading to the acquisition of autonomous and unregulated cellular proliferation. These signaling pathways involve a number of positive mediators of cellular proliferation, including the protein products of the c-*ras* gene family, c-*myc,* c-*fos,* various cyclins and cyclin-dependent kinases, and others.

Microarray-based studies of HCC and preneoplastic livers have resulted in the development of molecular signatures for this tumor and have potentially identified useful markers for disease initiation or progression. A comprehensive review of all these positive mediators of hepatocellular growth is beyond the scope of this review. Rather, the contributions of several cellular protooncogene products to hepatocarcinogenesis is considered, including the c-*ras* family, c-myc, and cyclin D1.

The expression of p21 ras is up-regulated in HCC and in preneoplastic livers (chronic hepatitis and cirrhosis), especially dysplastic hepatocytes and HBV-infected cells. Increased levels of expression of c-H-*ras* and c-K-*ras* have been documented in HCC, as well as some preneoplastic liver lesions. Similarly, some studies have shown c-N-*ras* to be overexpressed in HCC. However, other studies failed to detect overexpression of c-H-*ras* or c-K-*ras* in HCC. These findings may suggest that overexpression of a single member of the c-*ras* family is necessary for hepatocarcinogenesis, irrespective of which member of the family is up-regulated. Overexpression of c-*ras* family members may reflect amplification of the corresponding gene. Very few point mutations in the c-*ras* genes have been documented in HCC, suggesting that mutational activation of c-*ras* does not play a significant role in hepatocarcinogenesis. Nonetheless, the overexpression of p21 ras protein in nearly all HCCs examined suggests that the ras mitogen-activated protein kinase (MAPK) pathway is hyperactive in these neoplasms.

The nuclear transcription factor c-myc is overexpressed in ~50% of HCCs, and the c-*myc* messenger ribonucleic acid (mRNA) is overexpressed in more than 90% of HCCs. In some studies, the level of c-myc protein overexpression was 15-fold that of adjacent nontumorous liver. The level of expression of c-myc protein is also increased in chronic hepatitis and cirrhosis. Increased levels of expression of c-myc in HCC (and preneoplastic liver) may in part be a result of upregulation of the MAPK pathway in hyperproliferative liver. However, c-*myc* gene amplification and hypomethylation also contribute significantly to the overexpression of c-*myc* in HCC. The c-*myc* gene was found to be hypomethylated in 55% (15/27) of HCCs examined. In addition, hypomethylation of c-myc was detected in a significant percentage of cirrhotic livers adjacent to HCC, suggesting that hypomethylation of c-*myc* may reflect an early alteration leading to c-*myc* dysregulation in hepatocarcinogenesis. The c-*myc* gene was amplified in 31% (50/163) of HCCs evaluated. However, c-*myc* gene amplification was not detected in preneoplastic lesions associated with HCC.

The cyclins and cyclin-dependent kinases regulate the transit of cells through the cell cycle. Overexpression of these proteins can lead to unregulated cell cycle progression and uncontrolled cellular proliferation. Cyclin D1 protein is overexpressed in a significant fraction (~40%) of HCCs. The overexpression of cyclin D1 is related to amplification of the *cyclin D1* gene and overexpression of its mRNA in some cases.

Tumor-suppressor genes and hepatocarcinogenesis

A number of tumor-suppressor genes and other negative mediators of cellular proliferation have been implicated in the molecular pathogenesis of HCC. These tumor suppressor genes and tumor-suppressor–like genes include *p*53, retinoblastoma 1 *(Rb1), p73, mdm2,* adenomatous polyposis coli *(APC),* β-*catenin, E-cadherin,* phosphatase and tensin homolog deleted on chromosome ten *(PTEN), BRCA1,* fragile histidine triad *(FHIT),* and several others. Therefore, in the following sections the contributions of *p53* and *Rb1* to hepatocarcinogenesis is reviewed. The *p53* tumor-suppressor gene product is a multifunctional protein that is involved with numerous cellular processes, including cell cycle control, genomic stability and DNA repair, and apoptosis. The p53 protein is functionally inactivated in the majority of human cancers through one of several genetic or epigenetic processes, including mutation, allelic deletion, or interaction with inactivating proteins. In HCC, *p53* is frequently the target of chromosomal deletion (LOH) involving 17p. A review of a large number of studies showed LOH at the *p53* gene in ~41% of HCCs examined. A few studies have suggested that deletion of the *p53* gene occurs early in hepatocarcinogenesis as evidenced by loss of heterozygosity of the *p53* gene in nodular lesions of chronic hepatitis and cirrhosis.

The frequency of *p53* deletion was found to increase with increasing size of HCC, suggesting that loss of this gene is associated with tumor progression. Similarly, loss of heterozygosity of the *p53* gene is associated with higher tumor grade in HCC. Mutation of the *p53* gene occurs in conjunction with loss of heterozygosity of the *p53* locus in HCC, with most of the mutations following within the highly conserved region of the gene that includes exons 5–9. A summary of numerous studies of *p53* mutation in HCC suggests that mutations occur in ~27% (547/2029) of these tumors. However, the *p53* mutation frequency and mutational spectrum varies greatly in affected populations from various world regions, possibly reflecting specific exposures and risk factors.

Point mutation of codon 249 of the *p53* gene represents a hotspot for gene mutation in the liver, accounting for ~30% of *p53* mutations in HCC. This mutation, which results in a G to T transversion (AGG to AGT, arginine to serine), was first recognized in patients from Qidong, China but has also been recognized in HCCs from Africa and North America. The *p53* codon 249 mutation has been attributed to exposure to aflatoxin B_1. The mutational spectrum of the *p*53 gene in HCC differs significantly between geographic areas with high aflatoxin exposure and those with low exposures. Mutation of the *p53* gene can result in overexpression of the protein product (through stabilization of the protein) or lack of expression of the protein, depending on the nature of the mutation. Similarly, stabilization of the p53 protein can be effected through interaction with p53-binding proteins. The p53 protein is known to complex with the HBV X antigen, which can increase levels of the protein in cells while inactivating it.

Inappropriate overexpression of mdm2 could also result in the sequestration and functional inactivation of p53 protein, although studies to show this directly in HCC are lacking. Overexpression of p53 protein has been described in HCC, as well as preneoplastic liver lesions, including dysplastic hepatocytes and regenerative hepatocyte nodules in cirrhotic liver. In some studies, overexpression of p53 protein was noted in a higher percentage of more advanced HCCs, suggesting that p53 abnormalities may be associated with tumor progression.

Like *p*53, the *Rb1* gene product is a multifunctional protein that plays a central role in cell cycle control. The *Rb1* gene is deleted in a significant percentage of HCCs (~30–40%). In individual studies, the frequency of LOH at the *Rb1* locus was as high as 73%. In some studies, investigators examined LOH at the *Rb1* locus using specific probes that flank this gene, producing evidence suggesting that deletion of the *Rb1* gene is a frequent event in HCC. Deletion of *Rb1* (LOH) usually is accompanied by loss of expression of pRb. Deletion of *Rb1* has also been documented in nonneoplastic cirrhotic liver adjacent to HCC lacking this gene. In contrast, cirrhotic nodules adjacent to HCCs that exhibit no loss of *Rb1* also retain both *Rb1* alleles. These observations suggest that deletion of *Rb1* is an early event in hepatocarcinogenesis, occurring in preneoplastic cirrhotic livers. However, others have shown that HCCs that show loss of heterozygosity for *Rb1* can be closely associated with preneoplastic cirrhotic nodules that retain both *Rb1* alleles. This study, as well as others, suggests that deletion of *Rb1* may be a late genetic alteration in HCC, associated with tumor progression.

Concluding Remark

The major risk factors and etiologic agents responsible for development of HCC in humans have been identified, characterized, and described, including chronic infection with HBV or HCV, exposure to aflatoxin B1, and cirrhosis of any etiology (including alcoholic cirrhosis and cirrhosis associated with genetic liver diseases). Both chronic hepatitis and cirrhosis represent major preneoplastic conditions of the liver because the majority of HCCs arise in these pathologic settings. Hepatocarcinogenesis represents a linear and progressive, albeit slow, process in which successively more aberrant monoclonal populations of hepatocytes evolve. Regenerative hepatocytes in focal lesions in the inflamed liver (chronic hepatitis or cirrhosis) give rise to hyperplastic hepatocyte nodules, and these progress to dysplastic nodules, which are thought to be the direct precursor of HCC. In most cases, the neoplastic transformation of hepatocytes results from accumulation of genetic damage during the repetitive cellular proliferation that occurs in the injured liver in response to paracrine growth factor and cytokine stimulation. HCCs exhibit numerous genetic abnormalities, including chromosomal deletions, rearrangements, aneuploidy, gene amplifications, and mutations, as well as epigenetic alterations, including modification of DNA methylation. These genetic and epigenetic alterations together activate positive mediators of cellular proliferation, including protooncogenes and their mitogenic signaling pathways, and inactivate negative mediators of proliferation, including tumor-suppressor and cell-cycle control genes, resulting in cells with autonomous growth potential. However, HCCs exhibit a high degree of genetic heterogeneity, suggesting that multiple molecular pathways may be involved in the genesis of subsets of liver cancers. Nonetheless, comprehensive elucidation of the specific genes and molecular pathways involved in progression from preneoplastic lesions to frank neoplasia in the protracted process of hepatocarcinogenesis will facilitate development of new strategies for prevention and therapy. Identification of molecular pathways that drive the proliferation of neoplastic hepatocytes may enable development of drugs that can specifically target and kill those cells. Alternatively, chemopreventive agents may be developed that will impede the malignant conversion of dysplastic hepatocytes, impeding development of HCC in high-risk patients. Until molecular-based therapies of these sorts can be developed, the best hope for significant reductions in the worldwide incidence of HCC will require development of more effective anti-viral treatments or implementation of improved (more effective) strategies for preventing HBV and HCV infection.

6

COLON CANCER

Carcinomas of the colon and rectum (here summarized as colon cancer) are among the most prevalent cancers in Western industrialized countries. Together with lung cancer, breast cancer in females and prostate cancer in males, they constitute the majority of lethal cancers in these countries and a major public health problem. Like breast and prostate cancer, colon cancer is much less prevalent in the developing world, but also in the richer Asian countries and Southern Europe. These differences point to important life style factors in the etiology of the disease. Good evidence exists for the involvement of dietary factors.

Several distinct precursor stages can be distinguished in histology. The stages of cancer development thus range from hyperplasia through various benign adenomas and locally invasive carcinoma to systemic metastatic disease.

Several hereditary cancer syndromes increase the risk for colon carcinoma more or less specifically, among them *familial adenomatous polyposis* coli (FAP), *hereditary non-polyposis colon carcinoma* (HNPCC), *Peutz-Jeghers syndrome* (PJS), and Cowden's disease. The study of these moderately prevalent to very rare syndromes has greatly contributed to the understanding of sporadic colon cancer.

While it is a general tenet that human carcinomas arise by alterations in several distinct genes and regulatory pathways, in colon cancer, many of these alterations have actually been identified. Moreover, they can be assigned to specific stages of tumor development and related to specific histological changes. This molecular model of colon carcinogenesis has promoted understanding of the underlying biological processes. Attempts to transfer this model have often stimulated research on other cancers. In this sense, colon cancer has become paradigmatic for molecular oncology.

The fundamental '*gatekeeper*' step in colon cancer development leading primarily to adenomas is a constitutive activation of the WNT signaling pathway. It is usually caused by loss of function of the classical tumor suppressor APC, less frequently by mutations in *CTNNB1* oncogenically activating β-Catenin, and rarely by other changes in the pathway. The activation appears to confer a kind of '*stem-cell*' phenotype to the carcinoma cells.

Further steps in the progression of the cancer are associated with mutations activating KRAS, loss of function of TP53, and inactivation of the cellular response to TGFβ.

Colon cancer exemplifies that tumor development can be driven by several different mechanisms. Molecular research has revealed that the accumulation of molecular alterations in individual colon cancers can alternatively be driven predominantly by an increased rate of fixed point mutations, by chromosomal instability, or an increased rate of epigenetic alterations. These molecularly defined subclasses differ only moderately in their morphology and clinical behavior, but the classification should become very helpful for diagnostics and for definition of therapeutic targets.

Specifically, a subgroup of colon cancers is characterized by an increased rate of point mutations, which is most evident as frequent alterations in the length of microsatellite repeats. This '*microsatellite instability*' is caused by defects in the DNA mismatch repair system. It can arise spontaneously by genetic or epigenetic inactivation of genes encoding components of this system or as a consequence of inherited mutations in these genes in the dominantly inherited HNPCC syndrome.

Colon cancer also occurs in the context of chronic inflammatory bowel diseases such as ulcerative colitis. Non-steroidal antiinflammatory drugs diminish colon cancer risk in such patients, but seem to be efficacious also in others at risk for colon cancer. Thus, colon cancer also is also a pioneer example for chemoprevention.

Natural History of Colorectal Cancer

Colorectal cancer can develop in all segments of the large intestine. Although its location somewhat influences the prognosis and obviously the approach for surgical treatment, from a biological point of view, it can be considered under one heading, i.e. colon cancer. Interestingly, cancers of the small intestine are very rare and certainly represent a distinct disease.

There is good morphological and molecular genetical evidence that colon carcinoma develops through several precursor stages. The earliest recognizable preneoplastic changes result in hyperplastic or dysplastic crypts. There is some debate whether one or the other of these, or both can give rise to adenomas and carcinomas. In contrast, it is generally agreed that adenomatous polyps are a precursor stage for many carcinomas. They are usually found as single benign tumors protruding into the lumen of the bowel and consist of a thickened, more or less disorganized epithelium. Multiple polyps are found in certain circumstances, e.g., in the familial cancer syndrome '*familial adenomatous polyposis coli*' (FAP) discussed below. These polypous tumors are considered a type of adenoma and can be categorized into several substages according to the degree of growth and dysplasia.

Invasion of tumor cells through the basement membrane into the underlying mesenchyme is the diagnostic mark of carcinoma. Several tumor stages are distinguished in routine pathology according to the extent of invasion and the spread of the tumor mass. Localized colon carcinomas without metastases can often be cured by surgery. In many cases, '*adjuvant*' chemotherapy is applied after surgery to kill remaining tumor cells. The prognosis of colon carcinoma becomes worse and the treatment much more difficult, if the tumor has spread to local lymph nodes or metastasized to the liver, lung and other organs. Surgery and chemotherapy can still be curative, but often only prolong survival.

The incidence of colon cancer varies considerable across the world, with the highest incidences in Western industrialized countries. Colon cancer is usually a disease of older people. However, the incidence remains different between countries with on average younger or older populations even after adjustment for age. The causes for these differences in incidence are not really understood. The best evidence points to dietary factors being responsible.

Familial Adenomatous Polyposis Coli and the WNT Pathway

Familial Adenomatous Polyposis Coli (FAP) is the most prevalent of several related syndromes which carry a strongly enhanced risk for colon cancer. Related afflictions include Gardners syndrome, Turcots syndrome, and an attenuated form of FAP. These syndromes are distinguished from each other by the kind of tumors and developmental defects that appear in other organs besides the large intestine.

Patients with standard FAP characteristically develop hundreds of adenomatous polyps in their colon, rectum, and duodenum as well as gland polyps in the stomach, early in life. Congenitally, they display hypertrophy of the retinal pigment epithelium. Although the polyps are adenomatous, i.e. benign tumors, eventually one or the other progresses to malignancy and carcinomas develop, typically in the third or fourth decade of life. The life-time risk of carcinoma development approaches 100%. Therefore, removal of the colon is used as a preventive measure. FAP is inherited in an autosomal-dominant fashion. With its constellation of multiple tumors in the same organ, carcinoma development much before the usual age, and autosomal-dominant mode of inheritance, FAP is a prime example of an inherited tumor disease corresponding to the '*Knudson*' model.

The gene mutated in FAP was identified in 1991 and was named *APC*, for '*adenomatous polyposis coli*'. Positional cloning families with FAP and the related Gardner's syndrome was successful, strongly aided by a key patient with a cytogenetically recognizable deletion in chromosome 5q21 where the *APC* gene resides. *APC* turned out to be a large gene comprising binding several different proteins and of oligomerization. The oligomerization domain is located near the N-terminus. Several repeats are recognizable along the length of the protein, of which the catenin-repeats and the 20 aa-repeats are involved in assembling a protein complex containing β-Catenin, glycogen synthase 3β (GSK3β), and the scaffold protein Axin or its relative Conductin (or Axin2). This protein complex is involved in regulating WNT signaling. A basic region in APC located further towards the C-terminus interacts with microtubules. The actual C-terminal region binds EB1 and DLG, two proteins interacting with the mitotic spindle. There is some evidence that one function of APC lies in chromosome segregation. Loss of this function may favor the development of aneuploidy in colon cancer.

Patients with FAP inherit a mutation in one *APC* allele. Most are nonsense *C* mutations leading to a truncated or instable protein and almost all are located in the first half of the gene. As predicted by the '*Knudson*' model, adenomas and carcinomas either contain somatic mutations in the second allele as well or have lost the intact allele by 5q deletion or by recombination, as recognizable by LOH in the 5q21 region.

Not unexpectedly, the gene mutated in the Gardner and Turcot syndromes as well as in the attenuated variety of FAP is also *APC*. The various syndromes are in general distinguished by the location of the mutation, which appears to determine the spectrum of organs in which hyperplasia and tumors arise. For instance, truncating mutations between codons 463 and 1387 are associated with the congenital hypertrophy of the retinal pigment epithelium characteristic of standard FAP, while mutations between codons 1403 and 1578 are often found in families with Gardner syndrome. Interestingly, truncating mutations within the first 150 aa cause attenuated FAP, i.e. a milder phenotype. Nonsense mutations closer to the translational start would be expected to usually cause a complete loss of a protein, while mutations in later exons would be thought to more frequently yield truncated, but stable proteins. It is therefore conceivable that the truncated protein produced by mutations further downstream in the *APC* gene may somehow aggravate the disease, perhaps by interfering with the function of the normal APC protein encoded by the intact allele. Although these mechanistical relationships are still incompletely understood, cataloguing of such genotype-phenotype relationships is important to optimize the treatment and counseling of the affected patients and families.

Since deletions and LOH of chromosome 5q are among the most frequent alterations in colorectal cancer overall, following the identification of *APC* as the gene mutated in FAP, sporadic carcinomas were screened extensively for mutations in the gene. Today, it is assumed that both alleles of the gene are inactivated by point mutation and deletion/recombination, or occasionally promoter hypermethylation, in 70-80% of colon and rectal cancers, irrespectively of whether they are familial or sporadic. Moreover, the frequency of *APC* mutations is almost the same in early and late stage tumors. Thus, APC is a prototypic tumor suppressor. Since its inactivation appears to be almost mandatory for the development of colorectal tumors and most probably takes place at an early stage, the designation of '*gatekeeper*' is appropriate.

The crucial role of APC is underlined by the analysis of the 20% or so colon cancers, which retain a fully functional APC protein at normal expression levels. Almost all of these contain mutations in other components of the APC/β-Catenin/Axin/GSK3β complex. Most often, mutations in the *CTNNB1* gene encoding β-Catenin are found. More precisely, then, it is a disturbance of WNT signaling that is so crucial for development of colorectal cancers.

There are >23 different WNT proteins in man. They are usually produced and secreted by mesenchymal tissues and act on neighboring epithelial cells in a paracrine manner. Most are agonists, but some may be antagonists. In the canonical pathway, WNT factors bind to one of several cell surface receptors named Frizzled (FZD). These receptors belong to the large '*serpentine*' class of receptors characterized by seven transmembrane helices and interaction with trimeric G proteins. Activation of a FZD receptor activates the DSH (*dishevelled*) protein which in turn inhibits GSK3β. In a normal cell, this protein kinase is assembled together with Axin and APC in a cytosolic protein complex. This complex binds β-Catenin. In the absence of a WNT signal β-Catenin is phosphorylated by GSK3β at several sites near its N-terminus. This phosphorylation allows β-Catenin to be recognized by a ubiquitin ligase complex in which βTRCP performing the actual recognition.

Inhibition of GSK3β as a consequence of a WNT signal leads to accumulation of β-Catenin. The protein migrates into the nucleus, where it binds and activates TCF transcription factors, specifically TCF4 in colon cells. There are four known members of the TCF family, TCF1, LEF1, TCF3, and TCF4, which in the inactive state are complexed with transcriptional repressor proteins, usually from the Groucho family. This repression is alleviated by β-Catenin and transcription of TCF target genes resumes. Among these target genes are several that act directly on cell proliferation and survival, such as *CCDN1* and *MYC*.

Before becoming implicated in WNT signaling, β-Catenin had been known for a long time as a cytoskeletal protein binding to E-Cadherin which mediates homotypic cell interactions. Therefore, the concentration of active β-Catenin is also modulated by E-Cadherin. This may allow to integrate information from WNT signals and cell adhesion. Several further factors modulate WNT activity, e.g. SFRPs (*secreted frizzled-related proteins*), which interfere with WNT binding to receptors, and LRPs which support WNT binding to FZD receptors.

This intricate network is fundamentally disturbed in colon cancer. Obliteration of APC function, the most frequent alteration, causes a permanent WNT signal in the nucleus, since the regulatory protein complex cannot be assembled and β-Catenin does not become phosphorylated. As a result β-catenin accumulates and causes a constitutive activation of TCF target genes. Mutations in *CTNNB1* alter the amino acids in the recognition sequence of GSK3β prohibiting phosphorylation of β-Catenin, with essentially the same consequence. The rarer deletions of Axin likewise disturb efficient phosphorylation of β-Catenin by removing the platform on which the proteins interact. Inactivating mutations have also been reported for βTRCP impeding the ubiquitin ligase that initiates the proteolytic breakdown of β-Catenin. These central alterations in the WNT pathway may be compounded by alterations in modulating factors. During tumor progression many carcinomas lose E-Cadherin expression which may exacerbate the accumulation of β-Catenin. Likewise, WNT signaling may be further enhanced by down-regulation of SFRPs.

Many other cancer types besides colorectal cancer have meanwhile been investigated for mutations in *APC* and its interacting genes. Two important conclusions can be drawn.

1. Mutations in components of the WNT signaling pathway are found in many other carcinomas, with varying frequencies, although in none, it appears, with the same regularity. High to moderate prevalences are observed in hepatoma, medulloblastoma, and breast cancer, lower frequencies in prostate carcinoma, renal carcinoma and glioblastoma. Of note, some of these cancers are also more frequent in the context of the Gardners and Turcots syndromes. Clearly, however, some cancer types lack mutations in the pathway; although it is difficult to exclude the occurrence of mutations with current techniques. Moreover, one promoter of the *APC* gene tends to hypermethylated in many carcinomas; it is not clear, however, whether this an indication of differential promotor use or overall diminished transcription.
2. While *APC* is the major target in colorectal cancer, in other cancers mutations in *CTNNB1* predominate. It is not at all clear, why this is so. One possibility is that only colorectal carcinogenesis requires obliteration of other APC functions as well, such as the one presumed in mitosis. Another possibility is that the difference is related to the mechanisms involved in carcinogenesis in different organs. Distinct carcinogens involved may preferentially target certain positions in certain genes.

The requirement for constitutive activation of the WNT pathway in colon cancer may be closely related to the organization of this tissue. The colon epithelium is a constantly renewing tissue. The cells of the colon epithelium are derived from a small number – may be five or so of tissue stem cells located near the bottom of the crypt in a stem cell niche. When these cells divide asymetrically, one daughter cell retains the stem cell character while the other is committed to differentiation. It moves up the crypt, gradually differentiating and concomitantly losing its ability to proliferate. Cells that have arrived at the surface are sloughed off or die by apoptosis.

It appears that the WNT pathway is central to the regulation of this renewal strategy. WNT factors are produced by mesenchymal cells near the stem cell niche allowing reproduction and maintaining immortality of the stem cell population. As cells committed to differentiation move away from the growth factor source, differentiation and apoptosis programs are turned on. Cell-associated signaling proteins called Ephrins and their receptors are involved in establishing the differentiated state and are down-regulated by WNT signaling. Thus, colon epithelial cells not exposed to WNT signals may enter a default state of differentiation or apoptosis. Constitutive WNT signaling caused by APC loss of function or β-Catenin over-activity would prohibit differentiation and apoptosis and establish a stem-cell like state independent of position in the tissue.

A similar effect is thought to be exerted by activation of the Hedgehog pathway in basal cell carcinoma of the skin. It is tempting to speculate that the range of cancers in which mutations of the WNT pathway are observed may be related to the proliferation strategy of the respective tissues. There is still too little data on this question, though, for a judgement on this hypothesis.

Progression of Colon Cancer and the Multi-step Model of Tumorigenesis

As the FAP syndrome demonstrates, inactivation of both APC alleles is very likely sufficient for the formation of benign adenomatous polyps in the colon. For the transition to malignancy, i.e., invasion and metastasis, further genetic changes are required. Indeed, advanced colon cancers harbor a multitude of genetic and epigenetic alterations in addition to losses of chromosome 5q and mutations of *APC* or *CTNNB1*. Three of these alterations are consistent and well-characterized. In fact, they often seem to be associated with particular steps in the progression of colon cancer. They are (1) activation of KRAS by point mutations, (2) inactivation of TP53 by point mutation and allele deletion, (3) loss of responsiveness to TGFβ signaling, by loss of function of SMAD transcription factors or by mutations affecting the TGFβ receptor subunits.

1. RAS proteins act as signal transducers in several pathways. They relay signals from mitogenic growth factors via the MAPK cascade to the nuclus, regulate the structure of the cytoskeleton, and act on the PI3K signaling pathways augmenting cell growth and survival. In colon cancer, the *KRAS* proto-oncogene is activated by typical point mutations in codons 12, 13, or 61 that impede the

activity of the RAS GTPase and prolong the active state during which the protein relays signals. These mutations are found in 30–70% of all colon cancers and are more frequent in carcinomas than in adenomas. It is likely that these KRAS mutations further stimulate the proliferation of colon tumor cells, favoring the progression from adenoma towards carcinoma. Moreover, the effects of RAS signaling on the cytoskeleton and protein synthesis may contribute to the invasive potential of the transformed cells.

2. Inappropriate activity of genes like *RAS* and *MYC* is counterbalanced in normal cells by induction of cellular senescence or apoptosis. One important mechanism involves induction of $p14^{ARF1}$ by these and other oncogenes which leads to stabilization and activation of TP53. It is therefore not surprising that many advanced colon carcinomas have lost functional TP53. Usually, one copy of the *TP53* gene is inactivated by point mutations, predominantly in the central DNA binding domain of the protein, and the second copy is deleted or exchanged by allelic loss, detectable as LOH at 17p. Loss of TP53 function also compromises the cellular response to other types of cellular stress, including the responses to DNA damage, aneuploidy, and nucleotide imbalances. In colon cancer, loss of TP53 function appears to be associated with tumor progression. Likely, the loss of TP53 relieves a check on KRAS mutations and facilitates the development of increased genomic instability in advanced colon cancers.
3. In epithelial cells, the pathway activated by TGFβ decreases cell proliferation, e.g., by inducing CDK inhibitors, and promotes cell-matrix interactions. Accordingly, it is very frequently inactivated in highly invasive human cancers. In addition, secretion of TGFβ by carcinoma cells modulates their interaction with stroma cells and immune cells at the primary tumor site and during metastasis. In colon cancer, several genetic alterations may alternatively decrease TGFβ signaling. Truncating mutations of the TGFβRII receptor are frequent in the HNPCC subtype of colon cancer. In many advanced stage colon cancers, allelic loss is found at chromosome 18q in the region where the SMAD2 and SMAD4 genes reside. In fact, loss of 18q is one of the most consistent chromosomal changes in advanced colon carcinomas, together with loss of 5q and of 17p. In accord with expectations, point mutations and even deletions of the remaining SMAD2 and SMAD4 alleles have been found. However, their frequency seems rather low and questions remain about their importance in colon cancer.

So, during the progression of colon carcinoma to an invasive, metastatic cancer, a number of genetic alterations accumulate. The minimal requirements may comprise constitutive activation of the WNT pathway, activation of RAS signaling, loss of TP53 function, and inactivation of TGFβ signaling. Each of these changes may require more than one genetic or epigenetic alteration. For instance, WNT pathway activation in a sporadic colon cancer may require a point mutation in *APC* and loss of 5q, with additional changes in SFRPs or other modulators. Thus, a minimum of 5 - 7 genetic changes may be needed, but the actual number is likely higher.

Hereditary Nonpolyposis Colon Carcinoma

In FAP and related hereditary diseases, multiple polyps develop in the colon, from which individual carcinomas emerge. In other families with early onset colon cancer inherited in an autosomal-dominant fashion, no polyposis is observed. Moreover, the spectrum of associated tumors in other organs is distinct from that in the various syndromes resulting from inherited *APC* mutations. Instead, it includes endometrial and ovarian tumors in women as well as cancers of the stomach, liver, gall bladder and the upper urinary tract in both genders (in this approximate decreasing order). This syndrome was designated hereditary nonpolyposis colon carcinoma (HNPCC) and is now known to be considerably more frequent than FAP and its variant syndromes. Like FAP, its investigation has yielded important insights into the mechanisms of tumorigenesis not only in the colon, but also in other human cancers.

Colon cancers in the context of HNPCC are more often located in upper segments of the colon than in FAP and in sporadic cases and may - on average - have a more favorable prognosis. The major difference, however, lies in the type of mutations found in HNPCC carcinomas. Almost all genetic alterations in HNPCC carcinomas result from point mutations, base exchanges, small deletions and insertions, while chromosomal alterations are comparatively infrequent.

Mutations in this syndrome are most easily detected in microsatellite sequences which consist of repeats of one, two or three nucleotides. Since microsatellites are highly polymorphic, individuals are normally heterozygous for them at a given locus. Microsatellites can therefore be used as allelic markers in linkage studies, but also to follow chromosomal loss or recombination in tumor cells. Typically, allelic loss resulting from deletion or recombination is seen as loss or strongly diminished intensity of one band resulting from PCR amplification of a microsatellite. In HNPCC tumors, additional bands appear in addition to the two present in normal tissue. These result from the expansion or contraction of a microsatellite repeat, corresponding to an insertion or deletion mutation. This phenomenon has been termed '*microsatellite instability*' (abbreviated MSI).

Microsatellite instability and increased incidence of point mutations in HNPCC result from inactivation of genes involved in mismatch repair. Mismatches between DNA strands can occur as a consequence of several mechanisms and are repaired by according mechanisms. One repair system most active during DNA replication consisting of several different proteins recognizes base mismatches and differences in the number of bases between opposite DNA strands, such as occuring by base misincorporation or '*slipping*' of the DNA polymerase. These mismatches are first recognized by protein heterodimers consisting of MSH2 and MSH6 or MSH3 and MSH6, respectively. Further components of the complex, including PMS1, PMS2, and MLH1, are then directed towards the mismatch and remove the mismatched nucleotides. A repair DNA polymerase is recruited to synthesize the correct sequence and a DNA ligase seals the corrected strand.

Patients with HNPCC carry mutations in one gene encoding a component of this repair system. Mutation in the *MSH2* and *MLH1* genes are most frequent, more rarely the *PMS1*, *PMS2* or *MSH6* genes are mutated. In rarer cases, the *6 MYH* or *MBD4* genes are affected, but in ≈30% of all patients showing the characteristics of HNPCC, the underlying mutations are not known. Obviously, they could affect additional, still unknown components of the repair system.

Importantly, the mutation inherited in one allele is not sufficient to confer the MSI phenotype. Rather, mutation or epigenetic inactivation of the remaining allele has to take place before the function of the repair system is seriously compromised. So, the first step in tumor formation is probably the accidental loss of this second allele. In the affected cell, this creates a state of greatly enhanced mutability, specifically a strongly enhanced rate of point mutations. Eventually, these point mutations will affect genes crucial for the development of colon cancer. This sequence of events would explain convincingly why only single or a few carcinomas arise in HNPCC and the process does not stop in most cases at the stage of adenomas as in FAP.

Interestingly, MSI is also observed in sporadic cancers arising in patients without a family history. These cancers are also defective in mismatch repair. In many such cases, the inactivation of the mismatch repair system is caused by inactivation of the *MLH1* gene through promoter hypermethylation. Conceptually, one can consider the genes harboring inherited mutations in HNPCC as '*caretaker*' tumor suppressors, since mutations in these genes do not lead to tumor growth directly, but increase the risk of mutations in genes that control cellular proliferation, differentiation and survival. To some extent, therefore, HNPCC cancers contain mutations in the same genes as other colon carcinomas. For instance, the tumor suppressor genes *APC* and *C* *TP53* are inactivated and the protooncogenes *KRAS* and *CTNNB1* are activated by point mutations.

However, some genes are preferential mutation targets in colon cancers arising in the context of HNPCC and of sporadic MSI compared to other colon cancers. A prominent example is the *TGFBRII* gene which contains eleven successive adenines in its coding regions. Typical slippage mutations in this minirepeat leading to frameshift mutations are highly prevalent in HNPCC cancers. Another gene frequently affected by frameshift mutations encodes the pro-apoptotic protein BAX.

Genomic Instability in Colon Carcinoma

It is estimated that about 15% of all colon carcinomas overall, familial and sporadic together, display an MSI phenotype. Development and progression of these tumors are driven by an increased mutation rate. Importantly, only one particular type of mutations occurs at an increased frequency in these cancers, i.e. point mutations, which would be removed in normal cells by the mismatch repair system.

In contrast, chromosomal aberrations in MSI cancers are less frequent than in many other human carcinomas and some MSI cancers even remain diploid. One (hypothetical) explanation for this observation is that illegitimate recombinations are suppressed in these cancers. Such recombinations often involve homologous, but not identical sequences. Therefore, during recombination, small mismatches between these sequences appear. Unless these are corrected by mismatch repair, recombination may be inefficient.

In contrast, other colon cancers become aneuploid early during progression, losing or gaining whole chromosomes or chromosome parts. These changes result in increased or decreased gene copy numbers as well as chromosomal rearrangements that drive tumor progression, together with a smaller number of point mutations. This type of genetic instability is called chromosomal instability and sometimes abbreviated CIN. It is the predominant type of genetic instability in colon cancer, but also in many carcinomas of other organs. Nevertheless, the mechanisms causing CIN are not as clearly understood as those causing the MSI phenotype. In colon cancer, specifically, loss of APC function may contribute to the CIN phenotype, since the protein is associated with the mitotic spindle and the domains near the APC C-terminus involved in these interactions are often deleted by the prevailing truncating mutations. If correct, this explanation would account for the predominance of mutations in *APC* over those in *CTNNB1* in colon cancer. Intriguingly, a function in the control of mitotic segregation has also been postulated for RB1. Of course, loss of TP53 is at least '*permissive*' for aneuploidy.

So, there are at least two types of genomic instability in colon carcinoma and other human cancers, one leading to an increased rate of chromosomal alterations and one leading to an increased rate of point mutations. An important hypothesis states that the multistage development of human tumors requires some sort of increased mutation rate, a '*mutator phenotype*', which in these two types of cancer would be provided by an increased rate of point mutations or chromosomal changes, respectively. After all, at least 5 – 7 genetic alterations in one cell line are mandatory for colon cancer development, and this is likely a very conservative estimate.

An interesting addition to this story has emerged more recently. Upon studying DNA methylation changes in colon cancer, it was noted that these were much more prevalent in individual colon cancers than in others. So, a subset of colon cancers showed a sort of '*hypermethylator*' phenotype. The mechanism causing this phenotype is unknown. Moreover, the pattern of genes affected by mutations in this subset of colon cancers again seemed to be particular. In addition to a high frequency of *KRAS* changes, a high rate of inactivation of the *CDKN2A* gene by promoter hypermethylation was observed. This gene is otherwise not as frequently altered in colon cancers as in other human cancers. This type of colon cancers has been designated CIMP+ for CpG-island methylator phenotype. Of note, this subset is not really distinct from MSI and CIN cancers. The reason for this is that hypermethylation can inactivate genes required for mismatch repair or chromosomal stability. Notably, the MLH1 gene is a frequent target of hypermethylation.

The classification of colon cancers according to the mechanisms of genetic – or epigenetic – instability is more than just intellectually appealing. It may identify different subclasses of cancers with different clinical prognoses. Thus, on average MSI cancers may be somewhat less aggressive than CIN cancers. However, the classification appears most meaningful in predicting the reaction of a particular cancer to therapeutic intervention. Thus, MSI and CIN cancers may differ in their response to chemotherapy and CIMP+ cancers would be predicted to be particularly sensitive to inhibitors of DNA methylation.

INFLAMMATION AND COLON CANCER

An increased incidence of colorectal cancer is also observed in patients with chronic inflammatory bowel diseases. The increase in risk of colon cancer in patients with colitis ulcerosa has been variously estimated to be 4 - 20-fold increased.

The reasons for the increase in risk in these diseases may be complex. For instance, chronic damage to the mucosa may accelerate the turnover of the epithelial cells. Enhanced proliferation activity of tissue stem cells likely augments their risk of malignant transformation. Facilitated accessibility for mutagens from the intestine could also be relevant. However, inflammation as such is usually considered the main culprit for the increased risk.

Inflammatory cells like activated macrophages and lymphocytes release potentially mutagenic reactive oxygen species and a plethora of cytokines, proteases and other enzymes that modulate local tissue structure, cell proliferation and apoptosis. It was therefore not entirely surprising when epidemiological studies showed that common antiinflammatory drugs like acetyl-salicylic acid (aspirin) diminished the incidence of colorectal cancer. However, the magnitude of the effect suggested, up to 40%, came as a surprise, and it emerged that it was not restricted to patients with chronic bowel inflammation.

The most important targets of acetyl-salicilitic acid and related drugs, summarized as non-steroidal antiinflammatory drugs (NSAIDs) are cyclooxygenases, enzymes which convert arachidonic acid to prostaglandins. These reactions also yields reactive oxygen species as a side product. Prostaglandins act as paracrine signaling molecules on stromal as well as epithelial cells.

In fact, there are two kinds of cyclooxygenases. COX1 is a constitutively active enzyme, whereas COX2 is the enzyme induced by cytokines during inflammation. The promoter of the *COX2* gene is activated, a.o., by JNK and p38 MAPK and by NFκB pathways. COX2 can also be induced by mutated RAS. Drugs targeting specifically the inducible COX2 isozyme have turned out to be most effective. COX2 has been found to be induced in colon cancers, mostly in stromal cells like monocytes, fibroblasts and endothelial cells, but also in some carcinoma cells. Strong expression of COX2 appears to alter cell adhesion and to decrease apoptosis of emerging and established colon carcinoma cells. This effect may be mediated by paracrine effects.

Newer drugs such as sulindac and celecoxib have proven remarkably efficacious in diminishing the incidence of colorectal cancer and to slow down its progression in populations at risk including FAP patients. The action of sulindac is, however, not only due to its inhibition of COX-2, as it induces apoptosis in colon carcinoma cells that lack the enzyme. These relationships are under intense study, which is understandable given their potential for prevention.

This line of research is clearly not at an end and may yield even better means of intervention in the near future, although the results from ongoing trials are already very promising. Another interesting notion from studies on anti-inflammatory drugs and colon cancer is that plants may contain compounds that act in a similar fashion to NSAIDs, e.g., the bright yellow spice component curcumin. So the protective effect of vegetables apparent from epidemiological studies might partly be due to their effect.

7

Blood Cancer

Leukemias and lymphomas are cancers arising from cells of the hematopoetic lineage (hence: *hematological cancers*). Leukemias originate from hematopoetic stem cells or cells at different stages of myeloid or erythroid differentiation which spread throughout the body. Lymphomas also develop from more differentiated lymphoid cells in lymphoid organs and may present as localized cell masses. Hematological cancers can be classified by their derivation from erythroid, myeloid, or lymphoid cells at specific stages of development as determined by their morphology and by protein markers.

Hematological cancers are also often characterized by recurrent chromosomal aberrations, which in their initial stages may represent the only evident genetic change. These aberrations also comprise chromosome gains and losses, but specific translocations are most distinctive.

Translocations cause hematological cancers by either of two mechanisms. They activate a proto-oncogene by destroying its negative regulatory elements and/or by placing it under the influence of activating enhancers or they fuse two genes from the translocation sites that yield fusion proteins with novel properties. Either way, the gene product from the translocation site drives tumor development. During tumor progression, such as during the blast crisis of chronic myelogenous leukemias, further genetic and epigenetic changes accumulate, as commonly seen in carcinomas.

Chronic myelogenous leukemia (CML) is a disease of hematopoetic stem cells characterized by hyperproliferation of often immature cells of the myeloid, megakaryocytic and erythroid lineages. Its diagnostic chromosomal change is the '*Philadelphia chromosome*' resulting from a translocation between chromosomes 9 and 22 that creates the BCR-ABL fusion gene. The gene product is a fusion protein that retains the protein kinase activities of both original proteins, but is deregulated and mislocalized to the cytosol. There, the BCR-ABL protein activates several signaling pathways that promote cell proliferation, block apoptosis and decrease cell adhesion, thereby blocking maturation and causing release of immature cells into the blood. After several years, CML turns into blast crisis, a rapidly lethal disease resembling acute leukemias. This progression is promoted by interference of the BCR-ABL protein with the control of genomic stability. The acute phase of the disease is characterized by more pronounced chromosomal instability, with loss of tumor suppressors such as TP53 and $p16^{INK4A}$.

CML is treated by interferon therapy, chemotherapy and allogeneic stem cell transplantation. An important component of current therapy is a specific inhibitor of the ABL kinase, imatinib, which represents one of the great successes of molecular cancer research. Cytogenetic and molecular methods which detect the BCR-ABL translocation are helpful in diagnosis and in monitoring of treatment.

The efficacy of interferon therapy and allogeneic stem cell transplantation in CML have implications extending beyond this specific disease. They suggest that tumor cells can be recognized and kept under control through surveillance by the immune system. Highly sensitive molecular methods corroborate this assumption by proving the presence of Philadelphia chromosomes in healthy humans.

Burkitt lymphoma (BL) is an aggressive cancer derived from B-lymphocytes endemic in certain tropical areas of the world, and sporadically occuring in immuno-compromised individuals. These lymphomas have an extremely high proliferation rate which is not compensated by a high rate of apoptosis. Three alternative, diagnostic chromosomal aberrations invariably bring the *MYC* proto-oncogene on chromosome 8q24.1 under the influence of immunoglobulin gene enhancers from chromosome 14 (major translocation), 22, or 2 (minor translocations). Often, these translocations also destroy negative regulatory elements constraining this potent oncogene. MYC activity can be further augmented by point mutations.

Epstein Barr Virus (EBV), present in a few cells in most humans, but in the majority of BL clones, acts as a cofactor in this disease, perhaps by decreasing apoptosis. Additional genetic alteration in BL that diminish apoptosis severely aggravate the disease by counteracting the tendency of MYC to induce apoptosis in addition to cell growth. Beyond chemotherapy and stem cell transplantation, no specific treatment is available for BL.

In contrast, *promyelocytic leukemia* (PML), an *acute leukemia* (hence also: APL), is an example for successful targeted molecular therapy. It arises most often from a translocation involving chromosomes 15 and 17, t(15;17) (q22;q21), that creates a fusion protein from the nuclear coordinator PML and the retinoic acid receptor α (RARα). The fusion protein blocks differentiation and apoptosis of partially differentiated myeloid cells from which the tumor is derived. Unlike RARα, it does not respond to physiological levels of retinoic acid. Fortunately, pharmacological doses of retinoic acid activate the fusion protein, eliciting tumor differentiation and apoptosis. This '*differentiation therapy*' is not efficacious in cases of PML caused by fusion of RARα with the chromatin repressor PLZF. However, since PLZF acts by recruiting histone deacetylases, combined treatment with retinoids and histone deacetylase inhibitors may be possible. PML illustrates the importance of chromatin alterations in the development of human cancers and the therapeutic potential of understanding tumor pathophysiology at the molecular level.

Common Properties of Hematological Cancers

Hematological cancers comprise leukemias and lymphomas which arise from the hematopoetic lineage. All cells in this lineage originate from stem cells which in humans, after birth, are located in the bone marrow, after residing in the liver during the most of the fetal period. Here, stromal cells and an appropriate extracellular matrix support stem cell maintenance and help to regulate differentiation. Hematopoetic stem cells in the bone marrow and circulating in the blood can be identified by their expression of the surface antigen CD34.

The first step of differentiation of the rare pluripotent hematopoetic stem cells distinguishes the lymphoid lineage and the myeloid/erythroid lineage and leads to a larger population of '*committed*' progenitor cells. The lineages split further and lead to the various types of differentiated cells such as the B-cell and T-cell subtypes in the lymphoid branch, as well as the erythrocytes and platelets (*erythroid* and *megakaryocytic lineage*) and mast cells, granulocytes, monocytes and macrophages (myeloid lineage).

Proliferation and differentiation of hematopoetic cells are directed and controlled by a panoply of growth factors present in the bone marrow environment, and intracellularly by networks of lineage- and cell-type transcription factors. In each branch of the lineage, the options for differentiation are progressively restricted and cells become more and more committed towards a specific fate. In parallel, as a rule, their proliferative potential becomes more and more restricted, most obvious in case of erythrocytes which even lose their nuclei. Especially the later stages of differentiation in the myeloid and erythroid lineages are characterized by a tight coupling between differentiation and loss of proliferative potential, so that the number of cells produced is limited. For cancers to arise in this lineage, this dependency must be broken or the stimuli must be mimicked. Moreover, since differentiation diminishes proliferative potential, a carcinogenic change must block or at least substantially diminish the rate of cell differentiation.

The relationship between proliferation and differentiation is somewhat different in the lymphoid lineage since mature lymphocytes still remain competent for proliferation in response to infections. Their multiplication, however, is normally dependent on stimulation by antigens and by paracrine factors, mostly cytokines. Moreover, when an infection abates, lymphocyte numbers are restrained by apoptosis and only memory cells survive for longer periods. Controlled apoptosis is also involved in the selection procedure against self-reactive lymphocytes. Thus, cancers in the lymphoid lineage can arise not only in immature cells by failure along the path to differentiation, but also in differentiated cells by acquired independence of external proliferation stimuli or by evasion of apoptosis, or in the worst case both.

The phenotype of individual leukemias and lymphomas is therefore strongly dependent on which stage in which lineage is primarily affected. A hematological cancer may be derived from a stem cell such as in chronic myelogenous leukemia, a partially differentiated cell as in acute promyelocytic leukemia, or a cell at an advanced stage of differentiation as in multiple myeloma (a B-cell lymphoma). The many different subtypes of B-cells and T-cells, in particular, with different functions and tissue distributions, can give rise to a large variety of lymphomas.

The name of a hematological cancer often indicates the dominant cell type. Obviously, the cell of origin cannot always be straightforwardly identified, because cancer cells deviate from the original cell. In many types of leukemias and lymphomas, only the introduction of molecular markers in the last decades has allowed to determine their cell of origin and, in more than a few cases, to recognize morphologically similar diseases as different entities. Molecular markers used for this purpose comprise surface antigens characteristic for lineages and differentiation stages as well as typical chromosomal aberrations. An identification as precise as possible is, of course, necessary to predict prognosis and to choose appropriate treatments.

Genetic Aberrations in Leukemias and Lymphomas

On average, leukemias and lymphomas contain fewer genetic aberrations than carcinomas. Very often, their karyotype is near-diploid with few chromosomes altered. Those aberrations that are present, however, are characteristic for the particular type of leukemia or lymphoma. Although chromosomal losses and gains are also found, many hematological cancers are characterized by typical translocations.

In some hematological cancers, these translocations are so characteristic that they allow to classify the disease accordingly. So, >90% of chronic myeloid leukemias contain a characteristic translocation between the long arms of chromosomes 9 and 22, t(9;22) (q34;q11). On the other hand, apparently similar diseases may result from disparate translocations. So, the same t(9;22) translocation is found in 25% of acute lymphoblastic leukemias as well. However, in this group of diseases, a variety of other translocations are found.

Unlike deletions such as those of 6q or 13q found in some leukemias, translocations do not simply destroy genes and their functions, but alter them. Two mechanisms can be distinguished.

1. The coding region of the gene at the translocation site remains intact, but its regulation is altered, since the translocation removes some of its own regulatory regions and/or brings the gene under the influence of novel regulatory elements. In most cases, this leads to ectopic or deregulated expression of a gene product acting as an oncogenic protein. Burkitt lymphoma with its translocations activating the MYC gene is a case in point. Another frequent translocation t(14;18) (q32;q21) leads to deregulation and overexpression of the anti-apoptotic regulator protein BCL2 in follicular lymphoma. Here, the *BCL2* locus is brought under the control of a heavy-chain immunoglobulin enhancer.
2. The translocation creates a fusion protein expressed from a novel gene formed from the segments of two genes flanking the translocation sites. The fusion protein may have a different expression pattern, intracellular localization, regulation, and activity (or a combination of these properties) compared to the original components. Not infrequently, the destruction of one or both original genes also matters. Two examples out of many for this mechanism

are the BCR-ABL fusion protein in chronic myeloid leukemia and the retinoic acid receptor fusion proteins in acute promyelocytic leukemia.

The characteristic translocations are causally involved in the development of each specific cancer subtype. An impressive illustration of this relationship is found in *acute myeloid leukemia* (AML). Translocations in AML often interrupt the genes encoding transcription factors involved in the differentiation of myeloid cells, such as that encoding C/EBPα, and create fusion protein, which instead of activating target genes repress them. Some cases lack these characteristic translocations. In these, point mutations in the *CBPA* gene have been found which lead to a truncated protein that acts as a dominant-negative inhibitor of the protein expressed from the remaining intact allele.

AMLs belong to those hematological cancers that behave quite heterogeneously in the clinic. The course of the disease and the response to therapy can to a certain degree be predicted from the type of translocation (or *mutation*) present. In general, determining the characteristic translocations in a leukemia or lymphoma is very helpful in the diagnostis and treatment of the disease.

It is not entirely clear, which further genetic changes in addition to the typical translocations are present in the initial stages of leukemias and lymphomas and to what extent they are required for their development. Certainly, however, many leukemias and lymphomas progress to a state of more generalized genomic instability with aneuploid karyotypes, additional point mutations and changes in DNA methylation. Genes affected at this stage also comprise some of the oncogenes and tumor suppressors important in carcinomas, such as *RAS* genes, *S TP53*, *RB1*, *CDKN2A*, and also *CDKN2B*. This genomic instability not only confers a more aggressive character, but also presents a significant obstacle to chemotherapy by allowing the development of resistant cell clones, e.g. through point mutations or gene amplification.

Molecular Biology of Burkitt Lymphoma

Burkitt lymphoma (BL) is an aggressive malignancy consisting of highly proliferative B-cells which infiltrate lymph nodes and other organs. The tumor cells are distinguished as B-cells by their expression of IgM and κ or λ light chains and by specific surface markers such as CD19 and CD20. The high proliferative rate is obvious from numerous mitotic figures. Staining for markers such as Ki67 or PCNA, which are characteristic of cycling cells, shows that almost all tumor cells are participating in proliferation. The rapid proliferation in this cancer is only partly compensated by a high apoptotic rate, evident most straightforwardly from interspersed macrophages phagocytosing the apoptosed tumor cells.

BL was first described as a tumor in young people in equatorial Africa where it is endemic in some regions. It is much rarer in Europe and North America, although more frequent in the context of AIDS and in other immunocompromised patients. In tropical areas, most BLs harbor *Epstein-Barr virus* (EBV), which is not as consistently associated with the disease in countries of the temperate zones. Treatment by chemotherapy and stem cell transplantation12 can be successful in some cases.

The three characteristic translocations in BL all involve the *MYC* locus at *C* 8q24.1. The most frequent, 'major' translocation joins the gene to the *IGH* locus at *H* 14q32 which encodes the immunoglobulin heavy chain. The 'minor' translocations involve the *IGL* (Igλ) locus at 22q11 or the *IGK* (Igκ) locus at 2p12. These loci encode the two immunoglobulin light chains, either of which can be used in B cells. One of these three translocations is found in each case of BL. The diagnosis of BL therefore is made contingent on their presence. The converse is not true, i.e. these translocations are also found in other lymphomas, all of which are also aggressive.

In each translocation, the MYC gene is brought under the influence of an immunoglobulin gene enhancer which is strongly active at this stage of B-cell differentiation. BL is thus an important example of the gene activation mechanism by translocations. The translocations in BL result in deregulation and overexpression of a potent oncogene, which normally ought to become down-regulated in mature B-cells. While the overall result is the same, the mechanisms leading to deregulation differ in detail between the various translocations.

In most major translocations, the translocation breakpoint lies at some distance upstream of the *MYC* gene, which remains intact. The translocated *IGH* locus is *H* oriented in inverse orientation, with the enhancer positioned towards the *MYC* gene. This configuration appears to result in a '*classical*' enhancer activation mechanism, in which the strong enhancer activates the unchanged MYC promoters.

In some of the major translocations, the breakpoints are located in the first intron of the *MYC* gene, so that the first exon with the P1 and P2 promoters is removed. The gene is transcribed from the otherwise '*cryptic*' (i.e. unused) P3 promoter located in the first intron. In this configuration, all elements in the *MYC* upstream region controlling transcription are deleted. Specifically, the translocation inactivates an attenuation mechanism in the first intron which makes transcription of the gene contingent on continuous stimulation. In these translocations, the placement of the *IGH* enhancer next to the gene does not seem to be absolutely essential for *MYC* activation, but the presence of an active *IGH* gene is required, perhaps to guarantee an open chromatin structure.

In the minor translocations, the breakpoints are located downstream of the *MYC* gene, sometimes at a considerable distance (>100 kb). The regulatory regions of the *MYC* gene remain largely intact, with the possible exception of a negative regulatory element presumed to lie downstream of the gene. The light chain loci are located in inverse orientation with their downstream enhancers oriented towards MYC. These seem to be mainly responsible for driving MYC over-expression. In the *IGK* locus, further elements may contribute, including an intronic enhancer.

In all translocations, the translocated *MYC* gene becomes susceptible to mutations that augment the effects of the enhancers. In translocations retaining the *MYC* regulatory regions, point mutations are found which inactivate negative regulatory elements in exon 1 and the first intron, thereby exacerbating overexpression. In all translocations, mutations are also found in the N-terminal coding region of MYC. In general, these stabilize the protein. For instance, a common mutation in Thr58 prevents a regulatory phosphorylation that targets the gene for proteosomal degradation. Interestingly, an according mutation is also common in the v-myc oncogenes of retroviruses.

The genetic alterations at the *MYC* locus found in Burkitt lymphoma can be understood as accidents during the maturation of B-cells. During the differentiation of B-cells, V(D)J recombination of the *IGH* and either *IGL* or *IGK* immunoglobulin genes is employed to generate the antibody repertoire necessary for the immune response to many different antigens. Later, a further recombination event accompanies the switch from expression of IgM to that of IgG. Furthermore, in the germinal centers of the lymphoid organs, somatic hypermutation is directed to the rearranged immunoglobulin genes to generate additional antibody variants with higher affinities and improved specifity towards the encountered antigens. These processes are recognizable in BL, although deviant.

The RAG recombinases mediating V(D)J rearrangements recognize particular sequence motifs in the immunoglobulin genes which are found in the vicinity of the breakpoints in the translocated immunoglobulin genes, although not usually in the *MYC* gene. It is therefore possible that the translocations are initiated by the physiological introduction of double-strand breaks into the immunoglobulin genes by B-cell specific recombinases. By accident, these breaks are then wrongly connected to the *MYC* gene. Likewise, placement of the *MYC* gene into an immunoglobulin gene cluster may set it up as a target for somatic hypermutation. The accidents that initiate BL are likely to be very rare, even if favored by the unknown agents that cause endemic BL. However, activation of *MYC* provides a strong proliferation stimulus that may provide a large pool of cells from which the lymphoma arises, likely by further alterations that are less conspicuous than the translocations. Since BL is more frequent in immunocompromised individuals, an immune defense may exist which normally eliminates B cells with aberrantly rearranged immunoglobulin genes.

Activation of *MYC* to an oncogene accounts for many of the properties of BL cells. MYC stimulates many aspects of cell proliferation and cell growth. In particular, in many cell types overexpression of MYC is sufficient to maintain them active in the cell cycle, independent of growth factors. It may therefore account for the high proliferative fraction and rate in BL. MYC, through its action on telomerase, may also contribute to immortalization. Moreover, some proteins regulated by MYC are involved in cell adhesion, e.g. LFA-1 in lymphocytes. This may lead to altered interactions of BL cells with other immune cells.

The oncogenic potential of MYC is normally restrained by two factors. (1) The gene and the protein are tightly regulated by a variety of mechanisms which are subverted by the translocations and mutations in BL. (2) MYC is a strong inducer of apoptosis. This induction is, at least partly, mediated by induction of p14^{ARF} by E2F1 which is a transcriptional target of MYC. p14^{ARF} then blocks HDM2/MDM2 activating TP53 to elicit apoptosis. The high apoptotic rate found in BL suggests that a mechanism of this sort may indeed be active, but not sufficiently so as to compensate for the increase in proliferation.

It is therefore thought that the development of BL requires at least one further genetic alteration which limits apoptosis. Different recurrent genetic alterations, each observed in a fraction of BLs, may account for this requirement. About one third of all cases have mutations

Table 7.1. Effects of MYC on various cellular functions

Function	*Some proteins regulated by MYC*
Cell growth	↑ RNA polymerase, nucleolar proteins, ribosomal proteins, splice factors, eIF proteins, CAD, polyamine biosynthesis (ODC, spermidine synthase), chaperones,
Cell proliferation	↑ Cyclin D2, Cyclin B1, CDK4, CDC25A, E2F1, CUL1, hTERT ↓ $p21^{CIP1}$, $p27^{KIP1}$, MYC
Cell differentiation	↓ cell-type specific bHLH transcriptional activators, ID proteins
Metabolism	↑ LDH , PFK, enolase
Adhesion	↓ LFA1, PAI1
Apoptosis	↑ E2F1 ($p14^{ARF}$), BAX

in *TP53* and LOH at 17p, others have lost TP73, a related protein and a potential mediator of TP53-induced apoptosis. The *BCL6* gene at 3q27 is affected in BL, as well as in other B-cell lymphomas, by translocations and mutations, which may also stem from somatic hypermutation. The function of the transcriptional repressor BCL6 is probably specific to B-cells at a certain stage of differentiation in germinal centers. It is down-regulated during terminal differentiation. The various translocations, which are typically promoter substitutions, appear to keep the gene active beyond its time. Importantly, BCL6 does not stimulate cell proliferation, but influences the expression of specific B cell proteins and decreases apoptosis.

Since EBV is found in so many BL, it is tempting to speculate that this herpes virus may provide a complementary function to that of MYC in the development of this tumor. The relationship has, however, emerged as more roundabout. EBV occurs in >90% of all adults, but only in a fraction of B-cells. It is capable of immortalizing cells of this type. This ability is therefore used in the laboratory to generate permanent lymphoblastoid lines. The virus exists as an episome, whose maintenance and replication require minimally the expression of the EBNA-1 protein. In lymphoblastoid lines and in long-term infected cells *in vivo*, further genes are expressed which down-regulate apoptosis and help to avoid immune detection. These genes are obvious candidates for synergizing with MYC in BL, but most of them are more weakly expressed in the actual disease than normally. The EBER RNAs of the virus are also good candidates for cooperating with MYC. Conversely, there is evidence that strong MYC expression may support the maintenance of the virus.

Several alternative plausible explanations are therefore considered for the evident association of the virus with the disease. For instance, EBV-infected cells may be more susceptible to accidents during attempted V(D)J recombination or the BL cells may be initially protected from apoptosis and elimination by the immune system by EBV proteins, while later on the same functions would be provided by other alterations such as translocations or mutations of *BCL6*.

Molecular Biology of CML

Chronic myeloid leukemia (also: *chronic myelogeneous leukemia*, commonly abbreviated CML) is a moderately frequent leukemia occurring in adults, most often in their 40's or 50's. While its causes are in general unknown, it has been observed following exposure to high doses of ionizing radiation.

CML originates from hematopoetic stem cells. As a consequence, the production of many different cell types is increased overall and mature cells as well as progenitor cells of many or all hematopoetic lineages are present in the blood, prominently the myeloid cells for which the disease is named. Almost all cases are caused by one specific genetic alteration, a BCR-ABL fusion gene, usually present in an aberrant, smaller appearing chromosome 22 termed the Philadelphia chromosome.

If left untreated, CML continues over several years with rather unspecific symptoms, but then progresses through an accelerated phase into blast crisis in which highly aberrant leukemic cells kill the patient within months.

Until recently, CML was treated by chemotherapy and/or by interferon α (IFNα) which lead to hematological remission, i.e. a normalization of the cell distribution in blood, in about 70% of the cases. In 10% of the cases, '*cytogenetic*' remissions are achieved, i.e. no metaphases with Philadelphia chromosomes are detected in bone marrow aspirates. However, these treatments do not usually lead to a cure and the cancer recurs eventually.

A better chance of a cure is provided by allogeneic stem cell transplantation. Here, hematopoetic stem cells from an HLA-matched donor are transplanted. These provide normal cells necessary for function of the blood and immune system, but also generate an immune response towards the tumor. However, in some cases the immune cells from the bone marrow graft attack not only the tumor cells, but also normal tissues, leading to chronic or acute *graft-versus-host-disease* (GVHD), which can be lethal. Therefore, although better selection of donors supported by genotyping helps, stem cell transplantation remains risky.

Stimulation of an immune response against the tumor cells also appears to be responsible for the efficacy of IFNα in the treatment of CML. Like the increased incidence of Burkitt lymphoma in immuno-compromised individuals, it points to a role of the immune system in prevention of cancer by some sort of immune surveillance. This effect can apparently be recruited for therapy in some cases. The evidence from CML for a tumor-specific immune surveillance is actually a bit stronger than that from BL, because a virus might be involved in the pathogenesis of the latter disease, so the immune response may actually be directed against an exogenous antigen. There is no evidence for an infectious agens in CML.

Many properties of CML can be explained as consequences of a single genetic change, i.e. the creation of the BCR-ABL gene by a translocation between chromosomes 9q34 and 22q11. The translocation creates a novel gene which expresses a fusion protein with properties different from those of the original genes.

In most cases of CML, the translocation is reciprocal and the resulting chromosomes 9q+ and 22q- (or Ph') are the only aberrations in the karyotype of many CML cells in the chronic phase. Of course, being balanced, the translocation creates two fusion genes, but for all we know only the *BCR-ABL* fusion is relevant. Here, the promoter of the *BCR* gene from chromosome 22 drives the expression of a fusion protein consisting of a large N-terminal region from BCR and most of the ABL protein originally encoded on chromosome 9. The breakpoints in *BCR* and *ABL* can be located in different exons leading to several different fusion genes and proteins of different molecular weights. They all, however, concur in retaining the serine/threonine kinase activity of BCR and the tyrosine kinase activity of ABL, while lacking domains that control the activities of these kinases in the original proteins. Moreover, the fusion proteins also localize primarily to the cytoplasm instead of to the nucleus. The functions of the normal BCR and ABL proteins are not overly well characterized. The ABL kinase is normally involved as a signaling molecule in DNA repair and apoptosis, interacting a.o with DNA-PK. Although the precise function is unclear, it is certainly not a growth-stimulatory protein. Of note, an abl gene has also been recruited by the Abelson leukemia virus as an oncogene. In this murine virus, the N-terminal domain of the cellular gene is replaced by a part of the viral gag protein.

The BCR-ABL fusion protein acts in a pleiotropic fashion changing the activity of several signaling pathways and protein complexes in the cell. It interferes with the control of proliferation, apoptosis, adhesion, and DNA repair. RAS is activated and the MAPK pathway stimulated by GRB/SOS binding to a phosphorylated tyrosine (Y177) in the BCR domain, which is generated by the activity of the ABL tyrosine kinase. This kinase also phosphorylates and activates JAK2 and thereby the STAT pathway which stimulates proliferation in the hematopoetic lineage. Phosphorylation of STAT5 may also contribute to inhibition of apoptosis. This effect may be enhanced by activation of PI3K which is otherwise inhibited by normal ABL.

An important factor in the pathogenesis of CML is decreased adhesion, which explains the appearance of hematopoetic precursors in blood. By being lost from their proper environment, the immature cells are removed from exposure to growth factors and interactions with the ECM of the bone marrow which guide their differentiation. Altered adhesion is caused by the misdirected activity of the ABL tyrosine kinase which in the cytosol is bound to actin and phosphorylates proteins that organize the cytoskeleton like paxillin and *focal adhesion kinase* (FAK). Integrin function is also impeded and CBL is activated leading to altered turnover of membrane proteins.

Moreover, there is evidence that BCR-ABL also interferes with DNA repair, acting largely in a fashion opposite to the normal ABL protein, i.e. down-regulating TP53 and ATM signaling. This last activity of the oncoprotein may tile the path towards progression of the disease to its accelerated phase and blast crisis.

If perhaps not the only genetic alteration in chronic phase CML, the formation of a *BCR-ABL* fusion gene is certainly a consistent event and likely obligatory. This is helpful in the diagnosis of the disease and even more for monitoring of its treatment. It also provides a clear target for therapeutic intervention.

Detection of BCR-ABL can be made by several techniques, with different sensitivities. Cytogenetically, the Ph' chromosome can be detected in metaphases or more sensitively by FISH (*fluorescence in situ hybridization*) showing a closed apposition of the normally separate genes in interphase nuclei. Molecular techniques are even more sensitive, especially detection of a fusion transcript by RT-PCR.

Prior to therapy, the billions of leukemia cells in the blood are obvious under the microscope. Following therapy, their number decreases and hematopoetic precursors disappear. This is called '*hematological remission*'. Unfortunately, it does not amount to a cure, because the cancer often recurs after some time, in CML after several years. Such patients harbor '*minimal residual disease*'. Indeed, cytogenetic methods often detect tumor cells in the bone marrow of patients with an apparent normalization of the cell numbers and composition in the blood. If this is not the case, one speaks of '*complete cytogenetic remission*'. However, even this does not signify a certain cure, because millions of descendents of the tumor stem cells in the bone marrow may remain hidden among the normal cells in the blood. Descendents of these cells are detectable by RT-PCR in peripheral blood samples. So, the notion of '*molecular remission*' has entered modern hematology denoting the situation in which even this sensitive method detects no more leukemia cells. CML patients with '*molecular remission*' are usually cured.

So, very sensitive methods have been developed which are capable of detecting very few cells with Ph' chromosomes. Surprisingly, they reveal their presence in persons without evidence of disease and no evidence of their numbers increasing. The interpretation of this finding is controversial. It may mean that a second genetic event is needed for CML development after all, or provide further evidence for successful immune surveillance.

The elucidation of the role of BCR-ABL in CML has also led to the development of a specific drug, an inhibitor of the ABL kinase, imatinib (STI-571, marketed under the name of '*Gleevec*' or '*Glivec*'). This drug has recently proven very efficacious against CML, inducing remissions even in blast crisis CML and used as first-line therapy in chronic phase patients. However, while remissions are long-lasting in a large proportion of chronic phase patients (the cure rate will only be ascertained after longer observation periods), resistant tumors develop in many acute phase patients. Importantly, the mechanisms underlying this resistance show that the target was well chosen. In some cases, the resistance is caused by point mutations in the ATP binding domain of the ABL kinase in the BCR-ABL fusion protein which diminishes the impact of the inhibitor. In other cases of resistance, the fusion gene has become amplified.

The different rates of resistance against imatinib in blast crisis patients vs. chronic phase patients illustrates the development of genomic instability during the progression of CML towards blast crisis. Blast crisis cells are aneuploid with multiple chromosomal aberrations including chromosomal losses, gains, further translocations and amplifications.

Among the genes affected by these changes are *RB1* and *TP53* as well as *CDKN2A* which are inactivated by gene loss, mutation or, in the case of *CDKN2A*, also by promoter hypermethylation. Loss of TP53 by mutation and deletion certainly contributes to resistance against chemotherapy in this disease, as in cancers in general. Another remarkable instance of hypermethylation is that of the remaining intact *ABL* gene, underlining the tumor suppressor function of the normal gene. In contrast, the *MYC* gene is over-expressed as a consequence of trisomy 8 or outright gene amplification in blast crisis, but not in the chronic phase.

Acute myeloid leukemias other than those developing from CML also display characteristic translocations that lead to fusion proteins. One of them is a t(3;21) event which creates the AML/EVI1 fusion gene and protein. This translocation is also prevalent in blast crisis leukemia developing from CML. Like MYC overexpression, it is thought to further stimulate proliferation, but also to exacerbate the block to differentiation, which is relatively weak in chronic CML. Finally, a typical indicator of the acceleration phase that precedes blast crisis is an increased copy number of the *BCR-ABL* gene itself, typically becoming evident as a duplication of the Ph' chromosome. Once again, this highlights the crucial importance of this genetic alteration in CML, even at its final stage.

Molecular Biology of Promyelocytic Leukemia

Promyelocytic leukemia is, like the final phase of CML, an acute leukemia and therefore alternatively abbreviated as APL or PML (or most systematically as AML M3). It is, however, not a disease of stem cells, but of cells from an intermediate stage of differentiation towards granulocytes, denoted promyelocytes. These cells are obviously arrested at this stage and continue to proliferate. Compared to CML, PML is a rare disease comprising only a fraction of all AML. Like CML, however, PML has become paradigmatic for the understanding of leukemias and beyond, primarily as an example of successful '*differentiation therapy*' and, more recently, of chromatin alterations in cancer.

A distinctive t(15;17) (q22;q21) translocation found in >90% of all PMLs fuses the *PML* gene at chromosome 15q22 to the *RARA* gene at 17q21. Variant translocations always include *RARA* as well, but fuse it to the *PLZF* (promyelocytic leukemia zinc finger) gene at 11q23, to the *NPM* (*nucleophosmin*) gene at 5q35, or *NUMA* (*nuclear matrix associated*) gene at 11q13.

This general involvement of the retinoic acid receptor RARα in PML translocations is striking, as already in the 1980's its ligand *all-trans retinoic acid* (ATRA) was found to induce often dramatic hematological remissions of PML. Responsiveness to ATRA is specific for PML, and not observed in other AMLs. PML also responds better to certain drugs which are more generally used in chemotherapy, such as anthracyclins. So, precise diagnosis is a prerequisite for optimal treatment of this disease. Moreover, as in CML, cytogenetic and molecular techniques are employed to monitor treatment, detect minimal residual disease and select patients for stem cell transplantation.

Both certain cytostatic drugs and ATRA are efficacious in PML, and are used in combination. Cytostatic drugs act through apoptosis and cell cycle arrest in PML, as in other leukemias. In contrast, ATRA relieves the block to differentiation in the disease, allowing terminal differentiation towards granulocytes, with a concomitant decrease in proliferation. Some degree of apoptosis also occurs. This type of treatment has therefore been called '*differentiation therapy*'.

The PML-RARα fusion protein in PML acts as an inhibitor of both proteins from which it originates. It may also have gained additional, novel functions. RARα, retinoic acid receptor α, belongs to a group of closely related receptors for retinoic acids which are part of the steroid hormone receptor superfamily. Retinoic acid is produced from vitamin A as a locally acting hormone regulating growth and differentiation of many tissues, prominently the skin, reproductive organs and some glands. Accordingly, the closely related RARβ and RARγ proteins are frequently inactivated in other cancers, e.g. RARβ in breast and prostate cancer.

The basic structure of RARα resembles that of steroid hormone receptors. An N-terminal transcriptional activation domain (AF-1) is followed by the DNA-binding domain, an hinge region, and the ligand binding domain (LBD) containing a second transcriptional activation function (AF-2), with a short C-terminal region. The LBD/AF-2 domain is the most crucial one in the protein, since the ligand bound in this region elicits heterodimerization and recruitment of transcriptional co-activators such as CBP in exchange for the co-repressor N-CoR/SMRT. The DNA-binding domain interacts with a specific recognition site in

DNA called RARE (*retinoic-acid responsive element*) which has the typical motif for steroid hormone receptor-like transcriptional activators, AGGTCA. RARE sites actually used consist of a direct repeat of this sequence separated by five arbitrary nucleotides. The second half-site is occupied by one of the more distantly related RXR receptors which form heterodimers with RARs, as they do with several other receptors of the superfamily. Binding of RAR to a gene promoter usually leads to opening of the chromatin structure by remodeling and histone acetylation as well as to transcriptional activation.

In hematopoesis, gene regulation by retinoic acid appears to be particularly important during granulopoesis at the stage of promyelocyte differentiation. At this differentiation step, growth-promoting genes such as *MYC* need to be down-regulated and inhibitors of the cell cycle such as $p21^{CIP1}$ must be up-regulated. The genes of transcription factors more specifically involved in myeloid differentiation such as C/EBPε and HOXA are also RARα targets. Most interestingly, the RARα gene is activated by its own product. This auto-regulatory loop may provide a crucial amplifying step for the signal that makes differentiation irreversible.

The PML protein, named after the disease, is normally localized in 10-30 '*PML nuclear bodies*', a subcompartment of the nucleus consisting of morphologically recognizable protein assemblies sized 0.2 - 1 μm. The assembly of ≈1,000,000 proteins in these nuclear bodies is dependent on PML which may be their principle organisator and regulator. The function of the nuclear bodies is not entirely clear. Most likely, they act as a reservoir and interaction structure for proteins involved in response to cellular stress, DNA repair, apoptosis and chromatin structure. Proteins found to associate with PML and nuclear bodies include the proapoptotic DAXX protein, the Bloom syndrome helicase BLM, and TP53, but also the mRNA-cap-binding protein EIF-4E. Interestingly, formation and function of nuclear bodies may involve SUMOlation, i.e. covalent attachment of a SUMO protein to PML and other constituents. Another regulator of nuclear bodies is the JNK1 kinase. PML itself may then mediate the SUMOlation of other proteins, including TP53. The function of PML is reflected in its structure which contains several motifs involved in protein-protein interactions, such as a RING finger and a coiled domain.

The PML-RARα fusion protein retains most parts from both partners. PML mostly lacks its C-terminal Ser-Pro rich domain, while RARα lacks part of the AF-1 interaction domain. However, these changes suffice to turn the fusion protein into a transcriptional repressor at physiological concentrations of retinoic acids, and to destroy nuclear bodies and interfere with their function. Transcriptional repression may be aided by dimerization of the fusion protein which then binds to a dimeric RARE promoter site and recruits co-repressors to repress rather than activate genes crucial for myeloid differentiation.

Fortunately, the variant protein can still be turned into a transcriptional activator by micromolar concentrations of retinoic acid, i.e. at pharmacological concentrations, 100-1000-fold above the physiological level. In response to ATRA treatment, the co-repressors dissociate allowing transcription of the genes required for granulocyte differentiaton. The fusion protein itself is rapidly degraded following ATRA treatment, so transcription may also or even predominantly be promoted by normal RARα, which is itself induced during differentiation. Like the function of RARα, that of PML seems also to become restored as evidenced by reappearance of nuclear bodies.

The overall effect of ATRA treatment at the cellular level is differentiation towards a more mature granulocytic cell, with arrest of proliferation, but also significant apoptosis. Of note, the ensuing differentiated cells are no more cancerous, but are not normally functioning and can pose problems to the host. Moreover, retinoic acid at supraphysiological concentrations has some side-effects. So, while differentiation therapy is efficacious and may seem more elegant than chemotherapy, it is strenuous and dangerous to the patient.

Like the predominant type of PML caused by t(15;17) translocations, those with the variant t(5;17) and t(11q13;17) translocations respond to ATRA treatment. However, the rare t(11q23;17) translocation, which creates the PLZF- RARα fusion gene, does not. The difference lies in the fusion partner. PLZF is itself a transcriptional repressor capable of recruiting co-repressors and histone deacetylases. Therefore, in this fusion protein, not only is RARα locked in a repressor conformation, but also its fusion partner contributes to repression to at least the same extent. At least experimentally, however, it has been possible to still reactivate RARα by a combined treatment with ATRA and inhibitors of histone deacetylases. These may obliterate the repressor function of PZLF. As more and better such inhibitors become available, there seems to be a chance of successful treatment for patients with this translocation as well.

Finally, the obvious question is whether the RARα translocations are sufficient to induce PML. This cannot be definitely answered at present. Since vitamin A deficiency and other maladies that cause inefficient function of RARα only moderately affect granulopoesis, with at most a mild hyperplasia of promyelocytes, not only the loss of retinoic acid responsiveness, but the formation of the fusion protein is certainly crucial. Although the details are controversial, a function of PML in the regulation of apoptosis and replicative senescence is generally accepted. Moreover, the fusion protein obviously has a dominant-negative effect on at least some aspects of PML function. So, inhibition of differentiation and of apoptosis could well be oncogenic effects provided by the fusion protein. This leaves room for a genetic change that causes hyperproliferation. The best candidate for this is mutation of *FLT3*. The FLT3 protein is a receptor tyrosine kinase activated by the hematopoetic growth factor M-CSF which is particularly active in the myeloid lineage. Mutations in the *FLT3* gene are observed in several different subtypes of AML and in at least a third of PML patients.

8

KIDNEY CANCER

Several cancer types originate from the adult kidney. In addition, the organ is a site for metastases from other tumors. Within the kidney, tumors can be derived from different cell types. Tumors of mesenchymal origin can be benign or malignant, e.g. angiomyolipoma vs. sarcoma,. In the renal pelvis, urothelial carcinomas resemble those in the bladder. Actual *renal cell carcinomas* (RCC) are derived from various segments of the nephron. They are distinguished by their histological appearance and accordingly designated chromophobic, chromophilic, clear-cell, papillary etc. The clear-cell variety is most common (hence also: '*conventional*' RCC). There is also a benign epithelial tumor, oncoytoma.

Molecular and cytogenetic studies have shown that different histological subtypes of RCC carry typical chromosomal alterations. This recognition has helped to sort out ambiguous cases. Thus, modern classification of renal cell carcinoma is based on a combination of histological and molecular parameters.

Several hereditary syndromes confer an increased risk for renal carcinoma, prominently *von-Hippel-Lindau* (VHL) disease and *hereditary papillary renal cell carcinoma* (HPRCC). Genes affected in these syndromes are in general tumor suppressors, but the mutation underlying standard hereditary papillary carcinoma activates the *MET* proto-oncogene. This is one of a few exceptional instances, in which a hereditary tumor syndrome in man is caused by a dominant oncogene mutation.

The *VHL* gene is not only involved in most inherited cases cf clear-cell carcinoma, but also in sporadic RCC of this subtype. It is therefore a '*classical*' tumor suppressor gene. While inactivation of

VHL alleles can occur through various mechanisms, including deletion, point mutation and promoter hypermethylation, as a rule one allele is deleted by loss of chromosome 3p. This loss is characteristic for clear cell RCC. Its consistency may be facilitated by the presence of a major site of chromosomal instability (*FRA3B*) at 3p14.1, but likely also indicates the presence of a second tumor suppressor gene on this chromosome arm.

The elucidation of *VHL* function has yielded important insights into tumor biology. The VHL protein is a pleiotropic regulator of cell physiology and growth. Most importantly, it is involved in the cellular response to hypoxia. Loss of VHL function causes a switch in cellular physiology and gene expression which normally occurs transiently during hypoxia to become constitutive. This explains many of the morphological and biological features of the clear cell carcinoma phenotype, including a metabolic switch to glycolysis and prominent angiogenesis. VHL is the target recognition module of a E3 ubiquitin-ligase protein complex, which becomes disfunctional in renal cell carcinoma. This finding emphasizes how crucial disturbances of protein degradation are for the development of human tumors.

RCC remains a challenge for therapy. While localized tumors can be cured by surgery, chemotherapy for metastasized cancers has proved woefully inefficacious. Cytokines like interferon and interleukin 2 induce remissions in some cases and, strikingly, spontaneous remissions have been documented in individual cases. Since these are thought to be caused by an immune response against the tumor, RCC is a major target of experimental immunotherapy.

Diversity of Renal Cancers

Cancers of the kidney account for a few percent of all human malignant tumors. There is a large variety of tumors in this organ, which can serve well to illustrate the diversity of human cancers.

Most cancers in the kidney are carcinomas, which have traditionally been distinguished by their histological appearance. The incidence of *renal cell carcinomas* (RCC) in industrialized countries is ≈10:100,000/year. Most are thought to originate from different parts of the nephron. Clear-cell carcinomas, the most frequent subtype, are thought to originate from proximal tubuli, which are located in the renal cortex. Because it is the most common subtype (70 – 80% of all cases), it is also called '*conventional renal cell carcinoma*'. Papillary cancers also arise from the same region, perhaps from nephrogenic rests persisting from fetal development. In this regard they resemble Wilms tumors, but papillary renal carcinomas are derived from more mature cells at a later stage of development.

Table 8.1. Some benign and malignant tumors found in the kidney

Tumor type (remarks)
Angiomyolipoma (benign)
Chromophobic carcinoma (malignant)
Clear cell renal carcinoma (malignant)
Fibrosarcoma (malignant, adult)
Hyperproliferative cysts (benign)
Lymphoma (malignant)
Medullary carcinoma (malignant)
Metastases (malignant)
Metanephric adenoma (benign)
Oncoytoma (benign)
Papillary carcinoma type I (malignant)
Papillary carcinoma type II (malignant)
Papillary-tubular adenoma (benign)
Rhabdomyosarcoma (malignant, pediatric)
Urothelial carcinoma of the renal pelvis (malignant)
Wilms tumor (malignant, pediatric)

Chromophobic carcinomas very likely originate from the distal tubuli, as do benign tumors named oncocytomas. The rare aggressive Ductus-Bellini carcinomas are derived from the collecting duct in the medulla of the kidney. Since the renal pelvis is lined by urothelium, like the bladder, urothelial cancers can also develop in the kidney. There are also tumors from mesenchymal tissues, such as moderately frequent benign angiomyolipomas and rarer malignant sarcomas. Moreover, as an organ with an extended capillary system, the kidney is a site for metastases from carcinomas from distant organs and for lymphomas.

The variety of cancers in the kidney creates a certain predicament for therapy. Kidney tumors are nowadays usually detected by physical imaging techniques such as ultrasound or computer tomography. These give a good indication of the extension of the tumor, but no definitive information on the tumor type. This has to rely on histological and molecular investigations. Since biopsies on kidney cancers are regarded as problematic, non-invasive molecular assays for this purpose would certainly be very helpful.

Traditionally, when a tumor was present, the entire kidney was removed. Today, partial nephrectomy is often performed, if histological and molecular markers indicate that a tumor recurrence is unlikely. This is evidently a good option for benign tumors like oncocytoma. Partial nephrectomy can also be performed in patients with small malignant tumors and an increased likelihood of failure of the other kidney, e.g. in the context of an inherited cancer syndrome. For the choice of treatment, precise identification of the tumor variety is, of course, imperative.

For localized renal carcinomas, removal of the tumor by surgery is usually curative. In contrast, chances for a cure become minimal, once renal carcinomas have metastasized, since all varieties responding badly to currently available chemotherapy. In individual patients, therapies directed at stimulating the immune system can lead to excellent responses, but in a rather unpredictable fashion.

Cytogenetics of Renal Cell Carcinomas

The various subtypes of *renal cell carcinoma* (RCC) were traditionally distinguished only by their histological appearance. Indeed, this is in many cases distinctive. Renal clear cell carcinoma is characterized by large, clear cells with small, densely stained nuclei, and an abundance of blood capillaries indicating pronounced angiogenesis. *Papillary carcinoma* is, as its name suggests, distinguished by its pattern of growth as finger-like connective tissue structures lined by strongly staining small epithelial tumor cells with prominent nuclei. *Chromophobic carcinoma* at first glance resembles clear cell carcinoma, but upon closer inspection the cells are more irregular, with more internal structure and less dense nuclei. Also, blood vessels are not as abundant.

Of course, these descriptions refer to textbook cases, and in everyday practice the distinction cannot be made for each case with such certainty. For instance, older RCC classifications distinguish a subtype characterized by spindle-shaped cells. This subtype is now thought to be generated from other types by an epithelialmesenchymal transition. Neither can other types of cancer (e.g. *metastases*) always be excluded without further molecular characterization.

In these circumstances it is helpful that cytogenetic investigations, corroborated by molecular assays, have revealed distinctions between the subtypes. Each type of renal cell carcinoma displays characteristic patterns of chromosomal losses and gains. Such a close correspondence between karyotype and histological subtype is remarkable in carcinomas, because characteristic chromosomal alterations in carcinomas are often obscured by a cornucopia of other changes. Evidently, recurrent diagnostic chromosomal alterations point to a causal relationship. Moreover, it follows as a corollary that pronounced chromosomal instability tends to be a relatively late event in renal carcinomas.

Table 8.2. Typical chromosomal alterations in different subtypes of renal cell carcinoma

Subtype	*Presumed origin*	*Chromosomal alterations*
Clear cell renal carcinoma	proximal tubules	-3p, others
Papillary carcinoma	proximal tubules (nephrogenic rests?)	+7, +17, +3
Chromophobic carcinoma	distal tubules	-1, -10 also -2, -6, -13, -17
Oncocytomas (benign)	distal tubules	-1, t(11;14)?
Ductus-Bellini carcinoma	collecting ducts	highly aneuploid

The characteristic change in clear cell RCC is loss of chromosome 3p, which is found in >90% of all cases. A typical site of breakage, albeit not the only one, is the major fragile site at 3p14.1 (*FRA3B*), which is prone to breakage under conditions suboptimal for DNA replication. Particularly during progression, 3p loss is accompanied by further chromosomal changes, both gains and losses.

In contrast, papillary carcinoma typically shows predominantly gains of specific chromosomes, prominently of 7, 17, and 3 (!), as well as 8, 12, 16, and 20, with loss of sex chromosomes.

Chromophobic carcinoma is characterized by a preponderance of whole chromosome losses affecting chromosomes 1, 2, 6, 10, 13, 17, and - in males - Y.

Oncocytoma, as a benign tumor that almost never metastasizes, would be expected to contain a limited number of genetic alterations. Indeed, the tumor is characterized by specific losses of chromosomes 1 and 14 and by translocations, like t(14;11). Some of these may activate the *CCDN1* gene.

Molecular Biology of Inherited Kidney Cancers

Several inherited syndromes in man predispose to kidney cancers, with varying degrees of penetrance. Likewise, there are substantial differences in how specifically these syndromes predispose to cancers of the kidney.

Autosomal Dominant Polycystic Kidney Disease (ADPKD)

ADPKD may represent the most frequent autosomally dominant hereditary disease throughout the world with an incidence of ≈1:1000 and is therefore a major cause of kidney failure. In the course of their life, the patients develop multiple fluid-filled cysts lined by hyperproliferative, aberrantly differentiated renal epithelial cells, which eventually lead to kidney failure. Defects are also found in the liver and the vascular system. Renal carcinomas arise at an increased frequency in this syndrome, but are only as one among several complications. The disease may predispose to RCC in an indirect fashion, i.e. it may increase the risk of renal carcinomas by its disturbance of the tissue architecture. Perhaps, the incompletely differentiated epithelial cells in the cysts provides a precursor cell population from which malignant tumors develop by further mutations.

Tuberous Sclerosis (TSC)

The kidney is often affected in tuberous sclerosis, although renal carcinoma is not as frequent as benign tumors such as angiomyolipoma and renal cysts. This autosomal dominant syndrome is caused by inherited mutations in the *TSC1* or *TSC2* genes. Their respective products '*hamartin*' and '*tuberin*' interact with each other and inhibit the activation of protein synthesis by the PI3K pathway which is required for increased cell proliferation.

Hereditary Papillary Renal Carcinoma (HPRC)

Unlike ADPKD and TSC, HPRC seems to predispose rather specifically to papillary tumors of the kidney. In this highly penetrant dominantly inherited syndrome, hundreds of papillary carcinomas may develop in both kidneys. They are, fortunately, not prone to early metastasis. It is therefore possible to watch them carefully and remove larger tumors by partial nephrectomy, thereby delaying the eventual removal of both kidneys and the ensuing requirement for regular dialysis.

The gene affected in this disease is *MET* located at 7q31. It encodes the receptor for *hepatocyte growth factor* (HGF) which is a receptor tyrosine kinase. Notwithstanding its name, HGF stimulates the proliferation not only of hepatocytes, but of many other cell types, in particular of epithelial origin. HGF is important during kidney organogenesis by stimulating the proliferation of epithelial precursor cells during the formation of renal tubuli. It remains essential in adult life for tissue maintenance and repair in the kidney. In fact, the therapeutic administration of HGF to prevent fibrosis after kidney injury is contemplated. However, while HGF can promote tubule formation and regeneration, under certain conditions it evokes the dissociation of epithelial cells from each other. This function has earned HGF the designation '*scatter factor*' (hence also: HGF/SF). It may likewise contribute to its function in tissue morphogenesis.

The diverse effects of HGF are all mediated through MET which activates different intracellular signaling pathways such as the MAPK pathway and the PI3K pathway. In addition, it also regulates proteins involved in cellular adhesion and motility, evidently more strongly than other receptor tyrosine kinases. The MET mutations found in HPRC are located in the kinase regulatory loop of the intracellular domain and lead to constitutive activation of its tyrosine kinase. This is a mechanism generally found in oncogenic mutated receptor tyrosine kinases.

In HPRC, activation of MET appears to block the terminal differentiation of renal tubular cells and creates instead the aberrant structures of connective tissue papillas lined by proliferating epithelial cells that characterize the disease. Because no 'hit' in the second MET allele is required, this is one of a few autosomaldominant cancer syndromes caused by mutations activating an oncogene. However, since in HPRC patients the kidneys (and all other organs) show essentially no developmental defects, it is likely that further events are needed to initiate tumor formation, in addition to the inherited MET mutation. Likely, one event is gain of chromosome 7 leading to an increased dose of the MET oncogene as well as of other growth factors and their receptors such as EGFR. Apparently, the effect of a single mutated *MET* allele can be largely overruled by other homeostatic signals. Gain of chromosome 7 is also frequent in non-papillary kidney cancers.

Hereditary Leiomyoma Renal Cell Carcinoma (HLRCC)

Several features distinguish HPRC from another syndrome, HLRCC. HLRCC also includes a risk for papillary carcinomas, but with a slightly different morphology. These are designated type II and are more aggressive. Importantly, they develop metastases at a much earlier stage. In HLRCC syndrome, type II papillary renal carcinomas are accompanied by frequent leiomyomas in the uterus. HPRC, in contrast, is largely specific for the kidney, with a somewhat enhanced risk of hepatomas. The gene at 1q42.1 mutated in HLRCC behaves as a classical tumor suppressor and its second allele is inactivated in tumors developing in this syndrome. Surprisingly, the HLRCC syndrome gene encodes fumarate hydratase, a citric acid cycle enzyme. It is not at all clear, why loss of function of this enzyme should lead to renal carcinomas and leiomyomas.

Burt-Hogg-Dube-syndrome (BHD)

In BHD syndrome, the kidney is one of several organs in which tumors arise at an increased rate. In families afflicted by the disease, carcinomas as well as oncocytomas have been observed. It is caused by mutations in a gene in the 17p11 pericentromeric region.

Hereditary Clear Cell Renal Carcinoma (HCCRCC or simply HRC)

Inherited susceptibility to clear cell renal cell carcinoma is typically conferred by mutations altering chromosome 3p, as one might expect. In some families and individuals, clear-cell RCCs are caused by inherited or congenital balanced translocations involving this chromosome, typically a t(3;8)(p14;q24). The translocation sites on 3p cluster at the fragile site *FRA3B*. This site is spanned by the *FHIT* gene which is therefore disrupted by the translocations. FHIT stands for fragile site hi f stidine triad, indicating its location and a characteristic motif in the protein. The FHIT protein resembles Ap_4A phosphorylases, which are enzymes responsible for metabolic switches in microorganisms. FHIT loss of function does seem to facilitate cell proliferation, but it is not well understood how. So, it is a moot point whether alterations of FHIT in renal cell carcinoma are causative events or '*bystanders*'. This question extends beyond RCC, because deletions and translocations of 3p involving FRA3B also occur in a range of other cancers, prominently in lung carcinomas. The 8q24 gene affected by the t(3;8) translocations is *TRC8*, which has similarities to *PTCH1*. Its altered function could well be relevant.

Alternatively to or in addition to changes in genes at the translocation site, tumor formation in HRC may involve an unusual mechanism: Since translocated chromosomes are more easily missegregated during mitosis, the frequency of 3p loss could be enhanced. Since loss of 3p appears to be a rate-limiting step in the formation of clear cell RCC, the translocation may accelerate the development of clear cell carcinoma simply by facilitating this chromosomal loss.

Von-Hippel-Lindau Syndrome (VHL)

In the kidney, this syndrome predisposes exclusively to clear cell carcinoma. Its elucidation has not only improved our understanding of renal carcinomas, but of human cancers in general.

Von-Hippel-Lindau Syndrome and Renal Carcinoma

Von-Hippel-Lindau (VHL) syndrome is inherited in an autosomal-dominant fashion, with high penetrance, but variability in its phenotype. The most distinctive lesions in this multi-organ syndrome are angiomas and hemangioblastomas in the retina and cerebellum, respectively. Frequently, the patients also develop adenomas and cysts of the pancreas, epididymis, and the kidneys. All these tumors are benign, but ≈30% of VHL patients develop RCC, which can be bilateral and multifocal. It is always of the clear-cell type. A subtype of VHL disease now designated 'type II' is distinguished by an enhanced risk of pheochromocytoma, a tumor originating from the adrenal medulla and retaining the ability to produce catecholamines. Uncontrolled secretion of adrenalin and noradrenalin by pheochromocytomas causes increased blood pressure and metabolic disturbances which can be life-threatening. Although a considerably variety of tumors can develop in von-Hippel-Lindau syndrome, they share characteristic common properties, i.e. strong vascularization and the emergence of a clear cell component characterized by an increased rate of glycolytic metabolism and enhanced storage of glycogen and lipids. These are evidently properties observed in clear-cell renal carcinoma in general, i.e. also in sporadic cases.

The von-Hippel-Lindau syndrome is caused by germ-line mutations in a gene located at 3p25, appropriately designated *VHL*. It behaves like a classical tumor suppressor gene. Thus, each individual tumor arising in the VHL syndrome has lost the function of the second *VHL* allele as well, either by mutation, promoter hypermethylation, recombination or, typical of clear-cell RCC, 3p deletion.

The *VHL* gene encodes in three exons 6.0 and 6.5 kb transcripts containing a much smaller coding region which is translated predominantly into a 213 amino acid protein. Shorter protein variants are formed through use of an alternative start codon and alternative splicing of exon 2.

The VHL protein forms an essential part of the substrate recognition module of a specific E3 ubiquitin ligase protein complex. Further members of the complex are Elongin B and Elongin C, Cullin 2, and RBX1, which binds the E2-ubiquitin component. There are several different E3 complexes in a cell, each specific for a different range of substrates. While all have a similar basic composition, their individual components vary, most decisively the substrate recognition module, after which they are therefore (usually) named.

The VHL E3 protein complex is by far not the only ubiquitin ligase important in human cancer. The SCF-β^{TRCP} E3 complex directs the breakdown of β-Catenin. Its failure is crucial in colon carcinoma and in many liver cancers. The proto-oncogene product HDM2 constitutes the recognition protein of the E3 ubiquitin ligase that degrades TP53 and its function is mimicked by the HPV E6 oncoproteins. The SCF^{SKP2} E3 ubiquitin ligase mediates the degradation of $p27^{KIP1}$ that relieves the inhibition of the CDK2/Cyclin E holoenzyme at the end of the G1 phase and allows progression of the cell cycle into S phase. Overexpression of either Cyclin E, SKP2, or MYC appears to increase its activity inappropriately in several human tumors (including renal carcinomas).

As far as we know, the main substrates of the VHL E3 ubiquitin ligase are two closely related proteins, HIF1α and HIF2α, where HIF stands for '*hypoxia-inducible factor*'. Missense mutations in the VHL protein cluster in two regions, i.e., in one face that makes contact with the HIFα proteins and in the opposite face that interacts with the Elongins. The type of mutations inherited in the VHL gene bears some relation to the disease subtype. For instance, pheochromocytoma (i.e. type II VHL syndrome) is only found in patients with certain point mutations, such as 505C>T or 712C>T. In contrast, insertion and deletion mutations (which would be expected to lead to frameshift mutations) increase the risk for RCC.

The HIFα proteins are transcription factors that induce a particular pattern of gene expression in response to low oxygen, i.e. during hypoxia. Under normal conditions, i.e. normoxia, HIF1α and HIF2α proteins undergo rapid turnover, with a half-life of a few minutes. The prevailing oxygen partial pressure is signaled through specific proline hydroxylases which hydroxylate one proline in the HIFα '*oxygen-dependent degradation domain*' (ODD). These kind of enzymes belong to the EGLN family and are different from those involved in collagen biosynthesis, but likewise contain ferrous iron and require oxygen and 2-oxo-glutarate as cosubstrates. With its proline hydroxylated, the HIFα ODD domain is recognized by VHL and the HIFα proteins are ubiquitinated and targeted for degradation by the proteasome.

If the oxygen partial pressure decreases, the proline in the ODD domain remains non-hydroxylated and the HIFα proteins accumulate in the cytosol. They combine with HIF1β, also known as ARNT, which is the dimerization partner for several nuclear factors, including the dioxin receptor AhR. The HIFα/ARNT heterodimer enters the nucleus and binds to specific recognition sites in promoters to activate genes whose products help the cell adapt to low oxygen supply and to increase oxygen availability. These HIF-binding sites are called hypoxia responsive elements or for short HRE. The activity of HIFα factors is further regulated by oxygen-dependent hydroxylation of an asparagine in their transcriptional activation domain, which prevents binding of the p300/CBP co-activator protein.

Table 8.3. Some ubiquitin ligases important in human cancers

Ubiquitin ligase	*Function*
CBL	degradation of receptor tyrosine kinases
CDH1	mitotic regulation (anaphase promoting complex)
MDM2/HDM2	degradation of TP53
SKP2	degradation of $p27^{KIP1}$
βTRCP	degradation of β-Catenin
VHL	degradation of HIFα proteins

When oxygen partial pressure normalizes, the HIFα proteins are degraded and the transcriptional response to hypoxia is terminated. In von-Hippel-Lindau disease, therefore, loss of VHL leads to accumulation of HIFα proteins and constitutive activation of a transcriptional program for hypoxia response, independent of oxygen supply. The genes that are activated by the HIFs are intriguing, when considered in the context of clear-cell carcinoma and other tumors arising in the VHL syndrome.

Oxygen Supply

Improved oxygen supply is achieved by several mechanisms. For instance, endothelin-1 and inducible NO synthase (iNOS) lead to increased blood flow and VEGF and PAI-1 stimulate angiogenesis. This provides a straightforward explanation for the enhanced vascularization in tumors arising in the VHL syndrome. Iron transport proteins like transferrin and its receptor are also induced. Moreover, hypoxia also stimulates erythropoetin production in suitable cells. This growth factor stimulates the proliferation and maturation of erythroid precursors in the bone marrow leading to '*polycythemia*'. Erythropoetin production is regulated by the kidney in response to changes in oxygen partial pressure, e.g., at high altitudes. Constitutive activation of the hypoxia response in renal tumor cells can therefore lead to increased erythropoesis, which is one of several '*paraneoplastic*' symptoms found in renal carcinoma patients. Such symptoms can be confounding in diagnosis, because they suggest completely different diseases.

Glucose and Lipid Metabolism

HIF transcription factors change the metabolism of glucose and of lipids. Target genes in this regard include the glucose transporter GLUT1 and many glycolytic enzymes, such as LDH, aldolase, and PGK. For many glycolytic enzymes, several isoenzymes are expressed in a tissue-specific fashion, depending whether the tissue performs glycolysis or gluconeogenesis. Hypoxia invariably induces the glycolytic over the gluconeogenic isoenzyme. The kidney, particularly in its proximal tubules, is capable of gluconeogenesis, like the liver and the intestine. Therefore, in VHL clear-cell carcinoma proximal tubule cells switch from gluconeogenesis to glycolysis as well as to glycogen and lipid storage. Much of this metabolic switch, like increased angiogenesis, can be accounted for by constitutive HIF activation.

Growth Factors

In addition to VEGF, active HIFs induce further growth factors acting in a paracrine fashion, e.g. on endothelial cells, as well as in an autocrine fashion on the producing cell itself. These include PDGF, TGFβ factors, and – perhaps most significant in renal epithelial cells -TGFα, an important ligand of the EGFR. Within the cell, the PI3K pathway may be activated, independent of growth factor signals.

Apoptosis

While hypoxia elicites potential growth signals, it also promotes apoptosis. The fate of a hypoxic cell may therefore be decided by the relative balance of these signals. TP53 is activated and would be expected to not only promote apoptosis via BAX upregulation, but also to antagonize the pro-angiogenic response. The proapoptotic NIX and NIP3 proteins may constitute specific mediators of hypoxia-induced apoptosis.

Regulation of pH

The carbonic anhydrases CA9 and CA12 are among the most strongly HIF1-inducible proteins. These proteins are mainly located at the cell membrane and regulate pH by accelerating the reaction between CO_2 and H_2O (in both directions). In a hypoxic environment, they favor the establishment of a low pH through the dissociation of carbonic acid.

Molecular Biology of Clear Cell Renal Carcinoma

The recurrent chromosomal alterations found in diverse subtypes of RCC indicate a causal relationship. Nevertheless, their significance is not really well understood. For instance, papillary RCC exhibit consistent gains of chromosomes which contain genes for growth factors and their receptors, such as HGF/MET, EGF-like growth factors/EGFR/ERBB2, located on chromosomes 7 and 17. However, in sporadic cases, these receptor tyrosine kinases are rarely mutated, unlike MET in HPRCC. So, one would have to postulate that increased gene dosage of both receptors and ligands could create autocrine growth factor loops that could drive the growth of papillary renal carcinoma. Thus, quantitative rather than qualitative changes in gene expression could be important for the development of this cancer. Quantitative changes as a cause of cancer are difficult to ascertain, but evidence from model systems also supports their importance. For instance, growth of several lymphoma types depends crucially on the dosage of *MYC* which itself may elicit quantitative rather than qualitative changes in gene expression.

In clear-cell renal carcinoma, the loss of 3p is evidently crucial, since it is found in $>90\%$ of all cases. One gene clearly targeted by this loss is *VHL*. Loss of 3p removes one copy of the gene. The second allele is inactivated in $\approx 80\%$ of sporadic cases of renal cell carcinoma by point mutations, small deletions, or by promoter hypermethylation. So, *VHL* is a classical tumor suppressor, even to the point that bilateral renal clear cell carcinoma is predominantly found in cases of hereditary VHL disease.

Moreover, the function of the VHL protein explains several conspicuous phenotypical aspects of this tumor type, in particular its intense vascularization and its distinctive clear-cell appearance. However, the relationship of VHL inactivation to other properties of clear cell RCC is not as straightforward. VHL loss of function does appear to impede cell cycle regulation. It may also lead to overproduction of TGFα and its receptor EGFR. Even MET has been suggested as a target of HIFα, or at least to be induced secondary to hypoxia-induced gene activation. However, it is far from clear whether these changes are sufficient to drive the proliferation of clear-cell carcinoma, especially its progression to advanced stages.

Likewise, HIFs affect the synthesis of the extracellular matrix and VHL appears to interact directly with fibronectin. Overall, however, loss of VHL may promote deposition of ECM. While ECM synthesis may aid vascularization, it would be thought to inhibit rather than to enhance invasion. By comparison, increased activity of membrane carbonic anhydrases like CA9 and CA12 may indeed aid invasion by altering the extracellular pH. One characteristic of clear cell RCC is a pronounced change in the pattern of cell adhesion molecules, which is difficult to fully ascribe to the changes in VHL/HIF only.

The perhaps most crucial issue concerns apoptosis. Since the cellular response to hypoxia involves the induction of pro-apoptotic proteins, its constitutive activation by VHL loss would be expected to eventually lead to cell death. In VHL tumors and sporadic renal cell carcinoma, this branch of the hypoxia response is evidently not fully effective.

Therefore, in the development of clear cell renal carcinoma, the loss of VHL and the constitutive expression of the cellular response to hypoxia are likely compounded by additional genetic and epigenetic alterations. Some alterations are known and target tumor suppressors. Frequent LOH at chromosomes 17p13 and 9p21 points to the involvement of *TP53* and *CDKN2A*, respectively, and additional mutations in these genes are indeed observed in advanced cases. Down-regulation and loss of PTEN, an antagonist in the PI3K pathway due to 10q loss may be another significant change in progressive cases. As in papillary RCC, certain chromosomal gains may lead to increased expression of growth factors and their receptors, especially of EGFR and MET. Conversely, responses to TGFβ are diminished, most likely through down-regulation of the TGFβRII. As a rule, in RCC anti-apoptotic proteins such as the IAP survivin are frequently over-expressed and death receptors like FAS/CD95 are down-regulated. However, the mechanisms underlying these changes in the apoptotic balance are not understood.

In spite of these changes, each in a fraction of clear cell RCC, the by far most consistent change in clear-cell renal carcinoma is loss of 3p. It is now thought unlikely that loss of one *VHL* allele is its only relevant consequence. Most researchers agree that the loss of 3p is not only a consequence of frequent breaks at *FRA3B*, but is also functionally selected for because it leads to the loss of a second tumor suppressor.

1. *FHIT* at the fragile site is an obvious candidate.
2. The *T RASSF1A* gene located at 3p21 encodes a protein activated by RAS which may limit the cellular responses to RAS activation, perhaps by blocking mitosis or as a feedback inhibitor of RAS-induced gene expression. It is transcriptionally inactivated in many different human cancers, including RCC, by promoter hyper-methylation. The RASSF1 locus is complex. In addition to the

RASSF1A protein it encodes RASSF1B and RASSF1C which may counteract RASSF1A.

3. The gene for the retinoic acid receptor RARβ2, closely related to the RARα protein crucially involved in acute promyelocytic leukemia, is located at 3p24. This member of the family appears to relay and amplify differentiation signals in epithelial cells by a typical autoregulatory loop. The *RARB2* gene contains a RARE sequence to which retinoic acid receptors can bind. Binding by a ligand-activated RARγ, e.g.,. can activate *RARB2* transcription which increases the concentration of the RARβ2 receptor, further increasing gene activity until target genes that induce terminal differentiation can be turned on. Like *RASSF1A*, *RARB2* is found hypermethylated in several carcinoma types. As in the case of RASSF1A, the locus is complex and other isoforms may also matter. Of course, until further clarification, the list of candidates does not end here.

Chemotherapy and Immunotherapy of Renal Carcinomas

Renal cell carcinomas are notoriously difficult to treat by chemotherapy or radiation therapy. Several factors may contribute to this '*primary*' resistance.

1. Renal cell carcinoma are not particularly fast growing, presenting poor targets for therapies targeting highly proliferating cells.
2. Excretion of toxic compounds is an important functions of the normal kidney. Tumor tissues from this organ retain some of the protective systems of the kidney and in particular the excretion system involving the '*PGP glycoprotein*' MDR1. MDR1 is an ATP-dependent transport protein ('ABC' transporter) which helps to exchange lipids between the inner and outer leaflet of the cell membrane. This reaction also allows the excretion of a broad range of lipophilic cytostatic drugs from the cell. In this fashion, the protein contributes to multi-drug resistance in many human cancers. In other cancers, its expression is acquired or induced only after exposure to chemotherapy, leading to '*secondary*' chemo-resistance. In the kidney, in contrast, the MDR protein is normally expressed at high levels, likely to support the excretion of toxic compounds from the body. Therefore, the protein is present right from the start in RCC and this cancer type displays '*primary resistance*'.
3. A crucial change in the development of RCC is decreased apoptosis. Although the underlying mechanisms are not completey clear, they

are likely to result in decreased sensitivity towards chemotherapy and radiotherapy.

4. In advanced renal carcinomas, loss of TP53 and PTEN functions are relatively frequent. These losses are in general associated with poor responses to chemotherapy and radiation, by diminishing apoptosis and enhancing tolerance to DNA strand-breaks.

Desperation is therefore certainly part of the explanation, why RCC has become one of the favorite objects for immunotherapy. Of course, there are more strictly scientific reasons as well. Most strikingly, '*spontaneous*' regression of renal carcinomas has been documented in individual cases. It is commonly attributed to a successful immune response. In accord with these very rare '*miracle*' cures, treatment with cytokines that stimulate cytotoxic T-cells has been reported to lead to partial or complete responses in 15-30% of clear cell renal carcinoma patients, although not in other subtypes. Therefore, treatment with interleukin-2 (IL2) and/or interferon α (IFNα) is one of the few therapeutic options available for patients with metastatic disease. This treatment occasionally leads to spectacular responses, but it is rarely curative. Moreover, the side effects can be quite intense, comparable to those experienced in a severe case of flu. They would, perhaps, be more acceptable, if one could predict in which patient the treatment is efficacious, but this is not yet possible. So, more experimental approaches to immunotherapy of renal carcinoma are being attempted.

In melanoma, another promising target for immunotherapy, immune responses are directed against proteins particular to melanocytes and to cancer-testis antigens ectopically expressed in the cancer. In renal carcinoma, oncofetal antigens, i.e. proteins normally expressed only during fetal development and down-regulated in adult kidney, may represent one type of target. More broadly, antigens recognized by immune cells in RCC are derived from proteins as part of the constitutive hypoxia response, particularly in the conventional type. For instance, a promising cell membrane antigen recognized by the monoclonal antibody G250 is expressed on the surface of essentially every renal carcinoma (of various subtypes), but is not at all detectable in normal kidney. This antigen has turned out to be part of the CA9 carbonic anhydrase, which is induced several-hundred fold in clear cell RCC as a consequence of constitutive HIF1 activation.

WILMS TUMOR (NEPHROBLASTOMA)

Wilms tumors are nephroblastomas arising in young children from nephrogenic rests, parts of the developing kidney that have failed to complete differentiation. Accordingly, the tumor mass consists of several components resembling tissue structures in the fetal kidney, such as blastema, mesenchymal stroma, and tubular structures. Most cases can be cured by a combination of chemotherapy and surgery.

Like retinoblastoma, Wilms tumors can be unilateral or bilateral, and the latter situation occurs more often with germ-line mutations. However, the disease is genetically heterogeneous and the '*two-hit*' model does not apply strictly.

Wilms tumors are normally rare, occuring in 1:10,000 children, but are more frequent in the context of syndromes which disturb the development of the genitourinary tract at large, such as the WAGR, Denys-Drash, and Beckwith-Wiedemann syndromes.

In many cases, a limited number of genetic changes are observed and the tumor cells remain near-diploid or diploid. Chromosomes 1, 11, 16, and 22 are most often affected. Tumors with multiple chromosomal aberrations are more prevalent in older children. In younger children, germ-line mutations are more often found. Mutations in TP53 characterize a small group of anaplastic (poorly differentiated) tumors.

Mutations at several loci predispose to Wilms tumors. The best characterized locus is *WT1* on chromosome 11p13 which possesses many properties of a classical tumor suppressor gene, although with incomplete penetrance. Germ-line mutations of *WT1* predispose to early and bilateral development of Wilms tumors, in which the second allele of the gene is also inactivated by loss or recombination. Some sporadic cases also show inactivation of both *WT1* alleles. However, due to low penetrance, *WT1* is responsible for only a fraction of familial cases. These are instead ascribed to loci on 17q and 19q which are not yet identified. Another apparent 'Wilms tumor locus' called *WT2* is located on 11p15.5.

WT1 encodes a transcription factor which is involved in the development and differentiation of the genitourinary tract. In particular, WT1 is expressed and its function is necessary at the time when the metanephric mesenchyme forms renal tubuli under the influence of the branching ureter bud. The understanding of the function of WT1 is complicated by the presence of several different isoforms resulting from differential splicing and translational initiation. Accordingly, consequences of mutations in the *WT1* gene vary depending on their location. While some mutations predispose to Wilms tumor only, others cause malformations in the genitourinary tract.

While *WT1* may already seem a complex locus, *WT2* may not be a single locus at all. *WT2* is related to a locus that causes Beckwith-Wiedemann syndrome, a condition of fetal overgrowth, metabolic disregulation, and predisposition to childhood tumors, although the precise relationship is unclear. Some cases of this syndrome are caused by translocations in the 11p15.5 region, others arise as a consequence of uniparental disomy or apparently independently of chromosomal changes. In either case, the expression of imprinted genes located in the region is disturbed. Actually, two different gene clusters are involved, one consisting of the *H19/IGF2* tandem locus and one comprising, among others, the *CDKN1C* and the *BWR1C* genes. Disturbances in the imprinting of IGF2 may be the relevant alterations causing Wilms tumor, while alterations in *CDKN1C* are likely more pertinent to other overgrowth symptoms in Beckwith-Wiedemann syndrome. However, the relationship is complex. Intriguingly, it cannot be excluded that some cases of Wilms tumor are initiated by epigenetic changes only.

Histology, Etiology and Clinical Behavior of Wilms Tumors

Development of the kidney is among the more unusual processes in mammalian ontogeny because it involves transition of a mesenchymal to a predominantly epithelial structure. The ureter bud invading the condensed metanephric blastema induces the formation of tubuli with progressively differentiating epithelial cells. Concomitantly, the ureter branches to form the segmented renal pelvis and the collecting ducts. This process involves a sequence of concerted gene expression changes in the blastema and the ureter cells regulated by paracrine factors and cell-cell-contacts which couple their further proliferation to step-wise differentiation. It is neither surprising that this marvellous reorganization is a favorite issue in developmental biology, nor that it occasionally goes wrong, in various ways. As a consequence, congenital malformations of the kidney and ureter are relatively frequent in man. Some appear to be accidential, while others are expedited by inherited gene defects. This statement applies to Wilms tumor in particular.

Wilms tumor is a '*nephroblastoma*' found in one of ten thousand young children, presenting very rarely after the age of 6 years. The tumor mass typically consists of an undifferentiated proliferating blastema (therefore '*nephroblastoma*') mixed to various extents with differentiated components, which are typically partly tubular epithelia and partly mesenchymal stroma. In some tumors the stroma contains ectopic structures recognizably resembling other mesenchymal tissues, e.g., muscle, cartilage, bone, and adipose tissue. Often, the tumors are associated with nephrogenic rests, i.e. residual metanephric blastema that has not differentiated. Thus, Wilms tumors are apparently caused by renal precursor cells which do not differentiate and instead continue to proliferate. Wilms tumors are more likely to arise in the context of several syndromes characterized by malformations of the genitourinary tract and inappropriate growth, underlining their origin as a consequence of defective development.

Histologically, one can distinguish different subtypes of Wilms tumor, depending on which tissue components they contain. The most prevalent subtype is triphasic, i.e. consists of blastema, stroma and tubular epithelia. This subtype arises more often in association with intralobular nephrogenic rests, as do stroma-rich tumors with ectopic mesenchymal tissues. Wilms tumors from perilobular rests probably originate at a later stage of development and consist mostly of blastema. Anaplastic tumors, the most aggressive subtype, show no indication of differentiation. Today, Wilms tumor is regarded as a separate entity from other pediatric renal cancers which develop from connective tissue components, such as rhabdomyosarcoma or clear-cell sarcoma. Like Wilms tumors these are characterized by failure to differentiate. For instance, rhabdomyosarcomas develop from precursors of muscle cells.

As a result of several large international studies, the treatment of Wilms tumors is based today on a combination of chemotherapy and surgery. More than 85% of all children can be cured, although the cancer remains lethal in some cases because of local complications and of metastases.

Like retinoblastoma, Wilms tumor can be unilateral or bilateral, i.e. develop in one or both kidneys. Also like retinoblastoma, some Wilms tumors occur in families, although familial cases constitute only a few percent overall. Conspicuously, the age vs. incidence curve appears biphasic with a first peak around 2 years and a second one around 4 years of age. Familial cases often fall into the first group. Despite such parallels to retinoblastoma, the molecular genetics of Wilms tumors is more complicated and the Knudson model applies only partly.

Genetics of Wilms Tumors and the WT1 Gene

One would presume that tumor development in a young child cannot result from an accumulation of multiple genetic alterations, unlike cancers in older people. Indeed, Wilms tumors as a rule contain a limited number of evident genetic aberrations. Many have diploid or near-diploid karyotypes. In the other cases, chromosomes 1, 11, 16, and 22 are most often affected. On chromosome 1, the short arm tends to be lost, while the long arm is often gained. This can be explained by the formation of an isochromosome 1q with loss of 1p. 16q and 22q are subject to losses. The mutations in *TP53* and loss of heterozygosity (LOH) at its locus at 17p are found in a few cases, usually with anaplastic histology. They bode a poor response to chemotherapy. Chromosome 11 is also affected by losses, while chromosomes 6, 7, 8, 12, or 13 are gained in some cases.

The causes of these chromosomal alterations are not known. Loss or gain of whole chromosomes points to defects in chromosome segregation during mitosis. The frequently afflicted chromosomes 1 and 16 are distinguished by harboring a particularly large proportion of the GC-rich satellite sequences (*SAT1 – SAT3*) in the human genome. They are arranged as tandem repeats in juxta-centromeric heterochromatin at 1q and 16q. The CpG-rich satellite DNA is normally highly methylated in somatic cells, but is hypomethylated in Wilms tumors, which may make it more susceptible to breakage and recombination.

Several individual loci are involved specifically in Wilms tumor, of which WT1 is best characterized. The WT1 gene is located at 11p13 and was first identified in patients suffering from WAGR syndrome. The acronym WAGR stands for Wilms tumor, aniridia (lack of an iris), genitourinary malformations, and mental retardation. The syndrome is caused by deletions of. several consecutive genes on chromosome 11p13 including *WT1*, which explains the genitourinary malformations and Wilms tumor, and the paired-box transcription factor gene *PAX6*, which explains aniridia. Specifically, aniridia patients in whom the deletion does not encompass the *WT1* gene do not develop Wilms tumors. In Wilms tumors from WAGR patients, the second allele of *WT1* is also inactivated, often by nonsense mutations.

The WAGR syndrome is rare, but in ≈15% of all Wilms tumors as well, both alleles of the *WT1* gene are inactivated. Most often, this occurs by mutation of one allele and loss of the second by recombination, which is detectable by LOH at 11p13. In at least one third of these patients, the first mutation is present in the germ-line and the patients tend to develop tumors in both kidneys. In the others, the first mutation is also somatic and their tumors are unilateral. Thus, in this regard *WT1* behaves like a classical tumor suppressor gene such as *RB1*. However, until now, tumors caused by *WT1* mutations have not been observed in successive generations. The main reason for this seems that *WT1* mutations show much lower penetrance than mutations of *RB1*. Also, germ-line mutations in WT1 do not imply an increased risk for other tumors.

The reasons for these differences are not understood. They may relate to the different functions of the proteins and a difference in the '*window of opportunity*' for the cancers to arise. The WT1 protein seems to be required at one specific stage in renal development, i.e. for the blastema to begin its mesenchymal-epithelial transition. Once the cells have moved beyond this stage, loss of WT1 function may not matter, and the gene is, in fact, down-regulated. So, in a carrier of a germ-line mutation, the second '*hit*' must have been acquired by that time. In contrast, the requirement for functional RB1 may be most crucial at the very end of retinoblast differentiation, to permit the permanent exit from the cell cycle, i.e. terminal differentiation. Accordingly, retinoblasts might have more time to acquire the decisive '*second hit*'. A second, more speculative explanation is that *RB1* hemizygosity - unlike that of WT1 - already increases tumor risk somewhat, perhaps because of its additional functions in maintaining genomic stability.

Like RB1, however, WT1 is crucially involved in directing differentiation, certainly in the developing kidney, but likely also in the gonads, spleen and mesothelium, where WT1 expression is also found. In the adult kidney, its expression is restricted to podocytes, epithelial cells which are an essential component of the glomerulus. Importantly, during development of the kidney WT1 expression is most prominent in the condensing nephroblastema at the onset of the mesenchymal-epithelial transition. In suitable mesenchymal cells, transfection of WT1 can induce a transition of this type. Thus, the time and place where WT1 is needed in development fit well with the morphological appearance and location of Wilms tumors that have lost its function.

The 50 kb *WT1* gene encodes transcription factor proteins with a four zinc-finger DNA binding domain that is similar to those in the widely distributed EGR transcriptional activators and recognizes the same DNA sequence motif. WT1, however, contains both an activator and a repressor domain. Moreover, the protein binds to RNA and may regulate splicing. There are, in fact, several isoforms of the WT1 protein which differ with respect to these abilities. Translation of WT1 can initiate at two different codons. In addition, two sites are used for alternative splicing. The presence or absence of exon 5 alters the size of the activation domain by 17 amino acids and likely its function, too. Use of two alternative splice donors 9 bp apart at the end of exon 9 leads to two isoforms which differ by three amino acids in zinc finger 3 and are denoted as +/-KTS. Moreover, the WT1 transcript is subject to editing. Thus, overall, the WT1 gene encodes up to 16 proteins with 52 – 56 kDa MW which differ in their ability to repress or activate transcription and with respect to DNA binding. They are also expressed in different patterns in different tissues.

The significance of many variants is unknown, but at least the KTS variant is important, since splice mutations causing loss of this sequence are found in children suffering from Frasier syndrome. Denys-Drash-syndrome, by comparison is caused by de novo germ-line missense mutations in exons 8 or 9 of the *WT1* gene. These lead to changes in those amino acids in the WT1 zinc fingers that interact with DNA. Characteristics of the syndrome are defects in the glomeruli causing kidney failure, incomplete differentiation of the genitals, and an increased risk of Wilms tumors. The developmental defects are caused by the germ-line mutation alone, whereas formation of Wilms tumors requires inactivation of the second allele as well. Missense mutation in the WT1 zinc fingers are also found in sporadic Wilms tumors, but in these truncating mutations are more prevalent. Conversely, truncating mutations are not found as a cause of Denys-Drash-syndrome, suggesting that the characteristic zinc-finger missense mutations in this disease act as dominant-negatives or by a 'gain of function' mechanism.

So, in summary, while WT1 mutations may be passed on in the germ-line in some families, and sometimes cause Wilms tumors, they are not responsible for the majority of familial cases. Instead, pertinent loci have been mapped by linkage analyses to chromosomes 17q12-21 and 19q13 and have been named tentatively *FWT1* and *FWT2* (for: familial Wilms tumor). Previously suspected loci at 16q and 11p15 have now been exculpated as a cause of familial Wilms tumors, but they are certainly important in some sporadic cases.

Epigenetics of Wilms Tumors and the 'WT2' Losuc

Beckwith-Wiedemann syndrome (BWS), which conveys an increased risk for Wilms tumors and other pediatric malignancies, is caused by genetic or epigenetic defects in the chromosomal region 11p15.5. This region comprises two clusters of imprinted genes, including the twin loci *IGF2/H19* and a larger gene cluster apparently controlled by an imprinting center (IC) located in the *KCQN1* gene. Children suffering from BWS are oversized and overweight at birth, often presenting with overgrowth of only one side of the body ('*hemihyperthrophy*') or of visceral organs such as the liver. Furthermore, glucose homeostasis can be dangerously deregulated perinatally (around birth). The syndrome is caused by one of several defects: (1) balanced translocations or inversions in the 11p15.5 region on the chromosome inherited from the mother; (2) uniparental disomy, in which this region is derived from the father on both chromosomes 11; (3) point mutations in the *CDKN1C* gene encoding the CDK inhibitor p57^{KIP2}.

Most changes found in BWS have in common that *CDKN1C* function is compromised. Since the gene is significantly transcribed only from the maternal allele, chromosomal aberrations and uniparental disomy strongly diminish its expression, whereas point mutations inactivate the gene product, the CDK inhibitor protein p57^{KIP2}.

However, the phenotype of BWS is very likely not only due to *CDKN1C* loss of function. Specifically, Wilms tumors do not occur in children in which BWS is caused by mutations in this gene. Indeed, most alterations affect other genes as well, often from both imprinted gene clusters at 11p15.5. For instance, some translocations separate the imprinting center IC2 in the *KCQN1* gene from the *CDKN1C* and other genes, disturbing their maternal imprinting pattern.

Overall, there are six or more imprinted genes in the *KCQN1/CDKN1C* cluster. Several of them may have functions which could contribute to the phenotype of BWS such as regulation of transcription (*ASCL2 /MASH2*), cell-cell-interaction (CD81), signal transduction (*TSSC3/IPL/BWR1C*), and regulation of apoptosis (*TSCC5/BWR1A*). Obviously, their interaction may be difficult to disentangle, even more so, since animal models are of limited use, because the imprinting patterns of some genes differ between mammalian species, in particular between mouse and man. Still, *CDKN1C* '*knockout*' mice show several developmental defects resembling those in BWS including overgrowth. The *IGF2/H19* genes are also disturbed in many cases of BWS. For instance, uniparental disomy with both chromosomes derived from the father leads to an increase in IGF2 expression, as would be expected for two active gene copies compared to one.

In Wilms tumors, loss of imprinting in the *IGF2/H19* cluster is frequent, not only in those tumors arising in BWS patients. The expression pattern becomes paternal for both alleles, with an increase in IGF2 peptides and a decrease in H19 RNA. Increased expression of IGF2, a potent growth and survival factor, could well account for the overproliferation of nephroblastoma cells. Moreover, *IGF2* may be a target gene of WT1 and vice versa, suggesting a kind of pathway involved in the genesis of Wilms tumor. However, the data in this regard are controversial and it is possible that the down-regulation of H19 may after all also be significant. For instance, overexpression of H19 RNA in a nephroblastoma cell line was found to arrest its growth.

There are further epigenetic events affecting the development and progression of Wilms tumor. (1) As mentioned above, a frequent genetic change in Wilms tumors is loss of chromosome 1p. While often the entire arm is involved, mapping of the common region of deletion, in Wilms tumor and other pediatric cancers, points to a tumor suppressor gene in the 1p36 region, where some genes are also imprinted. So, loss of a single copy of this region may be sufficient to inactivate a tumor suppressor gene. (2) While the *WT1* gene itself is not imprinted, it overlaps partly with an RNA gene named *WIT1* transcribed in the opposite direction, but only from the paternal allele. LOH involving chromosome 11p, at large, is biased towards loss of the maternal copy, which diminishes the function of the maternally imprinted genes at the tip of the chromosome. However, this also implies an increased dose of *WIT1*. Its functional significance is, however, unknown.

Since so many cases of Wilms tumors remain diploid, it is an interesting question whether epigenetic changes may in some cases be sufficient to cause formation of this tumor type. This is not known for sure, but if this mechanism occurs in any human cancer at all, it could be Wilms tumor.

Towards an Improved Classification of Wilms Tumors

The histology and clinical behavior of Wilms tumors vary, and its genetic and epigenetic causes are heterogeneous. While one would presume that the latter may explain the former, the relationship does not seem to be straightforward. Nevertheless, a consensus appears to emerge which may help to cure even more children and select an optimal treatment for each patient.

For a while already, it has been known, that an anaplastic histology is a bad prognostic sign and TP53 mutations presage a poor response to chemotherapy. The same seems to be true for cancers with monosomy of chromosome 22, for reasons that are not understood. It has also been claimed that tumors with WT1 mutations may be more aggressive than others, too, even though they tend to have fewer chromosomal alterations. It is, however, not clear, whether this is a property of tumors with WT1 mutations or not – more likely – a property of the subtype to which they belong. Mutations in WT1 are almost exclusively found in tumors with a high stromal content that are associated with intralobular nephrogenic rests. These tumors appear to fail epithelial differentiation completely and then, in a more or less stochastical fashion, differentiate into some mesenchymal lineage. They arise earlier than the blastema-rich tumors associated with perilobular nephrogenic rests. These are very often characterized by loss of imprinting and overexpression of IGF2 and appear to respond better to chemotherapy. In contrast to the former group, WT1 is normally expressed indicating that the block in differentiation is caused by a different defect.

Our understanding of Wilms tumors is certainly at present incomplete. However, researchers and clinicians in the field agree that the pieces of the Wilms tumor puzzle begin to fall in place. This implies the prospect that this once often lethal cancer may eventually be cured with still fewer side-effects in an even larger proportion of the afflicted children.

9

Bladder Cancer

'*Bladder cancer*' is a somewhat imprecise generic name for carcinomas of the urothelium, a specialized epithelium lining the urinary tract from the renal pelvis into the urethra. A more precise name is therefore urothelial cancer. Most bladder cancers retain markers of the characteristic transitional cells of the urothelium and are therefore called *transitional cell carcinoma* (TCC). One type of TCC forms papillary structures growing predominantly into the lumen of the urinary tract. Papillary TCC does not readily become invasive, but tends to recur. The more aggressive invasive TCC typically develop from the flat, dysplastic carcinoma in situ. A different histological subtype prevalent in countries with endemic schistosomiasis has lost urothelial differentiation and presents as squamous cell carcinoma. This is an example of metaplasia. Due to the diversity in the type and clinical course of bladder cancers, an important clinical problem is choosing the optimal treatment for each individual patient.

Urothelial cancers are often caused by chemical carcinogens, notably aromatic amines, whereas squamous carcinomas of the bladder typically arise in the context of chronic inflammation. Genetic polymorphisms in genes involved in carcinogen metabolism modulate bladder cancer risk dependent on exposure, whereas no high-risk hereditary syndrome is known that specifically predisposes to this cancer.

Urothelial cancers tend to develop at multiple sites, at the same time or successively. This is an example of '*field cancerization*'. In fact, several factors are responsible, including true oligoclonality, migration of cancer cells within the epithelium, and spreading through the urine.

Invasive bladder cancers show pronounced chromosomal instability and alterations in several '*cancer pathways*'. Almost invariably, two crucial regulatory systems are incapacitated. (1) Cell cycle regulation is disrupted by loss of RB1, loss of $p16^{INK4A}$, or amplification of *CCND1*, augmented by down-regulation of CIP/KIP CDK inhibitor proteins. (2) The control of genomic integrity by TP53 is disturbed through mutations in its gene, loss of $p14^{ARF1}$, or overexpression of HDM2. These changes appear already in carcinomata in situ or high-grade papillary cancers.

In contrast, well-differentiated papillary TCCs show a limited range of genetic abnormalities, e.g. loss of chromosome 9, RAS mutations, or mutations in the FGFR3 growth factor receptor that lead to its constitutive activation. Distinctive differences towards invasive cancers, in particular FGFR3 mutations, characterize tumors with a low risk of progression.

The most consistent genetic change throughout all subtypes of bladder cancer is chromosome 9 loss, which is found in more than half of all cases. This loss targets the *CDKN2A* tumor suppressor on 9p encoding the two important regulator proteins $p16^{INK4A}$ and $p14^{ARF1}$. However, LOH and deletions are also regularly found on chromosome 9q, strongly suggesting that additional tumor suppressor genes are located there. It has proven surprisingly arduous to identify them. This illustrates that the route from a recurrent chromosomal change to the identification of a relevant gene is not always straightforward.

Papillary bladder tumors may grow mainly as a consequence of overactivity of those pathways which stimulate the proliferation of normal urothelial cells during compensatory growth or tissue regeneration. In contrast, invasive bladder cancers have largely uncoupled their growth regulation from extrinsic signals. In addition, the mechanisms maintaining chromosomal stability during cell proliferation are upset in invasive bladder cancers. The differences in clinical behavior of bladder cancers are thus based on differences in their molecular characteristics.

Histology and Etiology of Bladder Cancer

From the renal pelvis through the urinary bladder into the urethra, the urinary tract is lined by a specialized '*transitional*' epithelium called '*urothelium*', whose structure is in several respects different from that of squamous epithelia in the skin and other organs. The urothelium forms a low permeability barrier that prevents the components of the urine, even water, from seeping back into the body.

In a transitional epithelium, cells from several layers retain contact with the basement membrane. This allows them to shift across each other depending on the filling state. The top cellular layer forms the actual barrier and consists of terminally differentiated '*umbrella*' cells linked by tight junctions. The low permeability in the urothelium is achieved by a dense protein array in their apical membrane composed of uroplakins. These proteins are specific markers of urothelial differentiation. The urothelium normally turns over very slowly, but can proliferate rapidly and extensively in response to injury or to bacterial infections to replace damaged areas.

Bladder cancer is a generic term for carcinomas developing from the urothelium. Indeed, most urothelial cancers grow in this part of the urinary tract, but as those in other segments have similar properties, the designation is often loosely used. Most carcinomas arising from urothelium retain morphological and biochemical markers of its original structure. In particular, they express urothelial differentiation markers such as uroplakins and specific cytokeratins (e.g. CK7). These cancers are accordingly categorized as transitional cell carcinomas (TCC).

Bladder cancer is the ≈fifth-most frequent cancer and more prevalent in males. Transitional cell carcinoma represents the predominant histological type in industrialized countries. In countries with endemic schistosomiasis, a second type of bladder cancer, designated squamous cell carcinoma, is more prevalent. Although originating as well from cells of the urothelium, this carcinoma consists of - sometimes well-organized - layers of cells that resemble a squamous epithelium. Accordingly, the cancer cells express markers of such epithelia, but not of urothelium, e.g. the cytokeratin CK14 or even involucrin. This is a clear instance of metaplasia, since no squamous epithelium exists in the normal urinary tract upwards of the distal part of the urethra.

Transitional cell carcinoma can be induced by chemical carcinogens. This was first realized by the surgeon Ludwig Rehn who at the end of the 19th century treated workers making azo-dyes in a chemical plant in a suburb of Frankfurt in Germany. These people were literally drenched in aniline, benzidine, and the dyes made from them, and developed bladder cancers early in life and at a high rate. Today, in spite of much better precautions, occupational risks for bladder cancer remain in the chemical industry and in other branches where workers are exposed to aromatic amines or their metabolizable derivatives.

Other chemicals such as nitrosamines, nitro-aromates, polyaromates, and the cytostatic drug cyclophosphamide, as well as arsenic are also established or very likely bladder carcinogens. A cocktail of carcinogens is inhaled with tobacco smoke and the risk of bladder cancer is consequentially increased approximately 4-fold in smokers. The rate of bladder cancer is also enhanced in Eastern Europeans who have incorporated radioactive cesium from the Chernobyl accident.

The fact that carcinogenicity by aromatic amines shows such a strong organ preference has facilitated its understanding. To become carcinogenic, aromatic amines must be activated by hydroxylation at the amino group. This reaction is performed by isoenzymes of the P450 monooxygenase family, whose genes are designated *CYP*. Protonation of this N-hydroxyl group leads to dissociation of a water molecule and formation of a highly reactive arenium ion. Hydroxylation at the amino group is prevented by its acetylation. This is catalyzed by N-acetyltransferases, mostly by NAT2 enzymes. Moreover, the efficiency of excretion of hydroxylated amines into the urine vs. the gut depends on the extent of glucuronylation and sulfatation performed by UDP-glucuronyl transferases and sulfotransferase, respectively.

As many of the enzymes involved in the metabolism of arylamines are polymorphic in humans, the carcinogenicity of aromatic amines in individual humans depends not only on their level of exposure, but also on their genetic constitution. In chemical workers exposed to aromatic amines, *NAT2* appears to constitute the dominant genetic factor. Depending on dozens of combinations of different alleles, humans display two different phenotypes, '*slow*' and '*rapid*' acetylators, which are also important in the response to a range of medical drugs. Rapid acetylators are much less susceptible to bladder carcinogenesis by aromatic amines, although they may excrete more metabolites into the gut, leading to a somewhat increased risk for colorectal cancer.

Among bladder cancer patients in general, the *NAT2* genotype tends to be a less dominant factor because other carcinogens and endogenous processes contribute. However, the risk of smokers to develop bladder cancer is even greater in those who lack the GSTM1 glutathione transferase, which metabolizes chemical carcinogens related to benzopyrene. This lack is caused by homozygosity for the deletion nullallele of the GSTM1 gene.

While transitional cell carcinoma is often induced by chemical carcinogens, squamous cell carcinoma typically arises after chronic inflammation of the bladder. This is most obvious in schistostomainduced bladder cancer. Schistosoma parasites enter the human body from contaminated water and establish themselves in the lung, liver, and urinary bladder. In the bladder, schistosoma mansoni causes a chronic inflammation (bilharziosis) with permanent tissue damage and regeneration. This prepares the ground for the development of squamous carcinoma. This relationship makes bladder cancer one of the most frequent cancers in warmer countries with endemic bilharziosis caused by this species of trematode parasites.

In industrialized countries of the North, ≈90% of all bladder cancers display transitional cell carcinoma histology, while most of the rest are squamous cell carcinoma. Transitional cell carcinoma comprises two subtypes with different properties. The most frequent type is a papillary tumor which grows predominantly into the lumen and remains well recognizable as being derived from urothelium. Although they are malignant, only ≈20% of these tumors actually progress to an invasive stage and further to metastasis. Most, but not all of the tumors that will eventually become invasive are less than well-differentiated initially. Papillary tumors can usually be removed by local resection, but tend to recur at different localizations in the urothelium, sometimes having progressed to a less differentiated or more invasive state.

The reasons for this behavior are not entirely clear. Bladder cancer is often regarded as an example of '*field cancerization*' because multiple tumors arise in different places at the same time or successively, i.e. synchronously or metachronously. This could mean that the entire tissue has been transformed towards a kind of preneoplastic stage, perhaps as a consequence of exposure to carcinogens, chronic irritation or inflammation, or as a consequence of factors released by the actual cancer cells.

Molecular comparisons between multiple synchronous and metachronous cancers using microsatellite markers indicate that several factors combine to yield the impression of a field change. (1) Some bladder cancers are indeed oligoclonal, i.e. tumors at different sites or different times have mutually exclusive genetic changes indicating an independent origin, in line with the original idea of a field change. (2) Some cancers have so closely related microsatellite patterns that they must represent descendents from the same clone. In this case, they may have spread by migration within the mucosa or through the lumen. (3) Specifically, some recurrent tumors can be shown to be identical to the original tumor, whereas others are clearly independent.

In the first group, resection may have been incomplete or the tumor may have been spread during the surgical procedure.

Recurrences can be partly prevented by instillation of cytostatic drugs like mitomycin C or of BCG, a tuberculosis vaccine. This consists of inactivated mycobacteria which appear to induce an immune reaction that kills residual tumor cells along with parts of the urothelium. The normal urothelium is then replaced by regeneration. In spite of such '*adjuvant*' preventive measures, patients need to be monitored for recurrences for many years after surgery.

A more aggressive form of bladder cancer is found in ≈20% of patients upon first presentation. In these, the tumor grows less extensively into the lumen and more into the deeper layers of the tissue and beyond them, with a propensity to metastasize. These invasive cancers likely develop from carcinoma in situ, a flat, severely dysplastic lesion. Dysplasia in this case relates to both the cell morphology, to the tissue structure, and to the nuclei, which are highly polymorphic and aberrant, suggesting a substantial degree of aneuploidy. Invasive bladder cancers need to be treated more radically by removal of the urinary bladder ('*cystectomy*'), as soon they have progressed into the muscular layers of the tissue. Cystectomy represents a major surgical intervention associated with a low risk of mortality, but a significant rate of complications ('*morbidity*') and often severe consequences for the quality of life. Still, it is not invariably successful in curing the cancer. In some cases, chemotherapy is applied in addition to surgery (i.e. adjuvantly). In some cases where surgery is unadvisable, it is administered as the only treatment. Overall, cytostatic chemotherapy in bladder cancer is moderately efficacious, and certainly not curative in cases of metastatic disease. So, compared to colorectal cancer, whose development by and large seems to follow a linear sequence, that of bladder cancer branches out into different varieties with quite different properties. In the clinic, this creates the question of how to treat each patient optimally. For cancer research, the challenge is to identify which biological mechanisms underlie the differences between the varieties. For '*translational*' research, the tasks are to identify markers for the different varieties and to predict their clinical behavior and response to therapy, but also to find out which molecular targets they present for novel therapies.

Molecular Alterations in Invasive Bladder Cancers

All invasive bladder cancers are apparently defective in two important regulatory systems, i.e., the regulation of the cell cycle by

RB1 and the control of genomic integrity by TP53. Combined, these two defects appear to allow uncontrolled proliferation, increased genomic instability and growth beyond the limits posed by replicative senescence. Indeed, telomerase is generally activated in invasive bladder cancers. This constellation of changes is typical of many advanced human cancers, i.e. the same statement could be made for lung cancer, pancreatic cancer, squamous carcinomas of the head and neck, or glioblastoma as well as to squamous cell carcinoma of the skin. Of note, it would not as generally apply to colorectal cancers. In the various cancer types, different mechanisms leading to inactivation of the two regulatory systems contribute to various extents.

In advanced bladder cancers, inactivation of the RB1 pathway is achieved by loss of RB1 or of $p16^{INK4A}$, less frequently by constitutive overexpression of Cyclin D1 due to *CCND1* gene amplification, and in rare cases by overexpression of CDK4 due to amplification of its gene. Of these changes, loss of RB1 itself, usually by loss of one allele and deletions or truncating mutations in the other one, appears to implicate the most severe consequences. Bladder cancers with loss of RB1 protein, as detected by immunohistochemistry, take the most aggressive course. Moreover, the CDK inhibitors $p21^{CIP1}$, $p27^{Kip1}$, and $p57^{KIP2}$, which are all expressed in normal proliferating urothelial cells and in many superficial cancers, tend to disappear in advanced bladder cancers. Their down-regulation likely exacerbates the defects in cell cycle regulation. The mechanisms underlying these disappearances are poorly understood, but are probably to a large degree epigenetic.

Loss of TP53 function in bladder cancers is most frequently caused by point mutations in its gene and loss of the second functional allele by recombination or deletion affecting chromosome 17p. The TP53 point mutations are spread out through the central part of the gene and do not present an obvious clue to the carcinogens involved, although typical '*tobacco*' mutations may be somewhat overrepresented. Overexpression of MDM2/HDM2 is observed in some cases. More frequently, $p14^{ARF1}$ is lost. Like loss of $p16^{INK4A}$, this occurs most often by homozygous deletions encompassing the *CDKN2A* locus. It is technically difficult to ascertain the true frequency of homozygous deletions in tumor tissues, but a reasonable estimate is 40% deletions of both *CDKN2A* alleles in advanced bladder cancers, in addition to smaller fractions of cases with missense mutations or promoter hypermethylation. Interestingly, loss of $p14^{ARF}$ and TP53 mutations are not mutually exclusive, but loss of $p16^{INK4A}$ and RB1 are. This has been observed in various human cancers, although the reasons are not understood. It is clear, however, that loss of RB1 causes upregulation of $p16^{INK4A}$ expression, because RB1 represses its promoter. So, increased expression of the cell cycle inhibitor $p16^{INK4A}$ in human cancers, as detectable by immunohistochemistry, is often a bad sign, since it reflects the (usually) more severe inactivation of RB1. Equally paradoxically, higher levels of TP53 protein in a cancer often indicate its inactivity, since only accumulated mutant protein can be detected by standard immunohistochemistry. Accordingly, bladder cancers with immuno-histochemically detectable TP53 appear to take a more aggressive course than the average. Clearly, the group with the worst prognosis is that with TP53 mutated as well as RB1 lost.

A notable feature of bladder cancer distinguishing it from colorectal cancer is the virtual absence of mutations activating the WNT/β-Catenin pathway. APC expression and function seem unaffected and mutations activating β-Catenin are very rare. Of course, target genes of the canonical WNT pathway such as *CNND1*, *MYC*, and *MMPs* are also induced in bladder cancers, but obviously by other means. There is, likewise, little evidence for an important role of the SHH pathway that is so crucial in basal cell carcinoma of the skin, although the *PTCH1* gene is often hemizygous. Instead, the genetic alterations in bladder cancer resemble those in squamous cell carcinoma of the skin.

There are two, not mutually exclusive hypotheses to account for these differences. (1) Colorectal cancer and basal cell carcinoma appear to arise from tissue precursor cells by the constitutive activation of the respective pathways that maintain their stem cell character. Bladder cancers may originate from more differentiated cells in which these pathways are not active anymore. This idea is, of course, compatible with the expression of markers of advanced urothelial differentiation such as uroplakins or the cytokeratins CK7 and CK20 in transitional cell carcinomas. Squamous cell carcinoma metaplasia remains enigmatic in this hypothesis. (2) The urothelium as a tissue is organized in a very different fashion from the gut and skin. While these tissues turn over continuously, urothelium proliferates significantly only in response to injury. The organization of proliferation and differentiation in urothelial tissue may therefore involve regulatory systems other than the WNT/β-Catenin and SHH pathways.

Nevertheless, loss of cell cycle regulation and of TP53 function are certainly not the only genetic alterations in invasive bladder cancers. Most invasive bladder cancers are highly aneuploid and almost every chromosome is subject to numerical or structural aberrations in one or the other case. In the nomenclature developed for colon cancers, they would be assigned to the CIN class. Dysfunction of cell cycle checkpoints as a consequence of RB1 and TP53 inactivation is certainly one factor favoring this chaotic behavior. Additional, more specific defects in the maintenance of chromosomal stability may be involved, but as in many other carcinomas, they are not clearly defined.

In bladder cancer, however, it is clear that genomic instability arises very early in a subfraction of tumors, since many changes are already detectable in carcinoma in situ and in early invasive stages. In contrast, many papillary cancers present with a limited number of chromosomal alterations. Compared to colon carcinoma, microsatellite instability is very rarely found in bladder cancers. Urothelial cancers do occur in HNPCC patients at increased rates, but somewhat mysteriously only in the upper urinary tract, i.e. in the renal pelvis and the ureter. There is no good explanation for this specificity, the more so, as genetic alterations in general are similar between cancers from different regions of the urothelium. Perhaps, the concentration of carcinogens or the length of exposure is higher in the renal pelvis and ureter.

As a consequence of widespread genomic instability in bladder cancer, it is difficult to define those alterations that are crucial for tumor development, as opposed to those that have occurred as a consequence of genomic instability and are propagated as '*passenger alterations*' in a successfully expanding tumor cell clone. One approach to this problem is to focus on those chromosomal alterations that recur in many different cases or characterize specific subsets of cancers. For instance, loss of 13q and 17p is frequent in advanced cancers, and is likely related to the inactivation of RB1 and TP53.

Further recurrent chromosomal losses during progression concern 8p, 3p, 16q, and 11p, each in a subset of cases. One can presently only guess at which genes might be affected by these losses. *CDH1* encoding E-Cadherin on 16q and *CDKN1C* encoding $p57^{KIP2}$ on 11p are good candidates. Conversely, frequent gains of chromosomes 7p and 8q may relate to *ERBB1* encoding the EGFR and *MYC*, respectively, since in rarer cases more selective amplifications of 7p12 and 8q24.1 are observed. The consequences of the often concomitant gains or amplifications at 5p, 6p, and 20q are again enigmatic.

There is a practical and conceptual problem involved here in bridging the gap between chromosomal alterations and identifying the crucial genes activated or inactivated by them. This problem is alleviated, if an inherited high-risk syndrome points the way and positional cloning can be used to limit the range of candidate genes. These can then be screened for inactivation mutations (in the case of a tumor suppressor) or activating mutations (in the case of an oncogene) in normal cells of patients from affected families.

In cancers where no such syndrome is available, the task is more difficult, and further exacerbated by genomic instability. In cancers with pronounced genomic instability like invasive bladder cancers, the first step involves sorting relevant from passenger alterations. This already involves a conceptual difficulty, because there may be a considerable '*grey zone*' of alterations that affect properties of the cancer, although they might not be essential for its growth. However, the main problems arise from the fact that genetic (and *epigenetic*) alterations in cancers are not only functionally relevant and selected by their functional impact on the expansion of a tumor cell clone, but are also determined and restricted by the mechanisms causing them, especially by the type of genomic instability present in a cancer. Two examples from invasive bladder cancers can serve to illustrate this quite complex argument.

1. The most frequent amplification in invasive bladder cancers concerns a region at chromosome 6p22. Gains of 6p are observed in a larger fraction of advanced tumors, and ≈25% display true amplifications of a smaller segment of 6p22. The segment that is amplified is still variable, typically comprising several genes. One of them encodes the transcriptional activator E2F3, which can activate genes during S-phase and is regulated by RB1. Therefore, its amplification could lead to overexpression and loss of cell cycle control by RB1. However, the amplified region in some cases also encompasses the gene *SOX4* which encodes a non-histone chromatin protein known to regulate cell fate and differentiation, or *DEK* encoding a protein kinase regulating chromatin structure and involved as a partner in oncogenic fusions in hematological cancers, as well as additional genes. So, which of these genes is responsible, or may be several?

   Similar questions have been encountered in other cases of amplifications in other cancers, e.g. the 12q13 amplicon encompassing *HDM2/CDK4/GLI1* and the 11q13 amplicon comprising *CCND1/GSTP1/FGF1*. The reason for the difficulty stems from the mechanism underlying amplifications. They are likely generated as a consequence of chromosomal breaks that do not arise completely at random. Following an initial break, a segment of the DNA is replicated, which must have a minimal size. The maximum size may, in fact, also be influenced by structural features; it is possible that the size of an amplicon corresponds to some sort of DNA replication unit. Typically, amplicons are several Mbp in size. Since in the human genome, there is on average one gene per 100 kb, this may correspond to several dozen genes. So, in a human cancer, amplification of a single gene earmarking it as an oncogene is the exception rather than the rule.

2. In bladder cancer, quite independently of its subtype, LOH at chromosome 9 occurs in >50% of all cases. Usually, it reflects chromosome deletions. Doubtless, these changes contribute to inactivation of *CDKN2A* located at 9p21. However, the long arm of chromosome 9 is no less frequently affected, suggesting strongly that at least one further important tumor suppressor gene resides there. However, it has not been identified to date.

Identification of a '*classical*' tumor suppressor presupposes consistent inactivation of both alleles of a gene. Since no familial syndrome is known for bladder cancer, changes in cancer tissues must be investigated. In many bladder cancers, LOH at 9q is caused by loss of one entire chromosome 9, i.e. monosomy, or of the whole arm. These cases are not helpful. Even limited LOH at 9q often stretches across a larger sequence, varying between different cancers. Ideally, a tumor suppressor gene would be located in the smallest region of overlap. However, since most regions of LOH are large, the actual definition of the region of overlap relies on the exceptional cases with small deletions, which could well be untypical. This type of strategy could lead to those sites where chromosome breaks occur most often rather than to those where the functionally most important gene is located, particularly in cancers with pronounced chromosomal instability.

The success of the strategy therefore depends crucially on finding alterations that activate the second allele of the presumed tumor suppressor. This means tedious searches for point mutations or promoter hypermethylation. Again, however, not all genes inactivated by promoter hypermethylation in a cancer may be functionally relevant.

Chromosome 9q in bladder cancer is certainly an especially obstinate case, but similar problems have dogged the identification of tumor suppressors in many human cancers. It is therefore advisable to regard the identification of '*novel*' tumor suppressors with due caution.

Finally, it is quite conceivable, that the two-hit model for tumor suppressor function does not apply for each case. Indeed, for chromosome 9q in bladder cancer, '*haploinsufficiency*' is discussed, i.e. that deletion of one allele of a gene suffices to promote tumor development. Another possibility is that the predominance of larger regions of LOH may have a functional reason. Perhaps, these larger deletions or recombinations target two or more genes at once. This would then be a case of '*tumor suppressor cooperativity*'.

Molecular Alterations in Papillary Bladder Cancers

In contrast to invasive bladder cancers, papillary transitional cell carcinomas contain a limited number of chromosomal aberrations. This is particularly true for well-differentiated tumors which are usually not invasive, although clearly hyperplastic and with diminished terminal differentiaton. On average, the number of genetic changes in this tumor type increases with tumor grade.

Independent of tumor grade, however, loss of chromosome 9 is very frequent. As a result, $p16^{INK4A}$ and $p14^{ARF}$ may not be functional, and the enigmatic tumor suppressor gene at 9q could be affected. Expression of Cyclin D1 as well as MYC is usually increased. These are more likely indicators of increased cell cycle activity than its cause. In a small percentage of cases, mutations activating HRAS are detected, which could be responsible for the evident hyperproliferation. TP53 mutations are much rarer than in invasive bladder cancers and are found predominantly in high-grade tumors on the brink of becoming invasive.

Normally, urothelium is a quiescent tissue with a very low turnover. Following tissue damage, regeneration is stimulated by growth factors produced by the underlying mesenchyme, e.g. FGFs. Urothelial cells also produce autocrine factors, predominantly heparin-binding epidermal growth factor and related peptides of the EGF family. These act in normal urothelium through the EGFR which is mainly expressed in basal cells. Members of the FGF family may also regulate the thickness of the epithelial layer during development of the tissue.

Many urothelial cancers overexpress the EGFR, e.g. as a consequence of chromosome 7p gain. The strength of EGFR over-expression rather closely parallels the rate of proliferation detected by immunohistochemical markers such as the DNA replisome subunit PCNA or the protein Ki67, which is thought to be needed for increased nucleolar activity in proliferating cells. In bladder cancers, the EGFR is rarely activated by mutation.

In contrast, ≈60% of papillary urothelial cancers contain missense mutations in the FGFR3 receptor leading to its constitutive activity. The mutations in FGFR3 occur at very specific sites and appear to prolong the half-life of the receptor and of its activated state. The mutations in the FGFR3 extracellular ligand-binding domain may also alter its specificity for the >20 members of the FGF family. Mutations in FGFR3 are otherwise only found in cervical cancers. However, these and further mutations have also been encountered in hereditary achondroplasia. In this syndrome, specific point mutations in the receptor lead to shortened bones, particularly in the thighs and upper arms, because over-activity of FGFR3 causes premature differentiation of cartilage tissue in the growth zones. The same mutations in bladder cancers increase proliferation rather than differentiation of urothelial cells.

Surprisingly, bladder cancers with FGFR3 mutations have a distinctly lower risk of progression than those without. Thus, these mutations can serve as molecular markers for cancers that can be treated conservatively, i.e. solely by resection and by monitoring. In fact, the discrimination can be improved by using molecular markers associated with the opposite behavior. Mutations of TP53, which in bladder cancer can relatively reliably be detected by accumulation of mutant protein, or the proliferation index as determined by PCNA staining have been proposed.

Comparison of Bladder Cancer Subtypes

So, what distinguishes superficial papillary from advanced invasive bladder cancer? For one, genomic instability. Once it has set in, tumors may continuously generate variant clones of which some acquire the potential for invasion and metastasis. Indeed, high-grade papillary tumors, particularly those with TP53 mutations, do accumulate multiple chromosomal aberrations and have a greater potential for invasion.

A second difference may lie in the mechanisms driving tumor cell proliferation. Many papillary tumors seem to grow by mechanisms very similar to those acting during development and regeneration of normal urothelial tissues. These appear to be predominantly stimulated by EGF-like peptides and members of the FGF family. Further factors may aid to induce differentiation. These same mechanisms appear to be over-active in papillary cancers. This mode of tumor growth, however, appears to be self-limiting or at least retain checks that limit growth to the epithelial layer. It is possible that limitations on proliferation imposed by TP53 and RB1 are only partly compromised in these cancers, i.e. by loss of function of $p16^{INK4A}$ and $p14^{ARF}$, but not of TP53 and RB1 themselves.

These checks are obviously lost in invasive tumors in which growth seems to occur more independently of exogenous signals and even of endogenous signaling from the cell membrane. This is at least partly a consequence of abolition of cell cycle checkpoints by loss of RB1 and perhaps TP53. The open questions are, whether this abolition is sufficient to drive tumor progression and which mechanisms prohibit invasion in papillary tumors that proliferate as a consequence of growth factor receptor activation. Constitutive activation of the PI3K pathway and decreased responsiveness to the TGFβ pathway are good candidates for these differences. Indeed, they appear to correlate with tumor progression in bladder cancer as they do in many other carcinomas.

Finally, it is not clear at all which changes direct urothelial cells to transdifferentiate during formation of squamous cell carcinoma. So far, no qualitative differences in genetic alterations have been found that might distinguish TCC and SCC.

In spite of these open questions, it appears that a molecular classification of bladder cancers allowing improved prognosis and treatment selection for many patients may have come within reach.

10

Prostate Cancer

Prostate cancer, called more precisely '*prostate adenocarcinoma*', becomes clinically significant in up to 10% of all males in Western industrialized countries. It is rare in younger males, but its incidence increases continuously with age. The clinical course of prostate cancer is variable, ranging from clinically insignificant tumors which grow slowly over decades to aggressive cancers which spread locally and metastasize to bone and other organs, killing the patient within a few years. The detection of prostate cancer has been improved by modern imaging methods and especially by use of the biochemical serum marker *prostate specific antigen* (PSA), a moderately specific and very sensitive serum marker. Molecular markers for the classification of prostate cancers are still urgently sought.

Androgens and the *androgen receptor* (AR) have been central issues in prostate cancer research for many years and represent major targets for therapeutic intervention. Most prostate cancers respond to treatment by androgen depletion and receptor blockade, apparently by apoptosis of better differentiated tumor cells. Unfortunately, this therapy is palliative and only marginally prolongs survival, because the cancer is repleted from cells with altered responses to androgens that are refractory to anti-androgenic treatment. Several mechanisms contribute, including mutations and amplifications of the *AR* gene as well as changes in signaling pathways acting on the AR.

The incidence of clinically significant prostate cancer is vastly different between North-Western Europe and South-East Asia. This difference can be partly ascribed to the aging of the population in industrialized countries and improved detection by PSA assays. A difference remains after adjustments for age and detection rate, and points to factors in the '*Western life-style*' fostering prostate cancer. One candidate is a diet rich in saturated fat and relatively low in vitamins and micronutrients from fruit and vegetables.

Genes associated with familial prostate cancer do not behave as classical tumor suppressors. A large number of polymorphisms in genes related to hormone metabolism and action, nucleotide metabolism, and cell protection may modulate risk for prostate cancer.

Initial changes in prostate cancer are predominantly chromosome losses and other mechanisms leading to down-regulation of gene expression. In particular, silencing of several genes by promoter hypermethylation coincides with the onset of malignancy. Detection of tumor cells by hypermethylation assays therefore appears particularly promising in prostate cancer.

Tumor suppressors and oncogenes involved in other cancers such as *TP53*, *PTEN*, *MYC*, and *ERBB1* seem to be predominantly important during the progression of prostate carcinoma. Initial changes in prostate cancer appear mainly to result in decreased apoptosis and altered interactions with stromal cells.

As potential tumor suppressors in familial cases, several tumor suppressor candidates in sporadic prostate cancers do not undergo genetic alterations in their second alleles. It is therefore possible that quantitative alterations by decreased gene dosage or epigenetic inactivation rather than qualitative alterations by mutation initiate prostate cancers.

Epithelial cells in the normal prostate interact tightly with the underlying mesenchyme which supplies growth factors, partly in response to androgens. Throughout much of their development, prostate cancers seem to retain a strong dependency on stromal cells, perhaps more so than other carcinomas. Intense epithelial-mesenchymal interactions are even maintained in bone metastases, where prostate cancer cells appear to find a suitable '*soil*' for survival and growth. Here, a vicious cycle may be established, in which the cancer cells stimulate the maturation and activity of osteoblasts and osteoclasts which in turn produce growth factors that promote growth and survival of the cancer cells.

Epidemiology of Prostate Cancer

Prostate cancer develops from the glandular epithelium of the small organ which secretes most of the seminal fluid in males. Most prostate cancers can be clearly identified as adenocarcinomas. The prostate is about as big as a chestnut in younger males and almost regularly increases in size after mid-life, mostly by expansion of the mesenchymal stroma. This leads to a benign tumor, '*benign prostate hyperplasia*' (BPH). BPH is rarely life-threatening, but by compressing the urethra which passes through the prostate, it can lead to more or less severe problems in passing urine, up to the point of complete obstruction.

Prostate carcinoma is also a disease of elderly men, but often develops in parts of the organ away from the urethra and therefore does not cause urinary obstruction early on. In contrast to BPH, it is a malignant disease. Although BPH and prostate carcinoma are often found in the same organ, the carcinoma is not thought to develop from benign hyperplasia, which is rather characterized by expansion of the mesenchymal component. Precursors of the carcinoma may be dysplastic changes of the glandular ducts such as prostate inflammatory atrophy and *prostatic intraepithelial neoplasia* (PIN).

Many prostate cancers grow slowly and do not become clinically relevant in the lifetime of an older man. In autopsy studies, up to 40% of males aged over 70 years who died from other causes have been found to harbor cancerous areas in their prostate. While most prostate cancers, thus, may not be '*clinically significant*', a significant proportion grow in a more aggressive fashion, expanding locally and metastasizing to lymph nodes, bone, and other organs. Cancers confined to the organ can be cured by removal of the prostate ('*radical prostatectomy*') or radiation therapy, but metastasized prostate cancer is incurable.

In the mid of the 1990's, the public in the Western industrialized countries realized with some horror that prostate carcinoma was about to become the most lethal cancer in males. This prostate cancer '*epidemy*' turned out to have three sources.

1. Of all cancers, that of the prostate may be the one with the strongest age dependency. Prostate cancer is a rarity below the age of 50, but increases exponentially thereafter. With life expectancy increasing, the overall incidence keeps rising and the lifetime risk for clinically relevant prostate cancer is consequentially estimated as around 10%.
2. The second cause of the apparent prostate cancer boom lay in an improved detection rate. Until the late 1980s, most cases of prostate cancer were detected by the clinical symptoms they caused. Prostate cancer became evident through symptoms caused by bone metastases, more rarely by obstruction of the urethra. Some cancers can be

detected by '*digital rectal examination*'. However, even these tend to be relatively advanced. So, formerly, the typical patient presented with pain in the lower back, where metastases most often reside, and with advanced, incurable cancer. In principle, the cancer can be detected much earlier, while still confined to the prostate, by histological investigation of biopsies. This is an unpleasant and slightly risky procedure and only performed, if there is some indication for a cancer being present. A main breakthrough in prostate cancer detection was, therefore, achieved by the introduction of the serum marker PSA.

Prostate specific antigen (PSA) is a protease from the kallikrein family, which is secreted into the seminal fluid by differentiated secretory prostate epithelial cells. These are separated from the blood by a basal cell layer and a basement membrane. Since PSA is almost exclusively produced in these cells, only tiny amounts are normally present in the blood. Most prostate cancers keep producing the protein, although its processing may be altered. Through loss of polarity in the cancer tissue and breakdown of the basement membrane separating the epithelium from the underlying connective tissue and from blood vessels, more PSA appears in serum. Modern ELISAs detect <0.1 ng/ml serum, below the level in healthy middle-aged men. In the serum of prostate cancer patients, concentrations range from 2 ng/ml up to more than 1000 ng/ml.

Unfortunately, PSA as a tumor marker is neither completely specific nor perfectly sensitive. On one hand, serum PSA levels can also be increased in benign prostate diseases and they tend to rise with age. This creates a '*grey zone*'. Thus, confirmation of the diagnosis by histological investigation of biopsies remains mandatory. Newer assays for PSA exploit its altered processing and binding to serum protease inhibitors to better discriminate between benign and malignant prostatic diseases. On the other hand, some prostate carcinomas secrete little PSA and thereby escape detection.

Although PSA is not a perfect tumor marker, it is good enough to have led to a markedly improved detection rate of prostate carcinomas, even in those countries where no large-scale screening of the male population was attempted. Improved detection methods for prostate cancer were parallelled by improvements in the treatment of organ-confined cancers by surgery or radiotherapy and even of metastatic cancers by drugs or radiotherapy. This may also have contributed to earlier detection of prostate cancers by encouraging patients with minor symptoms to follow them up, because a curative therapy was available. If so, one would expect that prostate cancer incidence and mortality would peak somewhere in the late 1990s, because many cancers in years to come were already discovered and cured, which would not have been possible, had they been detected at a more advanced stage. Current preliminary figures suggest that this may indeed be so.

There are, however, two problems with this potential success story. At present, there is no method to reliably distinguish whether an early stage prostate cancer will continue to grow slowly or become aggressive. Thus, some patients identified by PSA assays would not have developed clinically relevant prostate cancer, and may have been over-treated. Conversely, the methods for detection of micrometastases are not perfect either. So, some patients are treated by prostatectomy to no avail, because they will die from metastases.

3. While the apparent prostate cancer epidemy partly reflected the age dependency of the disease and may have been inflated by improvements in its detection, a real rise could be hidden in the statistical figures. Its cause is different to extract. Some pieces of evidence link prostate cancer to '*life-style factors*' in Western industrialized countries.

The incidence of prostate cancer is very different in these countries compared to that in East Asian countries or in the Mediterranean area, and remains so after reasonable adjustments for age and detection rate. More strikingly, second generation immigrants from these countries into the USA show a prostate cancer incidence similar to average Americans. The underlying causes have been much speculated on. The immigrant studies indicate that genetic differences are unlikely to be the dominant factor. Specifically, genetic polymorphisms in hormone metabolism have been investigated, but no consistent differences have been identified. Alternatively, different exposures to estrogenic compounds in the environment have been invoked. Plant ingredients called '*phytoestrogens*' have been considered as protective, and various synthetic chemicals rather carelessly released into the environment in the 1950s and 1960s have been discussed as '*endocrine disruptors*'. Studies on these compounds continue, but are not yet conclusive.

Good evidence points to a relationship between diet and prostate cancer. Several individual food items and specifically micronutrients have been convincingly found to be associated with prostate cancer risk. A diet high in saturated fat and in dairy products seems associated with an increased risk of prostate cancer. This same diet may lack protective micronutrients, vitamins, and plant ingredients such as selenium, folate, lycopene (from tomatoes), and genisteine (from soy beans), which have each individually shown to correlate with a decreased risk of prostate cancer. Obviously, it is everything but trivial to ascertain how strong their combined effect may be. Other life-style factors may compound the influence of an unhealthy diet. For once, smoking and alcohol do not seem to be overwhelmingly important, whereas some data suggesting a relationship between prostate cancer risk and lack of exercise look intriguing.

A question for molecular biology is by which mechanisms such life-style factors might affect cancer risk. There are no definitive exogenous carcinogens known in prostate cancer, and the disease may therefore often be caused by endogenous processes. Many individual findings point to an important role of reactive oxygen species. They include an association with a high-energy diet and low selenium, which is a crucial constituent of glutathione peroxidase. Likewise, weaker genotypes of the OGG1 glycosylase, which removes oxidized guanine from DNA may predispose to prostate cancer. Indeed, the content of oxidized DNA bases in the prostate may increase with age. Moreover, the GSTP1 isoenzyme which inactivates electrophilic metabolites is down-regulated early in prostate carcinogenesis by promoter hypermethylation.

A different sort of link could be mediated by insulin-like growth factors, whose levels depend on life-style, i.e. diet and exercise, as well as on genetic constitution. In a large longitudinal study, the risk of prostate cancer correlated well with high levels of IGF1 and low levels of its inhibitory binding protein IGFBP3 in midlife.

While such findings are intriguing, it is clear that carcinogenesis in the prostate is probably multifactorial and the mechanisms are incompletely understood. Current recommendations for prevention of prostate cancer are therefore relatively unspecific.

Androgens in Prostate Cancer

The prostate gland produces part of the seminal fluid. Almost all prostate cancers arise from the glandular epithelium, which consists of a basal and a secretory layer. In the normal gland, basal cells constitute the proliferative fraction. They give rise to intermediate cells which terminally differentiate into secretory cells that line the ducts and produce prostate-specific proteins such as PSA. They turn over slowly and are continuously replaced.

The secretory cells express high levels of the *androgen receptor* (AR) and their survival and function is dependent on androgens. The cells in the basal layer contain fewer or no androgen receptors. The androgen receptor is a member of the steroid hormone receptor family and closely related to the estrogen receptors. Its AF-2 domain binds androgens in the same fashion as that of the ESRs bind estrogens.

The main androgen present throughout the body is testosterone. In the prostate, it is locally converted to dihydrotestosterone which binds to the androgen receptor with a $\approx$10-fold higher affinity. This reaction is catalyzed by 5α-reductase. The androgen receptor is also present in mesenchymal stroma cells. These are stimulated by testosterone and dihydrotestosterone to produce FGF and IGF growth factors that regulate the proliferation and survival of the epithelium, particularly of those basal cells, which lack an active androgen receptor.

During fetal development and puberty, the maturation of the gland is also dependent on androgens. Castration before puberty prevents maturation of the prostate, and also prostate cancer. In grown-up men, likewise, removal of androgens causes an involution of the gland. Such observations prompted the idea to treat prostate cancer by androgen depletion. This can be done by surgical removal of the testes in which the cells of Leydig produce >90% of the androgen in the male body. Alternatively, androgen synthesis can be suppressed by interfering with the release of the pituitary hormone LH which stimulates the production of androgens in Leydig cells. This is most commonly done by using drugs similar to GnRH which act on receptors in the hypothalamus inducing their down-regulation, as in the treatment of premenopausal ER+ breast cancers. After a short burst of LH (and FSH), no further gonadotropins are produced and the Leydig cells cease to synthesize androgens. Alternatively or concomitantly, binding of androgens to the androgen receptor can be inhibited by antiandrogens which bind to the AF-2 domain of the receptor but do not support its interaction with transcriptional co-activators.

Antiandrogenic treatment is used in the clinic in addition to surgical removal of the prostate (*prostatectomy*) or for treatment of metastases. Most cancers indeed shrink, with signs of apoptosis in tumor cells. However, unless completely removed by surgery, almost all prostate cancers recur and then respond no longer to continued antiandrogenic treatment. By and large, antiandrogenic treatment reduces the overall tumor mass, often relieving pain and other symptoms, but does not prolong survival by a large margin.

The reason for this is that growth of advanced and certainly of recurrent prostate cancers is dominated by cells that proliferate and survive relatively or completely independent of androgens. It is the subject of a long and continuing debate where these cells come from. According to opinion #1, the androgen-dependent cells in the tumor are differentiated derivatives of the actual tumor stem cells, which are related to each other in a similar fashion as basal and secretory cells in the normal tissue. Under pressure of antiandrogenic treatment, the stem cells would take over. According to opinion #2, initially all prostate cancer cells are androgen-dependent for their survival and perhaps even for their proliferation. The pressure of antiandrogenic treatment then leads to selection of cell clones which manage to grow at very low levels of androgens. These cell clones could be pre-existent in the tumor or develop during treatment. Their emergence might be faciliated by genomic instability in the cancer cells. So, even the nomenclature is debated: Advanced prostate cancers are called '*androgen-independent*' by some, but '*androgen-refractory*' or even '*androgen-hypersensitive*' by others.

Indeed, advanced prostate cancers show a bewildering variety of alterations in androgen signaling.

1. Some cancers contain amplifications of the androgen receptor gene at chromosome Xq12. These increase the AR concentration and allow responses to very low levels of testosterone.
2. Other cancers contain mutations in the AR, typically in the ligand-binding activation domain AF-2 but also in the N-terminal AF-1 domain. These mutations increase the affinity of the receptor towards androgens or augment its transcriptional activation function. Some mutations alter receptor specificity, making it responsive to other steroids in the body such as progesterone, dehydro-epiandrosterone or even anti-androgenic drugs.
3. Like other members of the steroid hormone receptor superfamily, the androgen receptor activates transcription through interactions with different co-activator proteins. Some of these show over-expression in prostate cancer, which may imply more efficient androgen signaling with lower requirements for ligand-binding.
4. Co-activators and the receptor itself are targets of phosphorylation by kinases from several signaling pathways. Androgen receptor activity becomes more dependent on such '*cross-talk*' and less on

ligand-binding in many prostate carcinomas. In these, growth factors such as TGFα or KGF (a different name for FGF7) augment androgen signaling, likely through MAPK pathways. Cytokines may also be involved, especially IL-6 and factors produced by osteoblasts and osteoclasts in bone metastases. The canonical WNT pathway can activate the androgen receptor through β-Catenin.

In some cases, other pathways may completely take over the control of proliferation and survival of prostate carcinoma cells, obliterating the requirement for the AR. Consequently, some prostate cancers lack its expression, and the *AR* promoter can become hypermethylated.

In addition, several genetic changes in advanced prostate carcinomas could relieve the requirement for androgen signaling in cell survival. These include mutations and LOH of *TP53* and loss of *PTEN*. These changes may mainly act by diminishing apoptosis. Overexpression of BCL2 is also found in a subset of prostate cancers and appears to presage a more rapid development towards androgen-refractory disease. Interestingly, BCL2 expression in the normal tissue is restricted to basal cells.

In addition, most metastatic prostate carcinomas overexpress the EGFR and MYC, not infrequently as a consequence of gene amplification. These latter changes may go along with an increased rate of proliferation in addition to diminished apoptosis completing the switch from androgen-dependent to androgen-independent growth.

Of course, proponents of opinion #1 point out that with these changes prostate carcinoma cells end up more or less where basal epithelial cells in the organ were in the first place, i.e. with cell growth and survival driven by peptide growth factors rather than androgens. So, why not assume that prostate cancers are derived from these cells? They suggest that prostate cancers initially consist of a small stem cell fraction, which '*lurks*' behind the major tumor mass consisting of more differentiated cells resembling the secretory cells of the normal prostate. Unlike their normal counterparts, however, these do not cease to proliferate. Anti-androgenic treatment acts as a palliative by diminishing this more differentiated fraction, which is, however, repleted from the '*lurker cell*' fraction.

The raging of opinions may seem academic, but in fact has important implications for the development of prostate cancer therapies. Opinion #2 predicts that better antiandrogenic treatment, which takes the possible escape routes into account, will eventually become capable of curing prostate cancer. Opinion #1 predicts that this will not work and genes and instead proteins unrelated to androgen signaling need to be targeted for a curative therapy.

Genetics and Epigenetics of Prostate Cancer

Some of the tumor suppressors and oncogenes that are so crucially involved in other common cancers, *TP53*, *PTEN*, *N MYC*, *EGFR*, and *BCL2*, contribute also to the progression of prostate cancer towards androgen-independent growth and metastasis. However, they do not appear to be responsible for the initial development of this carcinoma. Likewise, mutations or polymorphisms in these genes certainly do not account for the ≈4-fold increased risk of first-grade relatives of prostate cancer patients to develop the same disease.

In other major cancers, studies of inherited cancer syndromes have helped to identify key genes involved. In prostate cancer, this approach is complicated by several factors. (1) There are very few cases of prostate cancer at a conspicuously early age. Rather, an exponential increase sets in around the age of 50. Specifically, there is no hereditary syndrome with an obvious predisposition towards prostate cancer. (2) With a cancer that appears late in life, it is difficult to investigate several generations within one family. (3) Prostate cancer may be often multifocal, but this is difficult to ascertain as the prostate is a small organ. So, multifocality cannot be used to distinguish familial from sporadic cases. (4) Prostate cancer is so frequent that familial '*clustering*' occurs by chance with appreciable frequency.

In spite of these complications, many studies have been performed world-wide. Most have looked at families with several cases of prostate cancer, preferably with one or several at comparatively younger age, by using markers across the entire genome to search for linkage disequilibrium. Regions in the genome identified in this fashion are then more closely investigated, candidate genes are seleceted and are screened for mutations which segregate with the disease.

In the case of prostate carcinoma, roughly a dozen different regions in the genome have been implicated in different populations across the world, but few were consistent between several studies. Most likely, this means that familial clustering of prostate cancer is not caused by the action of one or a few high-risk genes. Rather, different genes may confer some degree of risk, perhaps even by interacting with environmental factors which differ between populations and individuals.

In line with this idea, the regions to which candidate hereditary prostate carcinoma genes have been assigned are not those most frequently undergoing LOH in the cancers. Also in accord with this idea, a gene identified in the top candidate region at 1q24, named *HPC1* (hereditary prostate cancer 1), turned out to encode RNaseL, which is involved in regulating cellular responses to infectious agents. Inactivating mutations and certain polymorphisms in this gene appear to go along with an increased risk of prostate cancer. There is little evidence that the gene is a target for '*second hits*' in prostate cancer tissue. So, it is probably not a classical tumor suppressor gene.

It is, of course, conceivable that how individuals react to infections in the prostate influences their risk to develop a cancer in this organ, as evidenced by the etiology of liver and stomach cancers. However, at this stage, the precise relationship between *HPC1* and prostate cancer is unclear. For several other genes involved in hormone metabolism, DNA repair and nucleotide metabolism, a relationship between polymorphic variants and prostate cancer risk has been observed. Perhaps, the *HPC* genes are susceptibility genes with a particularly strong influence.

A second useful approach to identifying key genes in human cancers is following up on recurrent chromosomal changes. Indeed, chromosomes 17p and 10q, where the *TP53* and *PTEN* genes are located, often undergo loss in advanced prostate cancers, whereas segments of the chromosomes 7 and 8q, where the *ERBB1* (EGFR) and *MYC* genes reside, are gained or even amplified. In earlier stages of prostate carcinoma, chromosomal losses predominate. The most frequent chromosomal change overall is loss of chromosome 8p, with losses of 13q, 6q, and 16q being relatively prevalent. Mapping of common region of deletion has yielded several regions and various candidate tumor suppressors, but their role is not fully established. The problems encountered are similar to those in the case of the tumor suppressor locus suspected at 9q in bladder cancer.

The most convincing candidate is *NKX3.1* (also *NKX3A*) encoding a transcription factor with a homeobox domain. NKX3.1 is largely specific to prostate epithelial cells, is induced by androgens, and is very likely necessary for the proper differentiation of prostate epithelium. Knockout mice engineered to lack the factor fail to develop a functional prostate and hemizygous mice display hyperproliferation of the prostate epithelium. In these respects, *NKX3.1* is as good a tumor suppressor candidate as they come. The problem prohibiting its general acceptance as a tumor suppressor is that in most prostate cancers, including those with LOH or outright deletion of 8p, at least one allele of the gene remains functional and is often expressed at close to expected levels (i.e. 50% of normal). To accept *NKX3.1* as a tumor suppressor, one would have to postulate that diminuation of its expression to half the normal level suffices to inactivate its function. Such '*haploinsufficiency*' has also been postulated for other genes, but is, of course, very difficult to prove in the context of a real human cancer. This is particularly so for prostate carcinoma, which is thought to be unusually heterogeneous and to always contain substantial amounts of stroma. Therefore, the suspicion lingers that the crucial changes in a gene might have escaped detection for technical reasons.

The same sort of problem concerns other established or novel tumor suppressors in prostate cancers. So, *PTEN* is clearly inactivated in some prostate carcinomas by loss of one allele and mutation of the second one; even homozygous deletions have been observed. Nevertheless, in many prostate carcinomas, the gene is intact, but strongly down-regulated. It is possible that loss of one *PTEN* allele suffices to promote tumor progression in the prostate, while complete loss of function is a characteristic of very advanced cancers.

Similarly, *RB1* is located at 13q14 telomeric to a region that undergoes LOH and net loss in many prostate cancers, but the remaining *RB1* copy is intact, although its expression level is debated. So, perhaps, the '*classical*' concept of tumor suppressors demanding inactivation of both alleles may not apply in prostate carcinomas. There are indeed '*heretical*' concepts which attempt to explain cancer development by the overall changes in relative copy numbers, without an absolute requirement for mutational events. Perhaps they may be helpful to understand prostate cancer.

While these ideas are speculative, it is clear that epigenetic mechanisms are very important in prostate cancers and could account for some of the unexpected findings at the genetic level. Specifically, alterations of DNA methylation are unusually prevalent in prostate cancer. One of the most consistent alteration in prostate cancer is inactivation of the *GSTP1* gene encoding an enzyme protective against electrophilic compounds from exogenous and endogenous sources. Loss of expression occurs very early during cancer development and may help to sensitize the tumor cells to further genomic damage. Loss of GSTP1 is almost always caused by epigenetic mechanisms and usually accompanied by dense hypermethylation of the gene promoter. More than a dozen genes have now been reported to become hypermethylated in prostate cancer at significant frequencies. Several appear to become coordinately hypermethylated by a sort of '*epigenetic catastrophe*' at around the stage of initiation of the carcinoma, perhaps even in advanced prostate intraepithelial neoplasia. Other genes, including those encoding cell adhesion molecules like E-Cadherin and CD44 become hypermethylated later, and still others, including *PTEN*, seem to be down-regulated by epigenetic mechanisms without becoming hypermethylated.

These observations carry interesting prospects for diagnostics and therapy of prostate cancer. Hypermethylation of CpG islands, as in the *GSTP1* gene, can be comparatively easy detected with high sensitivity and specificity, since CpG islands are unmethylated in normal tissues. So, detection of *GSTP1* hypermethylation, and that of additional genes, is being developed to assay for the presence of prostate carcinoma. Also, since epigenetic gene inactivation is, in principle, reversible, prostate cancer may be a particularly good target for inhibitors of histone deacetylases, histone methylases, and DNA methyltransferases currently under development. In cell and animal models of prostate cancer at least, such compounds are efficacious, usually by induction of apoptosis.

Tumor-stroma Interactions in Prostate Cancer

In normal prostate tissue, proliferation and survival of epithelial cells are controlled by growth factors and matrix proteins supplied by the mesenchymal cells which surround the glands as well as on nutrients and oxygen supplied via blood vessels in the mesenchyme. The tissue structure of the prostate, like that of other organs, is dependent on mutual interactions between epithelial and stromal cells. As prostate cancers progress, these relationships change, most dramatically in metastases. In general, tumor progression is associated with increased growth autonomy. In some cancers, this growth autonomy is established by mutations in cell cycle regulators or by inappropriate activation of cancer pathways that control the cell cycle. In many cancers, including prostate cancers, autocrine growth factor loops contribute to growth autonomy. To various extents, however, all cancers remain dependent on interactions with stroma, and this relationship is particularly crucial during metastasis. In this respect, prostate cancer may be near one end of a spectrum, as a cancer which retains intense interactions with stromal cells at the primary site as well as in metastases. However, these relationships are really a caricature of those in the normal tissue, because they are distorted by genetic and epigenetic changes in the carcinoma cells, as well as in the stroma.

In the normal prostate, epithelial cells proliferate under the influence of growth factors such as FGFs and EGF-related peptides.

Receptors for these factors are present mainly at the basal surface of the basal cell layer of the epithelium. The insulin-like growth factor IGF1 may act as a survival factor through the IGFRI receptor. The IGF binding protein IGFBP3 may limit the action of IGF1. Luminal secretory cells appear to additionally require androgens for their survival.

Further negative regulator of epithelial cell proliferation are TGFβ factors produced at low levels by the epithelial cells themselves. These levels may be sufficient to support a low level of proliferation of mesenchymal cells necessary for maintenance of the tissue.

Another paracrine factor is the 21 amino acid peptide endothelin-1 (ET-1) which is mainly secreted into the seminal fluid by the secretory epithelial cells, but may also act on the normal prostate mesenchyme. Cells in the prostate stroma express the endothelin receptor A (ETA), which is a G-coupled receptor. It uses Ca^{2+} as a second messenger and is capable of cross-talk with receptor tyrosine kinases. Therefore, endothelin and similar peptides can act synergistically with EGF-like growth factors. Normal prostate epithelial cells, however, do not express the ETA, but rather a scavenger receptor, ETB, which binds and removes ET-1.

This orderly organization changes during carcinogenesis. Prostate carcinoma cells synthesize FGFs, particularly FGF1 and FGF2, and EGF-like factors, particularly TGFα. Receptors for FGFs and for EGF-like factors become more strongly expressed and are no longer restricted to basal cells, but are expressed throughout the cancerous epithelium. Insulin-like factors are produced at an increased rate, likely by both carcinoma and stroma. Specifically, IGF2 levels increase. Conversely, IGFBP3 becomes down-regulated at the transcriptional level and by proteolytic cleavage of the secreted protein. Together, these alterations support increased and autonomous proliferation and survival of the carcinoma cells. FGFs, in particular, also stimulate the proliferation of stromal cells and FGF2 is one of the most potent angiogenic factors.

Somewhat paradoxically, the synthesis of TGFβ factors increases in prostate carcinoma. However, the receptor subunits, specifically TGFβRII, are down-regulated in carcinoma cells. Therefore, the growth-inhibitory effects on carcinoma cells are diminished, while the proliferation of stromal cells is stimulated. Specifically, TGFβ induces remodeling of the extracellular matrix which is necessary for invasion and angiogenesis. Moreover, particularly at later stages of invasion, the immunosuppressive effects of TGFβ may be relevant.

Endothelin production is maintained in prostate carcinoma cells. However, compared to normal prostate epithelial cells, ETA is up-regulated and ETB is down-regulated. So, ET-1 now acts on both epithelial and stromal cells. At some stage of local tumor growth, an HGF/MET autocrine loop is established, as in many other carcinomas. In prostate cancers, the expression of both HGF and MET appears to increase gradually. It may be initiated by hypoxia. Activation of MET, more than that of other tyrosine receptor kinases, induces scattering of proliferating epithelial cells and a tendency to change their shape towards a mesenchymal cell type. Indeed, a switch of cadherin types may take place during prostate cancer invasion which is typically associated with an epithelial-mesenchymal transition. This means that some of the apparent stromal cells in a malignant prostate tumor may in fact be cancer cells. However, prostate cancer metastases typically consist of epithelial cells, which often express E-Cadherin. So, this transition may be transient or may concern only a fraction of the carcinoma cells.

Hypoxia also induces expression of VEGF which synergizes with FGFs and ET-1 to induce angiogenesis. Indeed, an increase in microvessel density and local blood flow is a diagnostic sign of prostate cancers. Finally, tumor invasion requires an increased expression of proteases which remodel the tissue, aid in tumor cell migration, and liberate latent growth factors from cell surfaces and the extracellular matrix. Many such proteases, especially matrix metalloproteinases (MMPs) are produced by stromal cells activated by the carcinoma cells. In the prostate, the carcinoma cells contribute uPA and, of course, kallikrein proteases like PSA. PSA is only one of several proteases of this class secreted into the seminal fluid, and is systematically designated as hK3. So, hK3 and other members of the family are secreted and activated in prostate carcinoma tissue.

Together, these changes prepare the way for prostate cancer cells to eventually grow beyond the organ and spread through lymph and blood vessels to other parts of the body. Lymph node metastases are usually the first to become established. The most frequent site for hematogenic metastases are bones where prostate cancer cells extravasate in their capillary-rich interior. Bones in the spine are the prime target, due to anatomy. However, anatomy is not sufficient to explain the pronounced preference of prostate cancer metastasis for bone tissue. Instead, this affinity is a case in point for the '*seed-and-soil*' hypothesis.

Bone metastases can be osteolytic or osteoblastic. In osteolytic metastases, the dominating effect of the tumor is dissolution of the bone, whereas in osteoblastic metastases, the dominating effect is stimulation of bone formation. Throughout life, bone is constantly being rebuilt by the combined action of osteoblast cells which deposit trabeculi of calcium apatite and osteoclasts which remove them. Tumor cells in the bone interact with these cells stimulating either cell type or both. Prostate cancer metastases are predominantly osteoblastic.

In bone tissue, prostate carcinoma cells establish a vicious cycle, predominantly with osteoblasts. Autocrine stimulation by FGFs and EGF-like growth factors remains important. Angiogenesis is also promoted in the metastatic tissue by FGFs and VEGF. However, the crucial property that allows prostate carcinoma cells to establish metastases in bones is their adaptation to the tissue by interaction with specific local cell populations, to the point of cellular mimicry. So, metastatic prostate carcinoma cells in bone behave in an '*osteomimetic*' fashion.

Prostate carcinoma cells secrete TGFβ factors and ET-1, which stimulate the proliferation and maturation of osteoblasts. They also secrete bone morphogenetic proteins (BMPs) acting on these cells. BMPs use similar intracellular pathways for signalling as TGFβ, but have distinct receptors. While prostate cancer cells lose their responsiveness to TGFβ, they retain responses to BMPs. So, prostate carcinoma cells in the bone resemble osteoblasts by responding to BMPs and ET-1, thriving in the same microenvironment.

Secretion of proteases by carcinoma cells remains important in bone metastases. Specifically, uPA and kallikrein proteases liberate latent growth factors and allow expansion of the tumor mass. In addition, the protease cleave and inactivate the parathyroid-hormone related peptide (PTHrP). As this is an important growth factor for osteoclasts, its inactivation may be the decisive step that tilts the balance between bone resorption and bone synthesis towards an osteoblastic phenotype. Breast cancer also often metastasizes to bone, but the metastases are more often osteoclastic than osteoblastic. This may be due to secretion of PTHrP by these cancer cells.

In prostate cancer metastases, both osteoclasts and osteoblasts remain active, since activated osteoblasts secrete factors that stimulate the proliferation and maturation of osteoclast precursors, especially the RANK-L protein. The overall effect therefore is an increased turnover, perhaps with osteoclasts allowing the spread of the cancer and liberating factors such as IGF1 which support the cancer cells. These, then, follow, stimulating osteoblasts to produce new bone mineral with a net increase in disorganized bone mass. Systemically, hypocalcemia may develop. Locally, pain ensues.

All these are major problems in patients with advanced prostate cancer, exacerbated by the effects of locally recurrent cancers and metastases in other organs, e.g. the lung. In urine and serum, biochemical markers of increased bone turnover can be detected. These were used to diagnose prostate before the PSA era in patients that accordingly had invariably cancers at an advanced stage and may now be useful to detect metastases. The progression of bone metastases can be slowed and many symptoms can be alleviated by '*bisphosphonates*', drugs interfering with bone resorption, or by local irradiation. However, the overall process is too robust to be cured by present therapies.

Prostate carcinoma metastases in bone exemplify how successful establishment of metastases depends on adequate interactions at multiple levels between cancer cells and the tissue at the metastatic site. Breast cancers exhibit a similar preference for bone metastases, but establish a different assortment of interactions. Of course, still other interactions are required for metastasis to tissues such as the liver, lung, and brain which are preferred localizations of metastases in other cancers. Which interactions precisely are involved, is to date poorly understood.

11

BREAST CANCER

Carcinoma of the breast is a major lethal cancer in females in the Western world, on a par with lung and colon cancer. Most cases occur in postmenopausal women, but a significant number of younger women are afflicted, often in families with a hereditary predisposition. Known risk factors include the length of the life-time exposure to estrogens, ionizing radiation, cigarette smoking, and a high-fat diet.

Between 10% and 20% of breast cancer cases are ascribed to hereditary factors. Inherited mutations inactivating the *BRCA1* and *BRCA2* genes lead to an up to 80% life-time risk of breast and/or ovarian cancers. Breast cancers also occur at an increased frequency in rarer dominantly inherited cancer syndromes including Li-Fraumeni or Cowden disease, affecting *TP53* and *PTEN*, respectively.

In addition to high-risk mutations in some families, prevalent genetic polymorphisms that confer smaller risk increments to individual women are thought to be significant in the overall population. Examples are variants of genes encoding steroid metabolizing enzymes and certain heterozygous mutations in the *ATM* DNA repair gene.

The genes *BRCA1* at 17q21 and *BRCA2* at 13q12 encode proteins involved in DNA repair and the control of genomic integrity. They behave as classical tumor suppressors of the '*caretaker*' class in many familial cases of breast cancer, with one defective copy inherited and the second copy inactivated by mutation, recombination, deletion or epigenetic inactivation in the tumors. Cancers in BRCA families tend to occur at an earlier age and are more often bilateral. Inactivation of either gene is infrequent in sporadic breast cancers. Since the *BRCA* genes are expressed and function ubiquitously, it is not clear why they predispose mainly to breast and ovarian cancer. Since mutations in these genes are comparatively prevalent, counseling, monitoring and prevention of cancer in potentially affected women are being actively developed, albeit not without controversies.

Estrogens and progesterone are important factors in the development of breast cancer. Approximately 70% of all breast cancers retain the estrogen receptor α (ERα, encoded by *ESR1*) and the progesterone receptor (PR). A second, distinct estrogen receptor β (ERβ encoded by *ESR2*) is often lost. In the other cases, ERα and PR are down-regulated, usually by epigenetic mechanisms including promoter hypermethylation.

Like normal breast tissue, many breast cancers remain dependent on estrogens and gestagens for growth and survival and therefore respond to hormone depletion. Hormone depletion in premenopausal women is achieved by surgical removal of the ovaries. In addition, and generally in postmenopausal women drugs are used which inactivate the estrogen receptor. These act in a tissue-specific manner, with different degrees of side-effects on other organs such as the uterus, the cardiovascular system, and bone. The selective effect of such 'SERMs' (*selective estrogen receptor modulators*) is mediated by interactions with co-activators and co-repressors expressed in a tissue-specific fashion. SERMs like tamoxifen appear also to be useful in the prevention of breast cancer in women at high risk.

A subset of breast cancers, which are on average more aggressive, do not express estrogen receptors. In many of these, and even in some cancers expressing the ESRs, tumor growth seems to be driven predominantly through receptor tyrosine kinases of the ERBB family. Gene amplification and over-expression of ERBB2, which forms heterodimers with ERBB1 or ERBB3, is prevalent in this group. Accordingly, specific inhibitors of this protein and the specific monoclonal antibody trastuzumab, marketed under the name '*herceptin*', are used in selected patients with ERBB2 overexpression, with some success.

The established classification of breast carcinoma, e.g. with respect to steroid hormone receptor status and other molecular markers, is being further refined by gene expression profiling. This method has substantiated presumptions that breast cancers fall into several classes. These may partly reflect their respective cell of origin. Moreover, subgroups with different prognosis and responses to therapy, and specific patterns in patients from families with *BRCA* mutations may be discernible. An individualization of treatment, which is aspired in many major cancers, may therefore be within reach in breast cancer.

BREAST BIOLOGY

In adult humans, structures like the epidermis and the colon mucosa undergo a constant turnover, whereas others like the liver parenchyma and urothelium only proliferate significantly for the purpose of repair after damage. Breast tissue is different from all of these.

First of all, the organ does not develop fully before puberty, so there is one additional growth phase during the second decade of life. During puberty, the immature ducts elongate into the surrounding connective tissue to form 15-20 lobuli. This process involves multiplication of the ductal cells and an expansion of its stem cell population. The connective tissue in the breast likewise expands.

Then, for a period of up to 45 years, the ductular tissue undergoes regular monthly cycles of proliferation and apoptosis. In some women as many as 500 cycles take place, before cessation of ovulation and estrogen production in the ovaries induces menopause.

This regular cycling is interrupted by pregnancies during which the ducts extend further into the underlying connective tissue, where they branch and widen into alveoli. Concomitantly, the secretory cells differentiate and the ducts mature. After parturation, the gland produces substantial amounts of carbohydrates, fat and proteins secreted in the milk, potentially over several years. The secreted proteins provide nutrients, but also include growth factors and immunoprotective proteins. Weaning induces a partial involution of the gland, again accompanied by apoptosis of glandular cells, particularly the luminal secretory cells in the alveoli. Once again, the tissue, epithelia and stroma alike, is remodeled.

These cycles are controlled by a combination of hormones and locally produced growth factors. The pubertal growth phase is stimulated by estrogens from the ovaries, which become active at this time, and by growth hormone and its '*somatomedin*' mediators IGF1 and IGF2. The monthly cycles are controlled mainly by estradiol and progesterone, supported by insulin and further hormones. During the first phase of the monthly cycle, follicle cells secrete mostly estrogens. After release of the oocyte gestagens like progesterone are the major product. Unless fertilization takes place, the follicle degenerates and minimal estrogen and progesterone levels elicit an involution phase in the breast and, more pronounced, in the uterus endometrium. The pregnancy growth phase is stimulated by several hormones, including gestagens, estrogens, growth hormone and insulin, but also glucocorticoids and, of course, prolactin. As in other tissues, proliferation of epithelial cells in the breast is supported by the stroma. Stromal cells and epithelial cells both produce paracrine growth factors, partly in response to steroid hormones.

Estrogens represented by estradiol and gestagens represented by progesterone act on cells by binding to specific receptors which belong to the steroid hormone receptor superfamily. The superfamily encompasses a large number of DNA-binding proteins with a variety of ligands, e.g. the retinoic acid receptors. The estrogen receptors and the progesterone receptors belong to a group of more closely related receptors which also includes the androgen receptor. The members of this group are ligand-dependent transcription factors that bind as homodimers to specific symmetric binding sites on DNA. These are termed ERE (*estrogen-responsive element*), PRE (*progesterone-responsive element*), ARE (*androgen-responsive element*), etc.

The *estrogen receptor* α (ERα) is a typical representative. Its DNA-binding domain, which contains two zinc fingers, is located at the center of the primary amino acid sequence. It is flanked on the N-terminal side by a transactivation domain, designated as activation function 1, AF-1. A hinge region on its C-terminal side connects a second transactivation domain, named AF-2. The AF-2 domain binds the ligand and its activity is strongly dependent on ligand-binding. Moreover, protein interactions exerted by this domain control the receptor activity overall.

Inactive receptors are retained in the cytosol and become capable of entering the nucleus only after binding of the ligand and an ensuing conformation change. Some receptors are bound by heat shock proteins like HSP90, others are free, but are shuttled rapidly out of the nucleus, unless occupied by an agonistic ligand. After binding to their specific recognition sites on DNA, the receptor dimers recruit various co-activator proteins through their AF domains. The AF-2 domain of the ERα is known to bind at least five different co-activator proteins specifically. The best characterized of these is the SRC1 (*steroid receptor co-activator*) protein. Co-activators mediate the interaction between steroid hormone receptors and the general transcription apparatus and the modification of chromatin at the binding site. Binding of co-activators stimulates histone acetylation and the actual initiation of transcription. In addition, they integrate signals from several transcription factors binding to the regulatory regions of the same gene and from signal transduction pathways. For instance, certain co-activators interacting with the estrogen or androgen receptors are regulated by MAPK phosphorylation in response to growth factors of the EGF family. The receptor itself is also phosphorylated. While interactions with co-activators lead to gene activation, interactions with co-repressors can cause gene repression. Repression can be exerted by the ERα, but more pronounced by the progesterone receptor α.

A second mechanism of ERα action does not require binding of the receptor to DNA. Steroid hormone receptors can interact with several other transcription factors, either sequestering them or modulating their activity while they are bound to DNA. In this fashion, the receptors can regulate the activity of genes that do not possess canonical receptor binding sites. Specifically, the ERα can modulate the activity of AP1 transcription factors. This may be the main mechanism by which estrogens stimulate cell proliferation, i.e. by mimicking activation of MAPK pathways alone or synergistically with growth factors. Additionally, estrogens stimulate the production of EGF-like growth factors in breast tissue.

The regulation of breast tissue growth and function by estrogens is in reality more complex. Estrogen receptors can also influence gene activity through SP1 and NFκB sites by direct and indirect interactions. Moreover, ERα activity is modulated by protein-protein interactions with Cyclin D1 and, intriguingly, with BRCA1. In addition, estrogens – like several other steroid hormones – elicit very rapid effects at the cell membrane which may not be exerted through their canonical receptors, but through direct activation of ion channels. Most importantly, estrogens act on several different cell types in breast tissue, both epithelial and stromal.

There are two different estrogen receptors in man, estrogen receptor α and estrogen receptor β, which are encoded by two distinct genes, *ESR1* and *ESR2*. They exhibit only 30% homology overall, but almost identical DNA-binding domains, both recognizing the 'ERE' sequence AGGTCA NNN TGACCT. ERα mediates most of the proliferative effects in female reproductive tissues. In contrast, ERβ appears to act mostly as an inhibitor of ERα action, and perhaps even of the androgen receptor in males. The two estrogen receptors are expressed in different patterns throughout the human body.

Different subunits of the progesterone receptor (PRA and PRB) are translated from differently spliced mRNAs from the same gene. They can bind interchangably as homodimers or heterodimers. Expression of the PR is induced by ERα. PRA (also called PRα), in particular, appears to act as a feedback inhibitor of ERα. However, it is important to realize that PR action is dependent on gestagens, so its actual effect depends on the relative levels of gestagens.

Even more importantly, while estrogen receptors and progesterone receptors are present in many organs of the female (and even male), the effects of estrogens and gestagens are not the same in each tissue. Estrogens affect e.g. the brain and bone, but they do not stimulate proliferation in these tissues as in breast and endometrium. Even the effects of estrogens on breast and endometrium differ (like those of gestagens). Therefore, since many organs contain receptors, additional mechanisms ensure the tissue specificity of estrogen action.

One possible mechanism is differential expression of the two estrogen receptors. A second mechanism is provided by different expression patterns of co-activators, co-repressors and differences in their regulation. As a consequence, certain compounds with structural similarities to estrogens act as partial antagonists that inhibit estrogen activity to a different extent in different organs.

These are designated SERMs, for '*selective estrogen receptor modulators*'. Tamoxifen and raloxifene are examples of compounds in this class. Tamoxifen, e.g., blocks the stimulation of proliferation by estrogens in the breast, acting as an antagonist, but in the endometrium it rather behaves as an agonist, supporting proliferation. This difference may largely be caused by higher levels of the co-activator SRC1 in the endometrium, which is recruited by the tamoxifen-ERα holocomplex. In contrast, in breast tissue, this complex overwhelmingly recruits co-repressors.

Etiology of Breast Cancer

With colon cancer and increasingly lung cancer, breast cancer constitutes the trias of major cancers in females in Western industrialized countries. In these countries, the life-time risk of breast cancer is around 10% for women, and about 30% of them turn out to be lethal. Most breast cancers become apparent in women after their menopause, but a significant fraction is diagnosed earlier. In Western countries, the mean age at menopause is now ≈50 yrs, and menopause takes place in almost all women between 45 and 55. In females aged 40-60 years, breast cancer is the most frequent lethal cancer. In most countries, its incidence is rising, although the increase in mortality has been checked. There are several explanations for this phenomenon, invoking earlier detection and better treatment. In any case, it is generally agreed that certain aspects of the Western life style favor the development of breast cancer.

Table 11.1. Potential causes of human breast cancer

Potential factors causing breast cancer in humans
Length of exposure to estrogens
Ionizing radiation
Genetic predisposition (*BRCA1, BRCA2, others*)
Sedentary life style
High-fat diet
Alcohol
Tobacco smoking

Estrogen Exposure

One risk factor can be summarized as the life-time length of exposure to estrogens. Earlier menarche, later menopause, and fewer (as well as later) pregnancies associated with the Western life-style all lengthen this period. Each change singly is associated with an increased risk of breast cancer. The underlying mechanism could be simply probabilistic. With prolonged exposure to estrogen and a longer period of proliferation cycles, the number of cells that can contract mutations is increased and initiated tumor cells get more time to expand. Specifically, strong signals enforce differentiation of breast ductal cells during pregnancy and others elicit extensive apoptosis of alveolar and ductal cells after weaning. These cycles may help to remove initiated tumor cells and act to '*purify*' the tissue. Accordingly, a strong preventive effect is exerted by multiple pregnancies early in life with extended nursing periods.

A second, albeit not mutually exclusive explanation for the effect of estrogen exposure relates to the chemical structure of estrogens. Estrogens and their metabolites are phenolic compounds, after all. In particular, diphenolic estrogen metabolites can become partially oxidized to semiquinones which can react with macromolecules in the cell including DNA and induce mutations.

Semiquinones can, moreover, initiate a process called quinone redox cycling that produces highly reactive oxygen species. So, estrogens may act as chemical carcinogens. If so, the risk of cancers in organs with high estrogen concentrations may strongly depend on the individual ability to metabolize estrogens and to deal with quinone adducts to DNA and redox cycling. Many genes involved in estrogen biosynthesis and metabolism are polymorphic, as are some of the relevant protective enzymes. An interaction between genes and environment is therefore strongly suspected.

Exposure to Ionizing Radiation

Here, too, gene-environment interactions are suspected. They are particularly clear in the case of inherited defects in the repair of DNA damage caused by ionizing radiation. For instance, certain carriers of mutations in the *ATM* gene may be at increased risk for breast cancer. The relationship between exposure to radiation and breast cancer risk becomes specifically relevant, when discussing prevention of breast cancer mortality by early detection. There are concerns that population screening by frequent mammography might put susceptible individuals at increased risk.

High-fat Diet

The breast cancer incidence in a country is clearly correlated to the content of fat, particularly of saturated animal fats, in the diet. The biological mechanisms that underlie this epidemiologically clear-cut correlation are not really understood. One hypothetical chain of events also invokes estrogens. The adipose tissue of postmenopausal women contains aromatase, a key biosynthetic enzyme for estrogens. So, high-fat diets may lead to overweight with expansion of adipose tissue leading to increased aromatase activity leading to continued production of estrogens after menopause with inappropriate growth stimulation of breast epithelial cells.

Genetic Predisposition

The effects of all of the above factors may be dependent on genetic polymorphisms which modulate cancer risk in interaction with environmental factors. Polymorphisms in genes of steroid hormone metabolism, DNA repair, cell protection, and lipid metabolism, e.g. could all be relevant. While these polymorphisms may exert large effects on the overall incidence of breast cancer, they increase the risk only slightly for each individual woman and they are strongly dependent on other, notably environmental factors. In contrast, genetic factors predominate in the smaller fraction of (typically familial) cases that are caused by inherited mutations in one of a limited number of high-risk genes.

Hereditary Breast Cancer

At least seven genes are now known, in which inherited mutations in one allele conduce a high risk of breast cancer. Mutations in most tumor suppressor genes account for a small proportion of all familial cases, certainly less than 10%, while a larger fraction of familial breast cancers originates from mutations inactivating the *BRCA1* and *BRCA2* tumor suppressor genes.

The *PTEN* gene at 10q23.3 encodes a phospholipid and protein phosphatase which controls the activity of the PI3K pathway. It is mutated in Cowden syndrome. This rare dominantly inherited disease is characterized by multiple benign hamartomas and by thyroid cancers, but also includes an increased risk for breast cancer.

Table 11.2. Tumor suppressor genes implicated in hereditary breast cancer

Gene	*Location*	*Function*	*Other cancer sites*
BRCA1	17q21	DNA repair/control of homologous recombination	Ovary
BRCA2	13q12	DNA repair/control of homologous recombination pathway	Ovary
PTEN	10q23.1	lipid phosphatase/ regulation of PIK pathway	Several
TP53	17p13.1	Control of genomic integrity and DNA repair	Many
MLH1, MSH	3p21, 2p15-16	DNA mismatch repair	Several
LKB1	19p13.3	Mitotic control	Intestine

Mutations in the *TP53* gene are the cause of most cases of the rare Li-Fraumeni syndrome. In line with the general importance of the TP53 protein in the control of genomic stability, this is a generalized cancer syndrome which also includes a particularly high risk for breast cancer. A minority of cases might be caused by mutations in genes encoding the checkpoint kinases CHK1 and CHK2.

The more frequent HNPCC syndrome caused by mutations in DNA mismatch repair genes likewise leads to an increased incidence of various cancers, predominantly in the colon and rectum. Inherited mutations in the *MLH1* and *MSH2* genes have also been found in breast cancer patients.

Rare mutations in the *LKB1* gene, encoding a serine/threonine kinase that regulates mitosis, likewise cause predominantly cancers of the intestine and colon, but also increase the risk of breast cancer.

Up to 50% of familial breast cancers in some populations may be caused by germ-line mutations in the *BRCA1* and *BRCA2* tumor suppressor genes. These mutations predispose almost exclusively to cancers of the breast and of the ovaries, unlike many of those mentioned above. Notably, *BRCA1* and *BRCA2* are considered as '*caretakers*' like almost all other tumor suppressor genes in which mutations lead to a strongly increased risk of breast cancer. The obvious exception is *PTEN*.

BRCA1 and *BRCA2* have actually been named for their role in breast cancer, but they indeed exhibit further similarities.

BRCA1 is a ≈100 kb gene at chromosome 17q21 comprising 24 exons. Exon 11 of the gene is unusually large extending over >4.5 kb and accordingly contains a large part of the coding sequence. The BRCA1 protein consists of 1863 amino acids. Several centrally located nuclear localisation signal sequences identify it as a nuclear protein. There are several protein-protein interaction domains, including a RING-finger domain near the N-terminus. Near the C-terminus are two copies of a 110 amino acid sequence called BRCT motif. This motif was also detected in several other proteins involved in DNA repair and/or cell cycle regulation. BRCA1 also has a transcriptional activation function, unlike BRCA2.

The *BRCA2* gene is located at 13q12 and extends across ≈80 kb. Among 27 exons overall, exon 10 and 11 are – again – unusually large. The BRCA protein comprises 3418 amino acids. Nuclear localization signals are located C-terminally. Multiple protein interactions are supposed or documented. Most importantly, the central part of the molecule contains eight repeats of 'BRC' motifs, each consisting of ≈40 amino acids.

Germ-line mutations in both *BRCA* genes are spread out along almost the entire length of the genes. Most are small deletions or insertions resulting in frame-shift mutations. Nonsense mutations leading to truncated proteins are also prevalent. Splice-site mutations also occur as well as rare missense mutations. In each case, the mutations would be expected to inactivate the function of the proteins or – in some cases – perhaps to exhibit a dominant-negative phenotype.

In breast cancers arising in women with inherited mutations in a *BRCA* gene, the second allele is consistently inactivated as well, by deletion, recombination or point mutation. In this regard, therefore, *BRCA1* and *BRCA2* behave as classical tumor suppressor genes. However, mutations or deletions in these genes are almost never found in sporadic breast cancers. Instead, decreased levels of the proteins are often observed, which in some cases are associated with increased methylation of *BRCA1* regulatory sequences. In this respect, therefore, the BRCAs do not follow the standard scheme for tumor suppressors.

The BRCA1 and BRCA2 proteins are expressed in almost all tissues. They are important for DNA repair, prevention of chromosome breaks and checkpoint signaling. BRCA1 and BRCA2 have different, but related functions. Lack of either protein causes an increase in chromosomal aberrations in proliferating cells, including deletions and translocations, but even fragmentation and formation of multiradial chromosomes. All these aberrations are found in breast cancers with BRCA mutations. They are primarily due to a deficit in homologous recombination repair and secondarily to a failure to activate appropriate cellular checkpoints. Homologous recombination repair is the preferred mechanism for dealing with DNA double strand breaks during the S and G2 phase of the cell cycle in mammalian cells, when homologous DNA strands from sister chromatids are available. In contrast, non-homologous end-joining predominates during G1. This mechanism introduces a larger number of errors than homologous repair at the mended site, including small deletions and insertions. However, these errors do not seem to constitute the major problem in BRCA-deficient cells. Rather, non-homologous end-joining on its own appears insufficient to ensure chromosomal integrity.

The main function of BRCA2 in this regard appears to be control of RAD51. BRCA2 binds and inhibits RAD51 through its BRC repeats, keeping it from binding to DNA as a multiprotein filament. During homologous recombination repair, double-strand breaks must first be processed. Then, RAD51 is released from BRCA2, likely as a result of BRCA2 being phosphorylated, and mediates recombination between the strands that are to be repaired and the intact homologous double helix. This is followed by extension of the single strands by a DNA polymerase, ligation and resolution of the recombinant Holliday junction structure. At a later stage of this resolution, RAD51 is removed, apparently by reloading onto BRCA2. BRCA2 interacts with activated FANCD2 protein. This is activated via mono-ubiquitination by the FANC protein complex. It then moves to foci in the nucleus where BRCA2, RAD51 and the MRE11/RAD50/NBS1 (MRN) proteins reside and activates these. Homozygous germ-line mutations in *BRCA2* cause a form of Fanconi anemia and, conversely, breast cancer incidence is enhanced in this recessive cancer syndrome.

BRCA1 appears to have a still wider range of functions. In response to DNA double-strand breaks, it is phosphorylated by kinases sensing this damage, such as ATM, ATR or CHK2. It may also be activated by other types of DNA damage, since it interacts e.g. with the MSH2 and MSH6 proteins involved in mismatch repair, and perhaps also with the transcription-coupled nucleotide excision repair system. Following its activation BRCA1 mediates selected transcriptional responses, such as induction of the GADD45 repair protein, and at the site of damage aids in chromatin remodeling. A crucial function is regulation of the MRN protein complex that resects the DNA ends at double-strand breaks. In a similar fashion to BRCA2 directing and limiting the function of RAD51, BRCA1 may control this complex and keep it from overdigesting. An important function of BRCA1 is exerted through its RING finger domain. This domain characterizes substrate recognition proteins of ubiquitin ligases. BRCA1 heterodimerizes with a protein named BARD1. Together they may support monoubiquitination of FANCD2 by the FANC protein complex, but certainly help to relocate the activated protein to the nuclear foci where BRCA2 resides. In this fashion, BRCA1 mediates repair of DNA crosslinks and stalled replication forks as well as actual strand breaks.

So, both BRCA1 and BRCA2 are involved in regulating or executing homologous recombination stimulated by the FANC proteins and perhaps also in regulating the MRN proteins. In a sense, BRCA2 acts 'downstream' of BRCA1.

It is, of course, conspicuous that the functions of so many genes in which mutations convey an increased risk of breast cancer are closely related to DNA repair. On one hand, this has led to the conception of a sort of '*repairosome*' that includes the BRCAs as crucial components, but also proteins actually recognizing and removing DNA damage as well as signaling components. The mutations predisposing to breast cancer would have the common effect of impeding the function of this dynamic '*organelle*'. Its core structure may correspond to the nuclear foci in which BRCA2 resides.

On the other hand, the question arises why such mutations promote cancer of the breast in particular. In the case of BRCA mutations, the breast and the ovaries are the organs most susceptible to cancers by a large margin. A certain, but much lower increase of risk is observed for cancers of the pancreas, bile duct, stomach, colon, and prostate (in this approximate descending order). To date, the most likely explanation for this specificity seems that during the multiple cycles of growth and involution in the breast there is a high likelihood of incurring chromosomal aberrations unless the DNA damage surveillance and repair system works perfectly. This is plausible, but does not quite account for the increased risk of ovarian cancer as well and, even less, for the increased risk of male breast cancer in carriers of BRCA2 mutations. There are also continuing hints that some of the proteins in the '*repairosome*' interact in a more direct fashion with the estrogen response. BRCA1 and TP53, among others, have been shown to interact with the estrogen receptor, mutually regulating each other's activity. So, a second (and perhaps additional) explanation might be that these proteins limit the pro-proliferative and anti-apoptotic action of the activated estrogen receptor in mammary epithelial tissue. Accordingly, BRCA1, in particular, does seem to exert a direct effect on the growth of breast and ovarian cells.

Women with germ-line mutations in *BRCA1* and *BRCA2* have a 40-80% estimated life-time risk of breast cancer compared to the ≈10% risk in the female population in Western industrialized countries at large. The risk of ovarian cancers is roughly 20-fold increased, as they are otherwise less prevalent. The precise increase in risk depends on the particular mutation, on genetic modifiers, and likely on environmental factors. The 4-8-fold increase in life-time breast cancer risk caused by BRCA mutations may seem moderate, but is exacerbated by the typical effects of an inherited tumor suppressor gene mutation. In familial cases, the disease appears earlier and the risk of a cancer in the contralateral organ (breast as well as ovary) is hugely increased over that in sporadic cases.

It is estimated that up to 10% of all breast cancers develop as a consequence of a mutation in a high-risk gene. Within this group, mutations in *BRCA1* and *BRCA2* may each underlie approximately one quarter of the cases. Mutations in all other genes may account for another ≈10%. This leaves >40% of familial cases unaccounted for by mutations in known genes. As during the initial search for the *BRCA1&2* genes in the early 1990's, linkage studies are continuing in families with multiple cases of breast cancer, occuring at an younger than usual age and/or more often bilaterally. Today, such studies are greatly facilitated by the human genome sequence and technical advances allowing high-throughput analyses of genetic markers. It is therefore safe to conclude, even with research ongoing, that a "*BRCA3*" gene with the same impact as *BRCA1* and *BRCA2* will not be discovered. Instead, it is expected that mutations in several more individual genes conferring a very high risk will each be responsible in a small number of families. However, the majority of familial cases may result from mutations that increase the risk of breast cancer only moderately, but sufficiently so to cause an accumulation of cancers in some families that carry them. These same mutations will also be responsible for individual cases in other families that would be categorized as '*sporadic*'.

This line of thought thus suggests a gradualism in cancer predisposition, at least for breast cancer. Mutations in certain '*high-risk*' genes may confer such a pronounced increase in risk that they will regularly result in a clustering of cancers within families. They are highly penetrant and to a large degree independent of environmental modulators. Other mutations or polymorphisms in these same genes or mutations in '*low-risk*' genes may emerge as a series of cancer cases in some families, but contribute to the development of many more cases categorized as sporadic. At the other end of the spectrum, certain polymorphisms in genes of DNA repair, cell protection, lipid or hormone metabolism etc. may confer only small increments in risk for breast cancer which may be strongly dependent on environmental modulators such as a high-fat diet or exposure to ionizing radiation. Since these polymorphisms are common, in contrast to actual mutations in high-risk genes, their impact on breast cancer may overall be more important. However, these effects are much more difficult to discern than the mutations in high-risk genes.

Estrogen Receptors and ERBB Proteins in Breast Cancer

Estrogens and the estrogen receptors are key regulators of growth in the normal breast, together with a number of other hormones acting through nuclear or membrane receptors. Furthermore, in an incompletely understood fashion, they synergize with growth factors of the EGF family that activate receptor tyrosine kinases of the ERBB family to instruct proliferation and differentiation of the ductal and alveolar epithelia. Expression of the growth factors in stromal and epithelial cells and perhaps of the receptors as well is influenced by estrogens. Conversely, active ERBB receptors stimulate the MAPK cascade which leads to phosphorylation of the ERα and synthesis and phosphorylation of AP1 transcription factors with which the receptor interacts. In breast cancer, these same factors remain relevant, although in a distorted way.

At the time of presentation, in >70% of breast cancers the ERα can be detected by immunohistochemical staining or by biochemical assays such as ELISA. About half of these cancers also express the progesterone receptor. Since the *PR* gene is induced by the estrogen receptor, its expression is an indication that ERα is not only present, but also active. Only <5% of breast cancers express only the PR. The ERβ is usually down-regulated in breast cancer; quite often the *ESR2* gene is silenced by promoter hypermethylation. This underlines its function as a negative growth regulator that limits proliferative responses to estrogens.

The presence or absence of ERα/PR provides the basis for one type of classification of breast cancers. 'ER+' breast cancers are on average better differentiated, grow more slowly, are not as strongly aneuploid, and have a slightly better prognosis than ER- breast cancers. Moreover, as a rule, their growth remains dependent on estrogens. Thus, compounds that block estrogen action or diminish the level of endogenous estrogens are often efficacious against ER+ cancers, but not at all against ER- cancers. Several strategies to specifically treat ER+ cancers are in use or are being explored. Compounds such as tamoxifen and raloxifene are partial agonists/antagonists (SERMs) that interfere with estrogen binding and with some interactions of the receptor with co-activators. They are used for chemoprevention, neoadjuvant treatment, adjuvant treatment, or treatment of systemic disease with metastases. Newer full antagonists block the ERα more efficiently and induce its degradation. They are expected to become used mostly in actual tumor treatment rather than in prevention, because of adverse effects on other tissues, such as bones and heart.

In women before menopause, when endogenous estrogens are still produced at high levels, this production must be diminished for efficient treatment. This can be achieved by surgical removal of the ovaries ('*oophorectomy*') or by treatment with analogues of gonadotropin-releasing hormone (GnRH or LHRH). GnRH is a hypothalamic peptide that stimulates the release of luteinizing hormone (LH) in the hypophysis. It is secreted in a cyclic fashion and regulated by neuronal inputs and by steroid feedback inhibition. Most drugs used in therapy are GnRH receptor agonistic and induce an initial burst of LH. However, since their level during treatment remains steadily high, the GnRH receptors in the pituitary become down-regulated. As a consequence, the production of LH hormone ceases, the ovaries are no longer stimulated by LH and stop to produce estrogens. Since in postmenopausal women estrogen synthesis is no longer significantly controlled by LH, a different strategy is required. Usually, inhibitors of the estrogen biosynthesis enzyme aromatase are employed.

By and large, the growth of ER+ breast cancers appears to be promoted by overactivity of those mechanisms that stimulate normal breast epithelial cells to grow during the proliferative phase of the monthly cycle or during pregnancy. Of course, in the cancers, neither the cyclic regression phase nor the terminal differentiation of duct cells take place in an orderly fashion. In contrast, ER- tumors neither depend on nor respond to estrogens. The estrogen receptors are not expressed and the *ESR1* gene as well is quite frequently silenced by hypermethylation. In many ER- breast cancers, a large fraction of the proliferative stimulus appears to be provided through ERBB proteins.

In man, the ERBB family named after their first identified member, the retroviral v-erbB oncogene comprises four structurally related membrane receptors, ERBB1 - ERBB4. The designations HER1 - HER4 are also in use. Each receptor protein comprises an ≈600 amino acid extracellular ligand-binding domain, a 24 amino acid single-pass helical transmembrane domain and a >500 amino acid cytoplasmatic tyrosine kinase domain with multiple autophosphorylation sites and an autoinhibitory loop. ERBB1, also known as the EGF receptor, of course binds the epidermal growth factor, but also several further peptides that share with EGF a conserved motif with three cystine disulfide bridges, termed the EGF motif. In fact, in most physiological circumstances, the structurally related TGFα, amphiregulin, and heparin-binding EGF (HB-EGF) are probably more relevant than EGF itself. HB-EGF as well as betacellulin (BTC) and epiregulin (EPR) also bind and activate HER4. Neuregulins 1 - 4 (NRGs) are specific for ERBB3 and ERBB4, NRGs 1&2 being predominantly recognized by ERBB3 and NRGs 3&4 by ERBB4. This leaves ERBB2 with no known ligand and there may indeed be none. Rather, all ERBB receptors form dimers after ligand binding and all prefer to form heterodimers with ERBB2, although homodimers are also active.

Ligand binding induces a conformation change that relieves auto-inhibition of the tyrosine kinase by the pseudosubstrate loop to allow cross-phosphorylation with subsequent docking of adaptor and substrate proteins. Signals emanate from the ERBB receptors mainly through the MAPK, PI3K, and STAT pathways.

As ERBB2 is the odd member of the family with respect to ligand binding, ERBB3 is unusual with respect to kinase activity. Crucial residues in its active center are not conserved and ERBB3 may have no kinase activity at all. Thus, its tyrosine kinase activity is provided by its ERBB2 dimerization partner.

In normal breast epithelial cells, both proliferation and differentiation are influenced by several EGF-related peptides and each member of the ERBB family is involved, at least in a subset of the cells. Production of the peptide growth factors takes place in stromal and epithelial cells and is regulated by estrogens. Both their production and the cellular responses to the growth factors are influenced by cross-talk with other hormones and growth factors. For instance, release of HB-EGF requires proteolytic cleavage by metalloproteinases which are stimulated by endothelin-1 and bombesin acting through G-coupled serpentine receptors. Certain WNT factors also promote release of EGF-like factors. The relevance of WNT pathway activation in breast cancer may therefore have to be considered in this light. At the ERBB receptor step, cross-talk with cytokine receptors may be particularly important in breast tissue. Prolactin and growth hormone receptors induce phosphorylation of ERBB1 by JAK kinases.

With multiple growth factors and receptors distributed between several cell types and subject to cross-talk with further pathways, the precise relationships are extremely complex. In addition, they may substantially vary between different phases of breast growth and even segments of the ducts. In summary, it appears that activation of ERBB1, but even more of the ERBB2/ERBB3 heterodimer provides the main stimulus for proliferation. At least in the case of the ERBB2/ERBB3 unit, this stimulation may predominantly be exerted through the PI3K pathway, since ERBB3 after phosphorylation by ERBB2 provides several binding sites for the PI3Kα regulatory subunit. In contrast, the ERBB4 receptor which is activated by heregulins and perhaps by HB-EGF rather promotes the differentiation of mammary epithelial cells.

Approximately 50% of ER- and a smaller proportion of ER+ breast cancers overexpress ERBB2, as detected by immunohistochemistry. In most cases, strong positive staining is caused by amplification of the *ERBB2* gene. Measurements by biochemical assays reveal an inverse quantitative relationship between ERα and ERBB2 protein levels. There is thus a continuum, but in clinical routine, at most four classes are qualitatively distinguished, viz. ER+/ERBB2-, ER+/ERBB2+, ER-/ERBB2+, and ER-/ERBB2-.

Alternatively or in addition to ERBB2, ERBB1 is also overexpressed in some cases and may provide the crucial growth stimulus in some ER-/ERBB2- cancers. ERBB3 is not usually overexpressed, but is always present in ERBB2+ cancers. It is likely essential for the action of ERBB2 by providing the crucial binding sites for PI3Kα and other intracellular mediators. At normal concentrations of the receptors, they would be present as monomers and dimerization of ERBB2 and ERBB3 would be dependent on ligand-binding by ERBB3. Overexpression of ERBB2 may lower the concentration of ligand required or even obliterate it, thereby facilitating constitutive association and activity.

With increasing expression of ERBB2 or ERBB1, the estrogen requirement for growth of breast epithelial cells appears to be alleviated and eventually lost. Thus, while the normal cells require estrogens and EGF-like growth factors, and ER+ cancers retain these requirements at least to some extent, ER-/ERBB2 breast cancers need only the peptide factors and eventually even less of these. Estrogen action is, of course, partly, but not completely mediated through induction of growth factors and activation of ERBB receptors. Therefore, in addition to overexpression of ERBB receptors, some kind of '*rewiring*' must have occured in ER- cells. This is incompletely understood. Importantly, ER- cancers harbor a large number of further genetic and epigenetic alterations besides loss of the estrogen receptors and amplification of *ERBB2*.

Like the distinction between ER+ and ER- cancers, that between ERBB2+ and ERBB2- breast cancers has prognostic implications, because ERBB2+ cancers as a rule fare worse. It has also consequences for therapy. As for other tyrosine kinases, low molecular weight inhibitors of ERBB2 have been developed and are tested in clinical trials. A monoclonal antibody, named trastuzumab, is directed specifically against ERBB2. This antibody was originally generated in mice. To avoid immune reactions when applied to patients, it was humanized. The antigen recognition variable region derived from the mouse was retained, but the constant region was replaced by the human sequence. This biotechnologically produced antibody is now administered to breast cancer patients with metastatic disease, if and only if their cancers stain strongly positive for ERBB2 in immunohistochemistry. *ERBB2* gene amplification is additionally determined. The antibody drug indeed significantly prolongs survival in many of these patients, when administered with standard chemotherapy. In the future, it may also be used in adjuvant and neoadjuvant therapy of ER-/ERBB2+ cancers. Determination of ERBB2 gene amplification yields another piece of information. The *ERBB2* amplicon in most cases includes the *TOPO2A* gene encoding the α subunit of topoisomerase II. Its overexpression increases the sensitivity of tumor cells to cytostatic anthracyclins, providing another opening for targeted therapy.

Classification of Breast Cancers

Like other carcinomas, breast cancer is treated primarily by surgery. While formerly radical mastectomy with removal of all lymph nodes around the tissue constituted the standard approach, today's philosophy is to keep the surgical intervention as minimal as possible without risking a recurrence.

Breast cancer metastasizes to local lymph nodes as well as to distal organs such as bone, lung, and liver. At the time of surgery, the extent of distal metastasis is often difficult to determine, because many metastases are too small to be discovered by imaging methods and no reliable molecular assays are available for the detection of breast cancer micrometastases. Therefore, if any significant risk of metastasis is assumed, chemotherapy is applied following surgery. Such 'adjuvant' treatment very likely prevents recurrences in some patients, but constitutes an over-treatment for those without metastases. Nevertheless, it is not always efficacious, since some patients develop metastases or locally recurring tumors in the remaining breast tissue in spite of adjuvant treatment. As for other carcinomas, the therapeutic options for established systemic disease are limited.

The most important goal of breast cancer classifications is therefore to provide a basis for choice of therapy in each individual patient. The available choices include the extent of surgery, the administration of adjuvant therapy, and the selection of particular drugs. Several tools are already available for this purpose. '*Classical*' histological investigation distinguishes different subtypes such as Paget carcinoma, intraductal carcinoma, lobular carcinoma, and, importantly, precursors like ductal carcinoma-in-situ and benign tumors such as fibroadenoma. Of course, grading is applied and tumor staging is important. Specifically, the extent of lymph node involvement is a good indicator of the likelihood of metastases and recurrence.

Molecular markers have improved this classification. Today, determination of ER, PR, and ERBB2 status represents good standard practice. A diagnosis of ER+/PR+/ERBB2-, e.g., indicates a comparatively good prognosis and predicts a good response to anti-estrogenic drugs. By comparison, ERBB2+ cancers are on average more aggressive, but often respond to trastuzumab treatment in conjunction with chemotherapy. Breast cancers in patients with inherited BRCA mutations are special. They are as a rule ER-, and present histological markers of basal duct cells. Moreover, these patients have, of course, a relatively high risk of developing an independent cancer in the same or the other breast. Other molecular markers have been found by studying the correlation between the expression of proteins thought to be involved in tumor invasion and metastasis and the course of the disease. Several individual proteins constitute useful '*prognostic*' markers, e.g. high expression of uPA indicates a high probability of metastasis.

Further progress in the classification of breast cancer appears to emerge from gene expression profiles, which identify patterns in the expression of many genes that correlate with biological properties and clinical behavior of a tumor. Most widely, microarrays spotted with cDNA fragments or oligonucleotides corresponding to human genes are employed. Different types of arrays cover thousands to ten-thousands of human genes and their splice variants. RNA extracted from tumor or normal tissues are reverse transcribed and labeled to obtain cDNA mixtures that remain representative of the relative abundancies of mRNAs in the tissues. These are then hybridized to the microarrays. The measured hybridization intensities at each spot give an estimate of the expression level of each mRNA represented on the array.

These techniques allow the comparison of gene expression patterns between different samples, e.g. between tumor and normal tissue or between individual tumors. Because only a small number of measurements are taken on each sample and current microarrays have a limited dynamic range, measurements by microarrays are not very accurate. This means that the expression level of an individual gene in an individual tumor cannot be measured precisely. However, patterns defined by the expression of several hundreds of genes are robust and classify genes as well as samples into groups or '*clusters*'. These techniques can therefore on one hand serve to single out individual genes for closer investigation as tumor markers or therapeutic targets, or to identify particular pathways to be active in a certain subtype of cancer. On the other hand, they can provide a method to classify cancers by specific '*signatures*', sometimes in unexpected ways.

Investigation of breast cancers by this type of technique has yielded expected as well as unexpected results. ER+ and ER- cancers gave clearly distinct expression profiles. ERBB2+ cancers likewise presented specific signatures. Beyond corroborating current clinical practice, these signatures provide hints at which genes might be induced or down-regulated by estrogens or ERBB2 receptor activation in breast cancers and therefore might provide good targets for novel therapies in these subgroups.

Neither unexpectedly, cancers from patients with *BRCA* germline mutations formed part of a separate group. This group showed many characteristic markers of basal epithelial cells, such as the cytokeratins 5 and 6. Although lacking the signature of ER+ cancer profiles, these cancers were also clearly distinct from the ERBB2+ group. Thus, there seem to be at least two distinct classes of ER- cancers.

Interestingly, while one group of breast cancers showed expression profiles relating them to basal cells, the ER+ cancers displayed many markers characteristic of the luminal secretory cell phenotype. This finding substantiates previous speculations that different subtypes of breast cancers may derive from different stages of the mammary epithelial lineage, as already shown in other tissues, e.g. the skin.

The expression profiles also suggest that ER+ cancers can be divided into further subclasses, which is in line with their quite divergent clinical behavior. These results also underline that the properties of breast cancers are not determined by alterations in any single gene, but are multifactorial.

Expression profiling studies in breast cancer and in other carcinomas have also compared primary cancers and their metastases. In all such studies, individual primary cancers and their metastases proved to be more closely related to each other than primary cancers or metastases among themselves, clustering as separate pairs. This finding bears on an old controversy in cancer biology. Metastases could arise from the original tumor by gradual selection of cells that can manage each of the individual steps required for metastasis. Alternatively, the ability to metastasize could be determined by the pattern of genetic and epigenetic alterations present in the primary tumor. The close relationship between primary cancers and their metastases argues strongly for this latter hypothesis.

This conclusion is important in clinical practice, since the more the likelihood of metastasis is determined by the properties of the primary tumor, the better it can be predicted by analyzing the tumor tissue at the primary site. Moreover, a comparison of primary tumors that have metastasized to those that have not, may also yield a '*molecular signature*' that can help to identify metastatic cancers before overt metastases can be detected. Such a signature has been suggested and, intriguingly, includes not only properties of the tumor cells, but also gene expression patterns in the reactive stroma. This finding underlines current ideas on the crucial importance of both tumor and stromal properties for invasion and metastasis.

A specific aim addressed by gene expression profiling in breast cancer is the prediction of prognosis and of response to chemotherapy. Ideally, one would develop a smaller set of markers, detectable by analysis of DNA alterations such as gene amplification, by immunohistochemistry in a routine pathology lab, or perhaps by microarrays containing a smaller set of genes (a '*predictor gene set*') which are less expensive and easier to evaluate, but sufficiently robust for prediction. Several approaches have been taken towards this end. A typical approach involves a '*supervised*' analysis. Tumor gene expression profiles from patients that were cured by surgery or chemotherapy are compared to profiles from those in which the cancer recurred. The predictor gene set optimally distinguishing these groups is applied to a separate series of tumors for verification. Ideally, it would also classify patients with a favourable outcome or benefitting from a particular type of therapy. Breast cancerspecific microarrays of this type have been developed. It is hoped that they also prove successful in prospective studies.

The developments in expression profiling continue an established trend in breast cancer treatment towards an '*individualized*' treatment. This trend can also be observed in many other cancers which show great variation in clinical course and response to treatments. An obvious prerequisite is an actual choice of available treatments, as in breast cancer. In fact, the more sophisticated understanding of cancer biology and its molecular basis emerging in breast cancer has initiated a kind of paradigm shift in its therapy that is spreading to other tumor entities. Traditionally, the treatment of a cancer was adjusted according to its histological subtype, extension (as indicated by stage) and apparent biological aggressiveness (as indicated a.o. by grading). In the future, individualized treatment may be gauged by the particular molecular targets provided in a cancer. In breast cancer, this principle is already followed during anti-hormonal therapy contingent on the ER status and trastuzumab therapy contingent on ERBB2 expression. It is expected that identification of further molecular targets in breast cancer, by gene expression profiling or by other techniques, will boost this development.

12

Resource Center

Eukaryote Cell Primer

Life on Earth began 3.5 billion years ago in the form of single cells that appeared in the oceans. These cells evolved into ancestral prokaryotes and, about 2 billion years ago, gave rise to Archaea, bacteria, and eukaryotes, the three major divisions of life in the world. Eukaryotes, in turn, gave rise to plants, animals, protozoans, and fungi. Each of these groups represents a distinct phylogenetic kingdom. The archaea and bacteria represent a fifth kingdom, known as the monera or prokaryotes. Archaea and bacteria are very similar anatomically; both lack a true nucleus and internal organelles. A prokaryote genome is a single, circular piece of naked DNA called a chromosome, containing fewer than 5,000 genes. Eukaryotes (meaning "*true nuclei*") are much more complex, having many membrane-bounded organelles. These include a nucleus, nucleolus, *endoplasmic reticulum* (ER), Golgi complex, mitochondria, lysosomes, and peroxisomes.

The eukaryote nucleus, bounded by a double phospholipid membrane, contains a DNA (deoxyribonucleic acid) genome on two or more linear chromosomes, each of which may contain up to 10,000 genes. The nucleus also contains an assembly plant for ribosomal subunits called the nucleolus. The endoplasmic reticulum (ER) and the Golgi complex work together to glycosylate proteins and lipids (attach sugar molecules to the proteins and lipids producing glycoproteins and glycolipids), most of which are destined for the cell membrane to form a molecular "*forest*" known as the glycocalyx. The glycoproteins and glycolipids travel from the ER to the Golgi, and from the Golgi to the cell surface, in membrane-bounded vesicles that form by budding off the

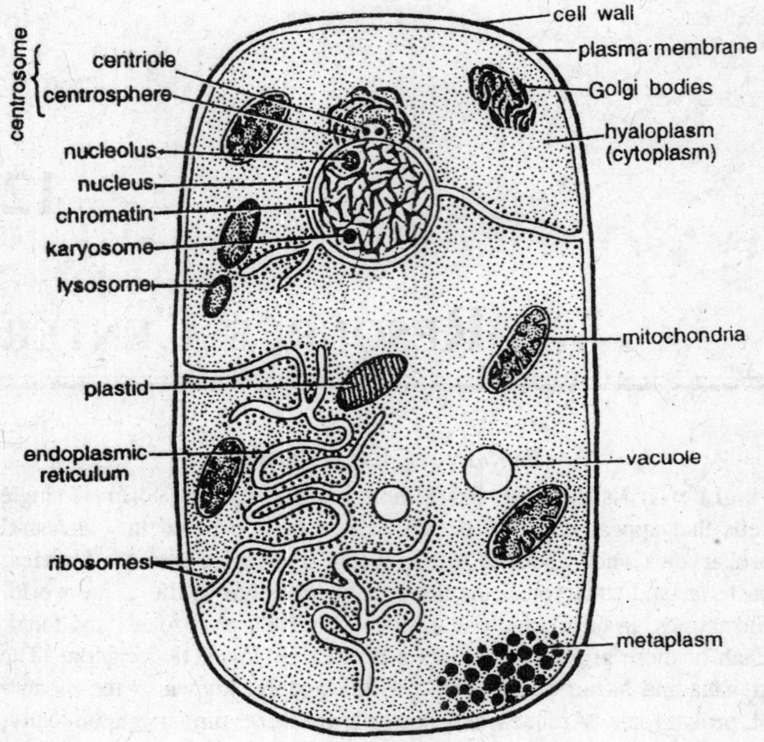

Fig. 12.1. Eukaryotic cell.

organelle by exocytosis. Thus,. the cytoplasm contains many transport vesicles that originate from the ER and Golgi. The Golgi vesicles bud off the outer chamber, or the one farthest from the ER. Mitochondria, once free-living prokaryotes, and the only other organelle with a double membrane, provide the cell with energy in the form of adenosine triphosphate (ATP). The production of ATP is carried out by an assembly of metal-containing proteins called the electron transport chain, located in the mitochondrion inner membrane. Ribosomes, some of which are attached to the ER, synthesize proteins. Lysosomes and peroxisomes recycle cellular material and molecules. The microtubules and centrosome form the spindle apparatus for moving chromosomes to the daughter cells during cell division. Actin filaments and a weblike structure consisting of intermediate filaments form the cytoskeleton.

Molecules of the Cell

Cells are biochemical entities that synthesize many thousands of molecules. Studying these chemicals and the biochemistry of the cell would be a daunting task were it not for the fact that most of the chemical variation is based on six types of molecules, which are assembled into just four types of macromolecules. The six basic molecules are amino acids, phosphate, glycerol, sugars, fatty acids, and nucleotides. Amino acids have a simple core structure consisting of an amino group, a carboxyl group, and a variable R group attached to a carbon atom. There are 20 different kinds of amino acids, each with a unique R group. Phosphates are extremely important molecules that are used in the construction or modification of many other molecules. They are also used to store chemical-bond energy. Glycerol is a simple three-carbon alcohol that is an important component of cell membranes and fat reservoirs. Sugars are extremely versatile molecules that are used as an energy source and for structural purposes. Glucose, a six-carbon sugar, is the primary energy source for most cells and it is the principal sugar used to glycosylate proteins and lipids for the production of the glycocalyx. Plants have exploited the structural potential of sugars in their production of cellulose and, thus, wood, bark, grasses, and reeds are polymers of glucose and other monosaccharides. Ribose, a five-carbon sugar, is a component of nucleic acids, as well as ATP. Ribose carbons are numbered as 1' (1 prime), 2' and so on. Consequently, references to nucleic acids, which include ribose, often refer to the 3' or 5' carbon. Fatty acids consist of a carboxyl group (when ionized it becomes a carboxylic acid) linked to a hydrophobic hydrocarbon tail. These molecules are used in the construction of cell membranes and fat.

Nucleotides are building blocks for DNA and RNA (ribonucleic acid). Nucleotides consist of three components: a phosphate, a ribose sugar, and a nitrogenous (nitrogen containing) ring compound that behaves as a base in solution. Nucleotide bases appear in two forms: A single-ring nitrogenous base called a *pyrimidine*, and a double-ringed base called a *purine*. There are two kinds of purines (adenine and guanine), and three pyrimidines (uracil, cytosine, and thymine). Uracil is specific to RNA, substituting for thymine. In addition, RNA nucleotides contain ribose, whereas DNA nucleotides contain deoxyribose (hence their names). Ribose has a hydroxyl (OH) group attached to both the 2' and 3' carbons, whereas deoxyribose is missing the 2' hydroxyl group. ATP, the molecule that is used by all cells as a source of energy, is a ribose nucleotide consisting of the purine base adenine and three phosphates attached to the 5' carbon of the ribose sugar. The phosphates are labeled α (alpha), β (beta) and γ (gamma), and are linked to the carbon in a tandem order, beginning with α. The energy stored by this molecule is carried by the covalent bonds of the β and γ phosphates. Breaking these bonds sequentially releases the energy they contain, while converting ATP to adenosine diphosphate (ADP) and then to adenosine monophosphate (AMP). AMP is converted back to ATP by mitochondria.

Macromolecules of the Cell

The six basic molecules are used by all cells to construct five essential macromolecules. These include proteins, RNA, DNA, phospholipids, and sugar polymers, known as *polysaccharides*. Amino acids are linked together by peptide bonds to construct a protein. A peptide bond is formed by linking the carboxyl end of one amino acid to the amino end of second amino acid. Thus, once constructed, every protein has an amino end and a carboxyl end. An average protein may consist of 300–400 amino acids. Nucleic acids are macromolecules constructed from nucleotides. The 5' phosphate of one nucleotide is linked to the 3' OH of a second nucleotide. Additional nucleotides are always linked to the 3' OH of the last nucleotide in the chain. Consequently, the growth of the chain is said to be in the 5' to 3' direction. RNA nucleotides are adenine, uracil, cytosine, and guanine. A typical RNA molecule consists of 2,000 to 3,000 nucleotides; it is generally single stranded, but can form localized double-stranded regions. RNA is involved in the synthesis of proteins and is a structural and enzymatic component of ribosomes. DNA, a double-stranded nucleic acid, encodes cellular genes and is constructed from adenine, thymine, cytosine, and guanine deoxyribonucleotides (dATP, dTTP, dCTP and dGTP, where "d" indicates deoxyribose). The two DNA strands coil around each other like strands in a piece of rope, and for this reason the molecule is known as the double helix. DNA is an extremely large macromolecule, typically consisting of more than 1 million nucleotide pairs (or base pairs). Double-stranded DNA forms when two chains of nucleotides interact through the formation of chemical bonds between complementary base pairs. The chemistry of the bases is such that adenine pairs with thymine and cytosine pairs with guanine. For stability, the two strands are antiparallel, that is, the orientation of one strand is in the 5' to 3' direction, while the complementary strand runs 3' to 5'. Phospholipids, the main component of cell membranes, are composed of a polar head group (usually an alcohol), a phosphate, glycerol, and two hydrophobic fatty-acid tails. Fat that is stored in the body as an energy reserve has a structure similar to a phospholipid, being composed of three fatty acid chains attached to a

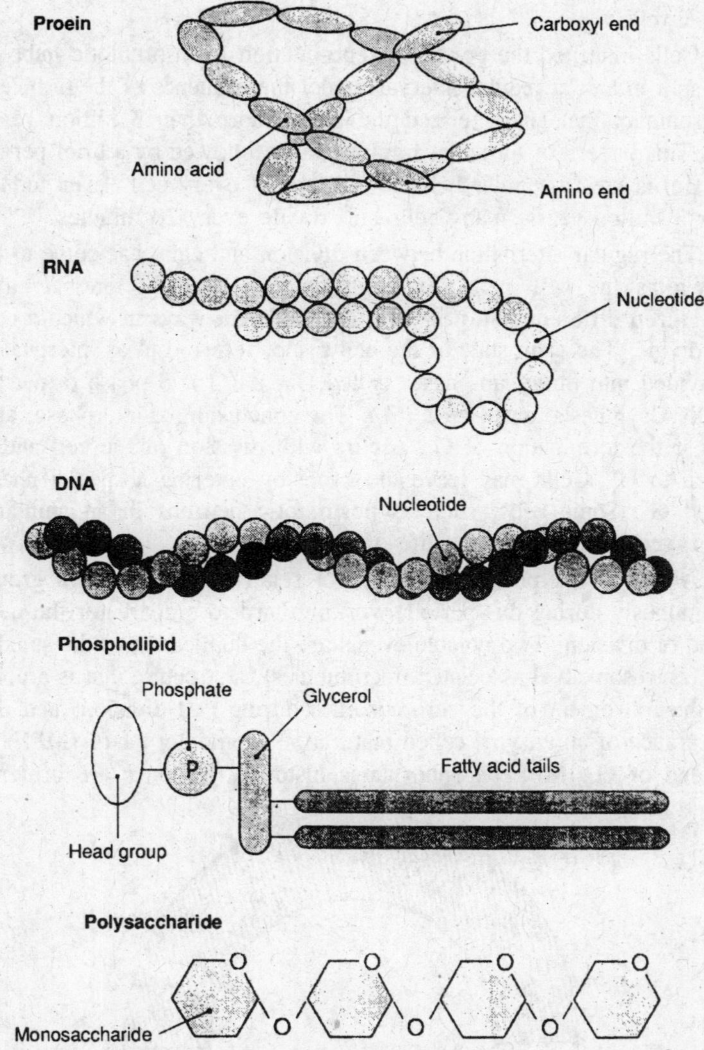

Fig. 12.2. Macromolecules of the cell.

molecule of glycerol. The third fatty acid takes the place of the phosphate and head group of a phospholipid. Sugars are polymerized to form chains of two or more monosaccharides. Disaccharides (two monosaccharides) and oligosaccharides (three to 12 monosaccharides) are attached to proteins and lipids destined for the glycocalyx. Polysaccharides, such as glycogen and starch, may contain several hundred monosaccharides and are stored in cells as an energy reserve.

Cell Cycle

Cells inherited the power of reproduction from prebiotic bubbles that split in half at regular intervals under the influence of the turbulent environment that characterized the Earth more than 3 billion years ago. This pattern of turbulent fragmentation followed by a brief period of calm is now a regular behavior pattern of every cell. Even today, after 3 billion years, many cells still divide every 20 minutes.

The regular alternation between division and calm has come to be known as the cell cycle. In studying this cycle, scientists have recognized different states of calm and different ways in which a cell can divide. The calm state of the cell cycle, referred to as interphase, is divided into three sub-phases called Gap 1 (G_1), S phase (a period of DNA synthesis) and Gap 2 (G_2). The conclusion of interphase, and with it the termination of G_2, occurs with division of the cell and a return to G_1. Cells may leave the cycle by entering a special phase called G_0. Some cells, such as postmitotic neurons in an animal's brain, remain in G_0 for the life of the organism.

Although interphase is a period of relative calm, the cell grows continuously during this period, working hard to prepare for the next round of division. Two notable events are the duplication of the spindle (the centrosome and associated microtubules), a structure that is crucial for the movement of the chromosomes during cell division, and the appearance of an enzyme called maturation promoting factor (MPF) at the end of G_2. MPF phosphorylates histones. Histones are proteins

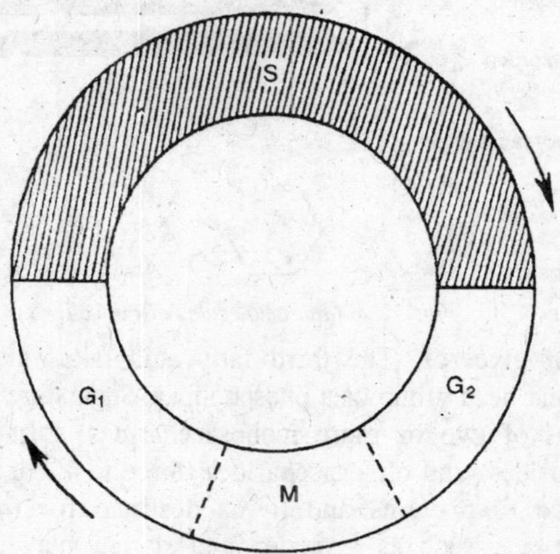

Fig. 12.3. Cell cycle.

that bind to the DNA, which when phosphorylated, compacts (or condenses) the chromosomes in preparation for cell division. MPF is also responsible for the breakdown of the nuclear membrane. When cell division is complete, MPF disappears, allowing the chromosomes to decondense and the nuclear envelope to re-form. Completion of a normal cell cycle always involves the division of a cell into two daughter cells. This can occur by a process known as mitosis, which is intended for cell multiplication, and by a second process known as meiosis, which is intended for sexual reproduction.

Mitosis

Mitosis is used by all free-living eukaryotes (protozoans) as a means of asexual reproduction. The growth of a plant or an animal is also accomplished with this form of cell division. Mitosis is divided into four stages: prophase, metaphase, anaphase, and telophase. All of these stages are marked out in accordance with the behavior of the nucleus and the chromosomes. Prophase marks the period during which the duplicated chromosomes begin condensation and the two centrosomes begin moving to opposite poles of the cell. Under the microscope, the chromosomes become visible as X-shaped structures, which are the two duplicated chromosomes, often called *sister chromatids*. A special region of each chromosome, called a *centromere*, holds the chromatids together. Proteins bind to the centromere to form a structure called the *kinetochore*. Metaphase is a period during which the chromosomes are sorted out and aligned between the two centrosomes. By this time, the nuclear membrane has completely broken down. The two centrosomes and the microtubules fanning out between them form the mitotic spindle. The area in between the spindles, where the chromosomes are aligned, is often referred to as the metaphase plate. Some of the microtubules make contact with the kinetochores, while others overlap, with motor proteins situated in between. Eukaryotes are normally diploid, so a cell would have two copies of each chromosome, one from the mother and one from the father. Anaphase is characterized by the movement of the duplicated chromosomes to opposite poles of the cell. The first step is the release of an enzyme that breaks the bonds holding the kinetochores together, thus allowing the sister chromatids to separate from each other while remaining bound to their respective microtubules. Motor proteins then move along the microtuble, dragging the chromosomes to opposite ends of the cell. Using energy supplied by ATP, the motor proteins break the microtubule down as it drags the chromosome along, so that the microtubule is

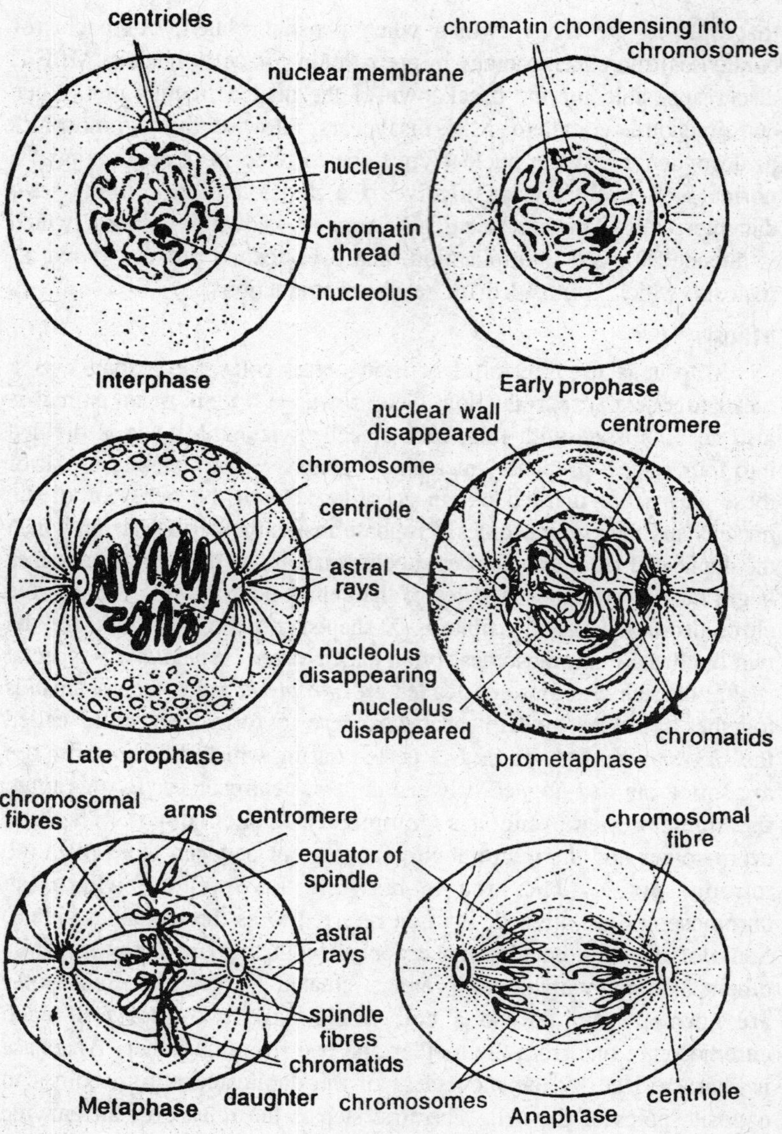

Fig. 12.4. Mitosis.

gone by the time the chromosome reaches the spindle pole. Throughout this process, the motor proteins and the chromosome manage to stay one step ahead of the disintegrating microtubule. The overlapping microtubules aid movement of the chromosomes toward the poles as another type of motor protein pushes the microtubules in opposite directions, effectively forcing the centrosomes toward the poles. This accounts for the greater overlap of microtubules in metaphase as compared with anaphase. During telophase, the daughter chromosomes arrive at the spindle poles and decondense to form the relaxed chromatin characteristic of interphase nuclei. The nuclear envelope begins forming around the chromosomes, marking the end of mitosis. During the same period, a contractile ring, made of the proteins myosin and actin, begins pinching the parental cell in two. This stage, separate from mitosis, is called *cytokinesis*, and leads to the formation of two daughter cells, each with one nucleus.

Meiosis

Unlike mitosis, which leads to the growth of an organism, meiosis is intended for sexual reproduction and occurs exclusively in ovaries and testes. Eukaryotes, being diploid, receive chromosomes from both parents; if gametes were produced using mitosis, a catastrophic growth in the number of chromosomes would occur each time a sperm fertilized an egg. Meiosis is a special form of cell division that produces haploid gametes (eggs and sperm), each possessing half as many chromosomes as the diploid cell. When haploid gametes fuse, they produce an embryo with the correct number of chromosomes.

The existence of meiosis was first suggested 100 years ago when microbiologists counted the number chromosomes in somatic and germ cells. The roundworm, for example, was found to have four chromosomes in its somatic cells but only two in its gametes. Many other studies also compared the amount of DNA in nuclei from somatic cells and gonads, always with same result: The amount of DNA in somatic cells is exactly double the amount in fully mature gametes. To understand how this could be, scientists studied cell division in the gonads and were able to show that meiosis occurs as two rounds of cell division with only one round of DNA synthesis. The two rounds of division were called *meiosis I* and *meiosis II*, and scientists observed that both could be divided into the same four stages known to occur in mitosis. Indeed, meiosis II is virtually identical to a mitotic division. Meiosis I resembles mitosis, but close examination shows three important differences: gene swapping occurs between homologous chromosomes in prophase; homologs (that is, two homologous chromosomes) remain paired at metaphase, instead of lining up at the plate as is done in mitosis; and the kinetochores do not separate at anaphase.

Homologous chromosomes are two identical chromosomes that come from different parents. For example, humans have 23 chromosomes

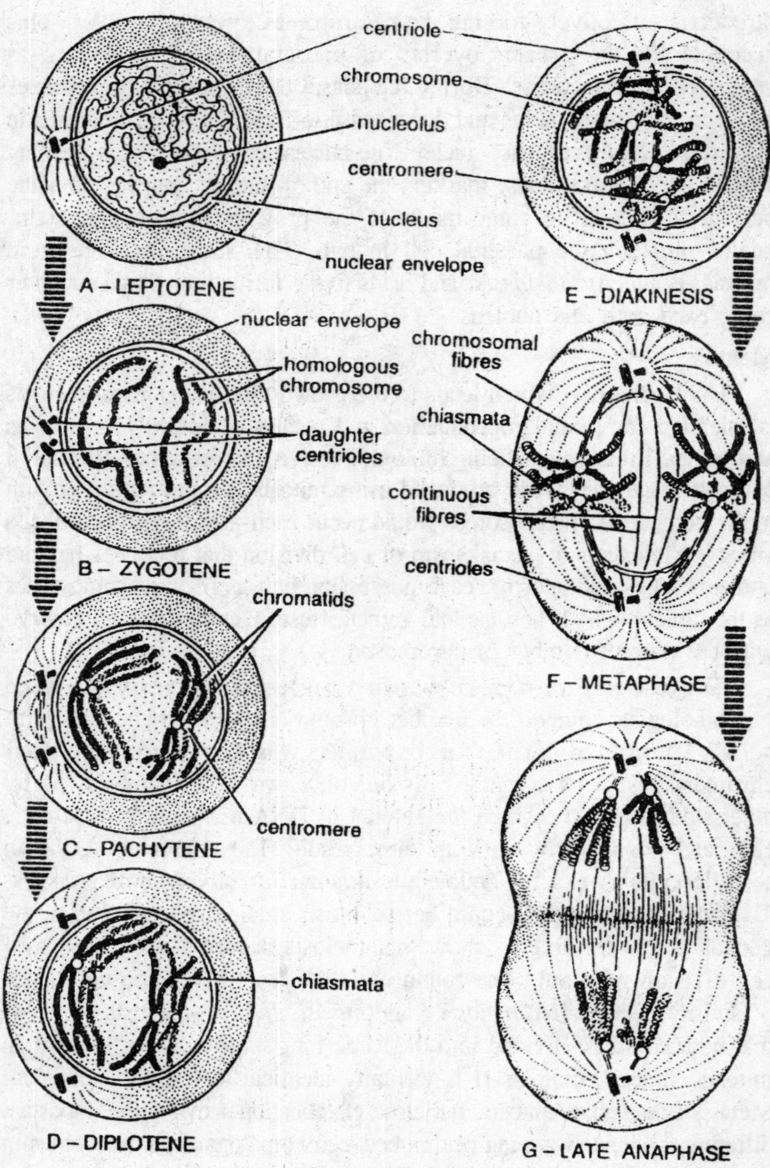

Fig. 12.5. Meiosis I.

from the father and the same 23 from the mother. We each have a maternal chromosome 1 and a paternal chromosome 1; they carry the same genes but specify slightly different traits. Chromosome 1 may carry the gene for eye color, but the maternal version, or allele, may specify blue eyes, whereas the paternal allele specifies brown. During prophase, homologous pairs exchange large numbers of genes by swapping whole pieces of chromosome. Thus one of the maternal chromatids ends up with a piece of paternal chromosome, and a paternal chromatid receives the corresponding piece of maternal chromosome. Mixing genetic material in this way is unique to meiosis, and it is one of the reasons sexual reproduction has been such a powerful evolutionary force.

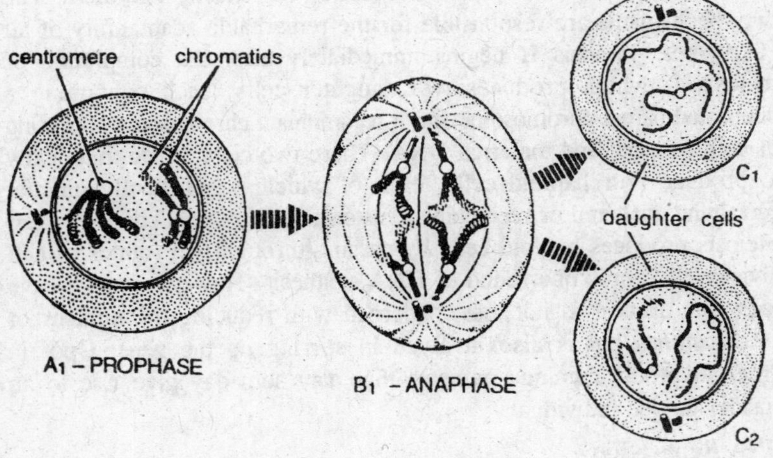

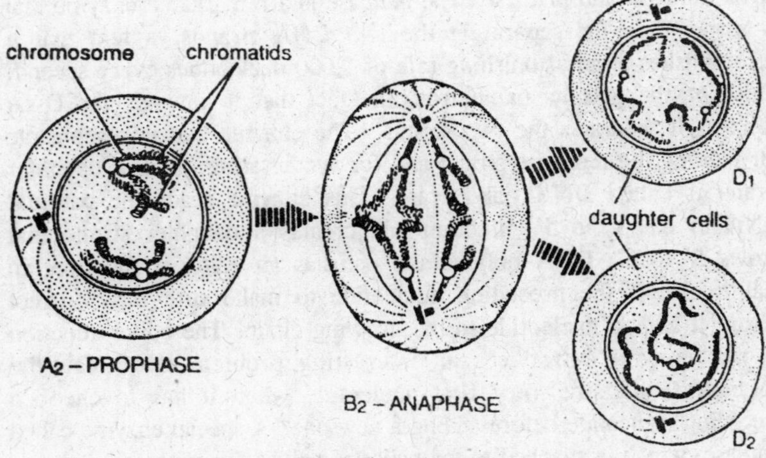

Fig. 12.6. Meiosis II.

During anaphase of meiosis I, the kinetochores do not separate as they do in mitosis. The effect of this is to separate the maternal and paternal chromosomes by sending them to different daughter cells, although the segregation is random. That is, the daughter cells receive a random assortment of maternal and paternal chromosomes, rather than one daughter cell receiving all paternal chromosomes and the other all maternal chromosomes. Random segregation, along with genetic recombination, accounts for the fact that while children resemble their parents, they do not look or act exactly like them. The two mechanisms are responsible for the remarkable adaptability of all eukaryotes. Meiosis II begins immediately after the completion of meiosis I, which produces two daughter cells, each containing a duplicated parent chromosome and a recombinant chromosome consisting of both paternal and maternal DNA. These two cells divide mitotically to produce four haploid cells, each of which is genetically unique, containing unaltered or recombinant maternal and paternal chromosomes. Meiosis produces haploid cells by passing through two rounds of cell division with only one round of DNA synthesis. However, as we have seen, the process is not just concerned with reducing the number of chromosomes but is also involved in stirring up the genetic pot in order to produce unique gametes that may someday give rise to an equally unique individual.

DNA Replication

DNA replication, which occurs during the S phase of the cell cycle, requires the coordinated effort of a team of enzymes, led by DNA helicase and primase. The helicase is a remarkable enzyme that is responsible for separating the two DNA strands, a feat that it accomplishes at an astonishing rate of 1,000 nucleotides every second. This enzyme gets its name from the fact that it unwinds the DNA helix as it separates the two strands. The enzyme that is responsible for reading the template strand and for synthesizing the new daughter strand is called DNA polymerase. This enzyme reads the parental DNA in the 3' to 5' direction and creates a daughter strand that grows 5' to 3'. DNA polymerase also has an editorial function, in that it checks the preceding nucleotide to make sure it is correct before it adds a nucleotide to the growing chain. The editor function of this enzyme introduces an interesting problem. How can the polymerase add the very first nucleotide when it has to check a preceding nucleotide before adding a new one? A special enzyme called primase, which is attached to the helicase, solves this problem. Primase

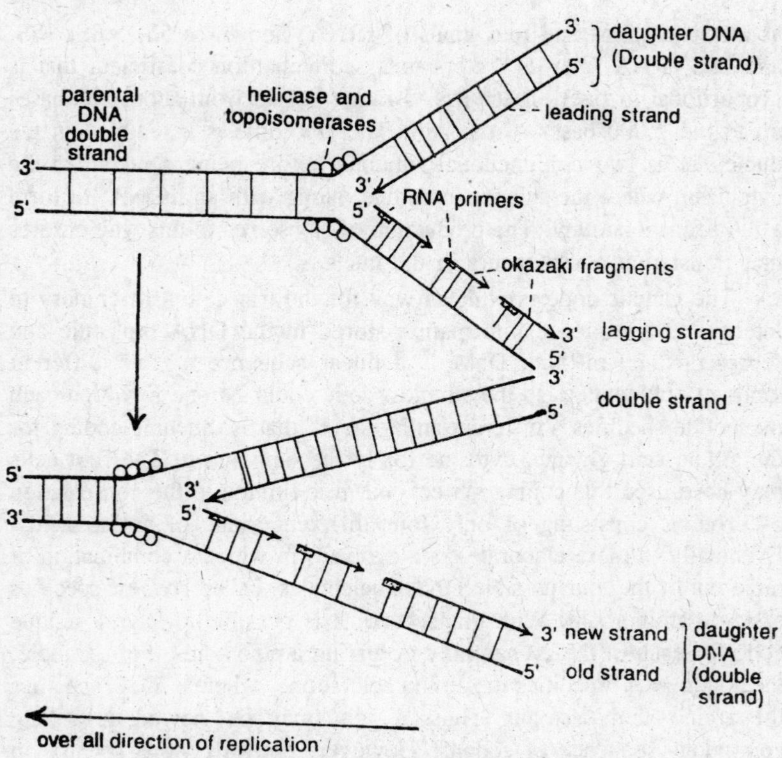

Fig. 12.7. Replication of DNA.

synthesizes short pieces of RNA that form a DNA-RNA double-stranded region. The RNA becomes a temporary part of the daughter strand, thus priming the DNA polymerase by providing the crucial first nucleotide in the new strand. Once the chromosome is duplicated, DNA repair enzymes remove the RNA primers and replace them with DNA nucleotides.

Transcription, Translation, and the Genetic Code

Genes encode proteins and several kinds of RNA. Extracting the information from DNA requires the processes of transcription and translation. Transcription, catalyzed by the enzyme RNA polymerase, copies one strand of the DNA into a complementary strand of messenger RNA (mRNA) or ribosomal RNA (rRNA) that is used in the construction of ribosomes. Messenger RNA translocates to the cytoplasm where it is translated into a protein by ribosomes. Newly transcribed rRNA is sent to the nucleolus for ribosome assembly, and is never translated. Ribosomes are complex structures consisting of about 50 proteins and four kinds of rRNA, known as 5S, 5.8S, 18S, and 28S rRNA (the "S" refers to a sedimentation coefficient that is proportional to size). These RNAs range in size from about 500 bases up to the 2,000 bases of the 28S. The ribosome is assembled in the nucleolus as two nonfunctional subunits before being sent out to the cytoplasm where the subunits combine, along with an mRNA, to form a fully functional unit. The production of ribosomes in this way ensures that translation never occurs in the nucleus.

The genetic code provides a way for the translation machinery to interpret the sequence information stored in the DNA molecule and represented by mRNA. DNA is a linear sequence of four different kinds of nucleotides, so the simplest code could be one in which each nucleotide specifies a different amino acid—that is, adenine coding for the amino acid glycine, cytosine for lysine, and so on. The first cells may have used this coding system, but it is limited to the construction of proteins consisting of only four different kinds of amino acids. Eventually, a more elaborate code evolved, in which a combination of three out of the four possible DNA nucleotides, called *codons*, specifies a single amino acid. With this scheme it is possible to have a unique code for each of the 20 naturally occurring amino acids. For example, the codon AGC specifies the amino acid serine, whereas TGC specifies the amino acid cysteine. Thus, a gene may be viewed as a long continuous sequence of codons. However, not all codons specify an amino acid. The sequence TGA signals the end of the gene, and a special codon, ATG, signals the start site, in addition to specifying the amino acid methionine. Consequently, all proteins begin with this amino acid, although it is sometimes removed once construction of the protein is complete. As mentioned above, an average protein may consist of 300 to 400 amino acids; since the codon consists of three nucleotides for each amino acid, a typical gene may be 900 to 1,200 nucleotides long.

Power Generation

ATP is produced in mitochondria from AMP or ADP and phosphate (PO_4). This process involves a number of metal-binding proteins called the *respiratory chain* (also known as the *electron transport chain*), and a special ion channel–enzyme called *ATP synthetase*. The respiratory chain consists of three major components: NADH dehydrogenase, cytochrome b, and cytochrome oxidase. All of these components are protein complexes that have an iron (NADH dehydrogenase, cytochrome b) or a copper core (cytochrome oxidase) and, together with the ATP synthetase, are located in the inner membrane of the mitochondria. The respiratory chain is analogous to an electric cable that transports electricity from a hydroelectric dam to our homes, where it is used to turn on lights or to power our stereos. The human body, like that of all animals, generates electricity by processing food molecules through a metabolic pathway called the *Krebs cycle*. The electricity, or electrons so generated, travel through the respiratory chain, and as they do, they power the synthesis of ATP. All electrical circuits must have a ground, that is, the electrons need someplace to go once they have completed the circuit. In the case of the respiratory chain, the ground is oxygen. After passing through the chain, the electrons are picked up by oxygen, which combines with hydrogen ions to form water.

Glycocalyx

This structure is an enormously diverse collection of glycoproteins and glycolipids that covers the surface of every cell, like trees on the surface of the Earth, and has many important functions. All eukaryotes originated from free-living cells that hunted bacteria for food. The glycocalyx evolved to meet the demands of this kind of lifestyle, providing a way for the cell to locate, capture, and ingest food molecules or prey organisms. Cell-surface glycoproteins also form transporters and ion channels that serve as gateways into the cell. Neurons have refined ion channels for the purpose of cell-to-cell communication, giving rise to the nervous systems found in most animal species. In higher vertebrates, certain members of the glycocalyx are used by cells of the immune system as recognition markers to detect invading microbes or foreign cells introduced as an organ or tissue transplant.

Recombinant DNA Primer

Recombinant technology is a collection of procedures that make it possible to isolate a gene and produce enough of it for a detailed study of its structure and function. Central to this technology is the ability to construct libraries of DNA fragments that represent the genetic repertoire of an entire organism or of a specific cell type. Constructing these libraries involves splicing different pieces of DNA together to form a novel or recombinant genetic entity, from which the procedure derives its name. DNA cloning and library construction were made possible by the discovery of DNA-modifying enzymes that can seal two pieces of DNA together or can cut DNA at sequence-specific sites. Many of the procedures that are part of recombinant technology, such as DNA sequencing or filter hybridization, were developed to characterize DNA fragments that were isolated from cells or gene libraries. Obtaining the sequence of a gene has made it possible to study the organization of the genome, but more important, it has provided a simple way of determining the protein sequence and the expression profile for any gene.

DNA-Modifying Enzymes

Two of the most important enzymes used in recombinant technology are those that can modify DNA by sealing two fragments together and others that can cut DNA at specific sites. The first modifying enzyme to be discovered was DNA ligase, an enzyme that can join two pieces of DNA together. It is an important component of the cell's DNA replication and repair machinery. Other DNA modifying enzymes, called *restriction enzymes*, cut DNA at sequence-specific sites, with different members of the family cutting at different sites. Restriction enzymes are isolated from bacteria, and since their discovery in 1970, more than 90 such enzymes have been isolated from more than 230 bacterial strains.

The name "*restriction enzyme*" is cryptic, and calls for an explanation. During the period when prokaryotes began to appear on Earth, their environment contained a wide assortment of molecules that were released into the soil or water by other cells, either deliberately or when the cells died. DNA of varying lengths was among these molecules, and was readily taken up by living cells. If the foreign DNA contained complete genes from a competing bacterial species, there was the real possibility that those genes could have been transcribed and translated by the host cell with potentially fatal results. As a precaution, prokaryotes evolved a set of enzymes that would restrict the foreign DNA population by cutting it up into smaller pieces, before being broken down completely to individual nucleotides.

Gel Electrophoresis

This procedure is used to separate different DNA and RNA fragments in a slab of agar or polyacrylamide subjected to an electric field. Nucleic acids carry a negative charge and thus will migrate toward a positively charged electrode. The gel acts a sieving medium that impedes the movement of the molecules. Thus, the rate at which the fragments migrate is a function of their size; small fragments migrate more rapidly than large fragments. The gel, containing the sample, is submerged in a special pH-regulated solution, or buffer, containing a nucleic acid–specific dye, ethidium bromide. This dye produces a strong reddish-yellow fluorescence when exposed to ultraviolet (UV) radiation. Consequently, after electrophoresis, the nucleic acid can be detected by photographing the gel under UV illumination.

DNA Cloning

In 1973 scientists discovered that restriction enzymes, DNA ligase, and bacterial plasmids could be used to clone DNA molecules. Plasmids are small (about 4,000 base pairs, also expressed as 4.0 kilo base pairs or 4 Kbp) circular mini-chromosomes that occur naturally in bacteria and are often exchanged between cells by passive diffusion. When a bacterium acquires a new plasmid it is said to have been transfected. For bacteria, the main advantage to swapping plasmids is that they often carry antibiotic resistance genes, so that a cell sensitive to ampicillin can become resistant simply by acquiring the right plasmid.

The first cloning experiment used a plasmid from *Escherichia coli* that was cut with the restriction enzyme *Eco*RI. The plasmid had a single *Eco*RI site, so the restriction enzyme simply opened the circular molecule, rather than cutting it up into many useless pieces. Foreign DNA, cut with the same restriction enzyme, was incubated with the plasmid. Because the plasmid and foreign DNA were both cut with *Eco*RI, the DNA could insert itself into the plasmid to form a hybrid, or recombinant plasmid, after which DNA ligase sealed the two together. The reaction mixture was added to a small volume of *E. coli* so that some of the cells could take up the recombinant plasmid before being transferred to a nutrient broth containing streptomycin. Only those cells carrying the recombinant plasmid, which contained an antistreptomycin gene, could grow in the presence of this antibiotic. Each time the cells divided, the plasmid DNA was duplicated along with the main chromosome. After the cells had grown overnight, the foreign DNA had been amplified, or cloned, billions of times and was easily isolated for sequencing or expression studies.

Genomic and cDNA Libraries

The basic cloning procedure described above not only provides a way to amplify a specific piece of DNA, but it can also be used to construct gene libraries. In this case, however, the cloning vector is a bacteriophage, called lambda. The lambda genome is double-stranded linear DNA of about 40 Kbp, much of which can be replaced by foreign DNA without sacrificing the ability of the virus to infect bacteria. This is the great advantage of lambda over a plasmid. Lambda can accommodate very long pieces of DNA, often long enough to contain an entire gene, whereas a plasmid cannot accommodate foreign DNA that is larger than 4 Kbp. Moreover, bacteriophage has the natural ability to infect bacteria, so that the efficiency of transfection is 100 times greater than it is for plasmids.

The construction of a gene library begins by isolating genomic DNA and digesting it with a restriction enzyme to produce fragments of 1,000 to 10,000 base pairs. These fragments are ligated into lambda genomes, which are subjected to a packaging reaction to produce mature viral particles, most of which carry a different piece of the genomic DNA. This collection of viruses is called a *genomic library* and is used to study the structure and organization of specific genes. Clones from such a library contain the coding sequences, in addition to introns, intervening sequences, promoters, and enhancers. An alternative form of gene library can be constructed by isolating mRNA from a specific cell type. This RNA is converted to the complimentary DNA (cDNA) using an RNA-dependent DNA polymerase called reverse transcriptase. The cDNA is ligated to lambda genomes and packaged as for the genomic library. This collection of recombinant viruses is a cDNA library and contains only genes that were being expressed by the cells when the RNA was extracted. It does not include introns or controlling elements, as these are lost during transcription and the processing that occurs in the cell to make mature mRNA. Thus a cDNA library is intended for the purpose of studying gene expression and the structure of the coding region only.

Labeling Cloned DNA

Many of the procedures used in the area of recombinant technology were inspired by the events that occur during DNA replication. This includes the labeling of cloned DNA for use as probes in expression studies, DNA sequencing, and polymerase chain reaction (PCR,). DNA replication involves duplicating one of the strands (the parent, or template strand) by linking nucleotides in an order specified by the template, and depends on a large number of enzymes, the most important of which is DNA polymerase. This enzyme, guided by the template strand, constructs a daughter strand by linking nucleotides together. One such nucleotide is deoxyadenine triphosphate (dATP). Deoxyribonucleotides have a single hydroxyl group located at the 3' carbon of the sugar group, while the triphosphate is attached to the 5' carbon. The procedure for labeling DNA probes, developed in 1983, introduces radioactive nucleotides into a DNA molecule. This method supplies DNA polymerase with a single-stranded DNA template, a primer, and the four nucleotides in a buffered solution to induce in vitro replication. The daughter strand that becomes the probe is labeled by including a nucleotide in the reaction mix that is linked to a radioactive isotope. The radioactive nucleotide is usually deoxycytosine triphosphate (dCTP) or dATP.

Single-stranded DNA hexamers (six bases long) are used as primers, and these are produced in such a way that they contain all possible permutations of four bases taken six at a time. Randomizing the base sequence for the primers ensures that there will be at least one primer site in a template that is only 50 bp long. Templates used in labeling reactions such as this are generally 100 to 800 bp long. This strategy of labeling DNA, known as random primer or oligo labeling, is widely used in cloning and in DNA and RNA filter hybridizations.

DNA Sequencing

A sequencing reaction developed by the British biochemist Dr. Fred Sanger in 1976, DNA sequencing is another technique that takes its inspiration from the natural process of DNA replication. DNA polymerase requires a primer with a free 3' hydroxyl group. The polymerase adds the first nucleotide to this group, and all subsequent bases are added to the 3' hydroxyl of the previous base. Sequencing by the Sanger method is usually performed with the DNA cloned into a plasmid. This simplifies the choice of the initial primers since their sequence can be derived from the known plasmid sequence. An engineered plasmid primer site adjacent to a cloned DNA fragment is shown in the accompanying figure. Once the primer binds to the primer site the cloned DNA may be replicated. Sanger's innovation involved the synthesis of artificial nucleotides lacking the 3' hydroxyl group, thus producing dideoxynucleotides (ddATP, ddCTP, ddGTP and ddTTP). Incorporation of a dideoxynucleotide terminates the growth of the daughter strand at that point, and this can be used to determine the size of each daughter strand. The shortest daughter strand represents the complementary nucleotide at the beginning of the template, whereas the longest strand represents the complementary nucleotide at the end of the template. The reaction products, consisting of all the daughter strands, are fractionated on a polyacrylamide gel. Polyacrylamide serves the same function as agarose. It has the advantage of being a tougher material, essential for the large size of a typical sequencing gel. Some of the nucleotides included in the Sanger reaction are labeled with a radioactive isotope so the fractionated daughter strands can be visualized by drying the gel and then exposing it to X-ray film. Thus, the Sanger

EXAMPLE OF A SEQUENCING REACTION

Tube	Reaction Products	
A	G-C-A-T-C-G-T-C	G-C-A-T-C-G-T-C
	C-G-T-**A**	C-G-T-A-G-C-**A**
T	G-C-A-T-C-G-T-C	
	C-G-T	
C	G-C-A-T-C-G-T-C	G-C-A-T-C-G-T-C
	C	C-G-T-A-G-**C**
	G-C-A-T-C-G-T-C	G-C-A-T-C-G-T-C
G	C-**G**	C-G-T-A-**G**
	G-C-A-T-C-G-T-C	
	C-G-T-A-G-C-A-**G**	

Fig. 12.8. The Sanger sequencing reaction is set up in four separate tubes, each containing a different di-deoxynucleotide.

method uses the natural process of replication to mark the position of each nucleotide in the DNA fragment so the sequence of the fragment can be determined.

The sequence of the daughter strand is read beginning with the smallest fragment at the bottom of the gel, and ending with the largest fragment at the top. The sequence of the template strand is obtained simply by taking the complement of the sequence obtained from the gel (the daughter strand).

Southern and Northern Blotting

One of the most important techniques to be developed, as part of recombinant technology, is the transfer of nucleic acids from an agarose gel to nylon filter paper that can be hybridized to a labeled probe to detect specific genes. This procedure was introduced by the Scottish scientist E. M. Southern in 1975 for transferring DNA and is now known as Southern blotting. Since the DNA is transferred to filter paper, the detection stage is known as filter hybridization. In 1980 the procedure was modified to transfer RNA to nylon membranes for the study of gene expression and, in reference to the original, is called northern blotting. Northern blotting is used to study the expression of specific genes and is usually performed on messenger RNA (mRNA). Typical experiments may wish to determine the expression of specific genes in normal versus cancerous tissue, or in tissues obtained from groups of different ages. The RNA is fractionated on an agarose gel and then transferred to a nylon membrane. Paper towels placed on top of the assembly pull the transfer buffer through the gel, eluting the RNA from the gel and trapping it on the membrane. The location of specific mRNA can be determined by hybridizing the membrane to a radiolabeled cDNA or genomic clone. The hybridization procedure involves placing the filter in a buffer solution containing a labeled probe. During a long incubation period, the probe binds to the target sequence immobilized on the membrane. A-T and G-C base pairing mediate the binding between the probe and target. The double-stranded molecule that is formed is a hybrid, being formed between the RNA target, on the membrane, and the DNA probe.

Fluorescent In Situ Hybridization (FISH)

Studying gene expression does not always depend on northern blots and filter hybridization. In the 1980s scientists found that cDNA probes could be hybridized to DNA or mRNA in situ, that is, while located within cells or tissue sections fixed on microscope slides. In this case the probe is labeled with a fluorescent dye molecule, rather than a radioactive isotope. The samples are then examined and photographed under a fluorescent microscope. FISH is an extremely powerful variation on Southern and northern blots. This procedure gives precise information regarding the identity of a cell that expresses a specific gene, information that usually cannot be obtained with filter hybridization. Organs and tissues are generally composed of many different kinds of cells that cannot be separated from each other using standard biochemical extraction procedures. Histological sections, however, show clearly the various cell types, and when subjected to FISH analysis provide clear results as to which cells express specific genes. FISH is also used in clinical laboratories for the diagnosis of genetic abnormalities.

Polymerase Chain Reaction (PCR)

PCR is simply repetitive DNA replication over a limited, primer defined, region of a suitable template. The region defined by the primers is amplified to such an extent that it can be easily isolated for further study. The reaction exploits the fact that a DNA duplex, in a low salt buffer, will melt (that is, separate into two single strands) at 75°C, but will reanneal (rehybridize) at 37°C. The reaction is initiated by melting the template, in the presence of primers and polymerase in a suitable buffer, cooling quickly to 37°C, and allowing sufficient time for the polymerase to replicate both strands of the template. The temperature is then increased to 75°C to melt the newly formed duplexes and then cooled to 37°C. At the lower temperature more primer will anneal to initiate another round of replication. The heating-cooling cycle is repeated 20 to 30 times, after which the reaction products are fractionated on an agarose gel and photographed. The band containing the amplified fragment may be cut out of the gel and purified for further study. The DNA polymerase used in these reactions is isolated from thermophilic bacteria that can withstand temperatures of 70°C to 80°C. PCR applications are nearly limitless. It is used to amplify DNA from samples containing, at times, no more than a few cells. It can be used to screen libraries and to identify genes that are turned on or off during embryonic development or during cellular transformation.

Gene Therapy Primer

When we get sick it often is due to invading microbes that destroy or damage cells and organs in our body. Cholera, smallpox, measles, diphtheria, AIDS, and the common cold are all examples of what we call an infectious disease. If we catch any of these diseases, our doctor may prescribe a drug that will, in some cases, remove the microbe from our bodies, thus curing the disease. Unfortunately, most of the diseases that we fall prey to are not of the infectious kind. In such case, there are no microbes to fight, no drugs to apply. Instead, we are faced with a far more difficult problem, for this type of disease is an ailment that damages a gene. Gene therapy attempts to cure these diseases by replacing or supplementing the damaged gene.

When a gene is damaged, it usually is caused by a point mutation, a change that affects a single nucleotide. Sickle-cell anemia, a disease affecting red blood cells, was the first genetic disorder of this kind to be described. The mutation occurs in a gene that codes for the β (beta) chain of hemoglobin, converting the codon GAG to GTG, which substitutes the amino acid valine at position 6, for glutamic acid. This single amino-acid substitution is enough to cripple the hemoglobin molecule, making it impossible for it to carry enough oxygen to meet the demands of a normal adult. Scientists have identified several thousand genetic disorders that are known to be responsible for diseases such as breast cancer, colon cancer, hemophilia, and two neurological disorders, Alzheimer's disease and Parkinson's disease.

Gene therapy is made possible by recombinant DNA technology (biotechnology). Central to this technology is the use of viruses to clone specific pieces of DNA. That is, the DNA is inserted into a viral chromosome and is amplified as the virus multiplies. Viruses are parasites that specialize in infecting bacterial and animal cells. Consequently, scientists realized that a therapeutic gene could be inserted into a patient's cells by first introducing it into a virus and then letting the virus carry it into the affected cells. In this context the virus is referred to as the gene therapy delivery vehicle or vector (in recombinant technology it is referred to as a cloning vector).

Commonly used viruses are the retrovirus and the adenovirus. A retrovirus gets its name from the fact that it has an RNA genome that is copied into DNA after it infects a cell. Coronaviruses (cause of the common cold) and the AIDS virus are common examples of retroviruses. The adenovirus (from adenoid, the gland from which the virus was first isolated) normally infects the upper respiratory tract, causing colds and flu-like symptoms. This virus, unlike the retrovirus, has a DNA genome. Artificial vectors called liposomes have also been used that consist of a phospholipid vesicle (bubble) containing the therapeutic gene.

Gene therapy vectors are prepared by cutting the viral chromosome and the therapeutic gene with the same restriction enzyme, after which the two are joined together with a DNA ligase. This recombinant chromosome is packaged into viral particles to form the final vector. The vector may be introduced into cultured cells suffering from a genetic defect, and then returned to the patient from whom they were derived (ex vivo delivery). Alternatively, the vector may be injected directly into the patient's circulatory system (in vivo delivery). The ex vivo procedure is used when the genetic defect appears in white blood cells or in stem cells that may be harvested from the patient and grown in culture.

The in vivo procedure is used when the genetic defect appears in an organ, such as the liver, brain, or pancreas. This is the most common form of gene therapy, but it is also potentially hazardous, because vectors, being free in the circulatory system, may infect a wide range of cells, thus activating an immune response that could lead to widespread tissue and organ damage.

The first gene therapy trial, conducted in 1990, used ex vivo delivery. This trial cured a young patient named Ashi DeSilva of an immune deficiency (adenosine deaminase deficiency) that affects white blood cells. Other trials since then have either been ineffective or were devastating failures. Such a case occurred in 1999, when Jesse Gelsinger, an 18-year-old patient suffering from a liver disease, died while participating in a gene therapy trial. His death was caused by multiorgan failure brought on by the viral vector. In 2002 two children being treated for another form of immune deficiency developed vector-induced leukemia (cancer of the white blood cells). Despite these setbacks, gene therapy holds great promise as a medical therapy, and there are currently more than 600 trials in progress in the United States alone to treat a variety of genetic disorders.

Matching Tissues

A molecular forest called the glycocalyx covers the surface of every cell and has a central role in the process of matching tissues for transplant operations. The glycocalyx consists of a diverse population of treelike glycoproteins and glycolipids that have "trunks" made of protein, or lipid, and "leaves" made of sugar. These molecular trees are embedded in the cell membrane much like the trees of Earth are rooted in the soil. A panoramic view of the glycocalyx, consisting of different kinds of glycoproteins and glycolipids, enhances the impression of a surrealistic forested landscape.

The exact composition of the glycocalyx varies with each individual, much in the way that an Earth forest located at the equator is different from one located in the Northern Hemisphere. The human immune system uses the spatial arrangement of the exposed sugar groups to decide whether a cell is foreign or not. Thus the glycocalyx is like a cell's fingerprint, and if that fingerprint does not pass the recognition test, the cell is destroyed, or forced to commit suicide. Immunologists refer to the glycoproteins and glycolipids in the glycocalyx as cell-surface antigens. The term *antigen* derives from the fact that cell-surface glycoproteins on a foreign cell can generate a response from the immune system that leads to the production of antibodies capable of binding to and destroying the foreign cell.

An extremely important pair of cell-surface glycolipids is known as the A and B antigens. These glycolipids occur on the surface of red blood cells and form the ABO blood group system that determines each individual's basic blood type. The A and B antigens are derived from a third antigen called H, which all individuals possess. Blood type A is produced by the *A* gene, which codes for a glycosyl transferase that adds an N-acetylgalactosamine to the H antigen. Blood type B is produced by a different transferase that places a galactose molecule on the H antigen. Some individuals have both A and B transferases and thus are said to have blood type AB. Individuals with blood type O have neither transferase. In North America, blood types A and O dominate, with A occurring in 41 percent of the population and O in

45 percent. Blood types B and AB are rare, with B occurring at a frequency of 10 percent and AB at only 4 percent. An individual that is blood type A will form antibodies against the B antigen, and therefore cannot receive blood from a type B individual, but can receive blood from type O individuals. Similarly, a type B individual cannot receive blood from someone with blood type A, but can receive it from someone that is type O. Individuals that have blood type AB can receive blood from individuals that have blood types A, B, or O, and therefore such individuals are called universal recipients. On the other hand, people with blood type O can only receive type O blood since they will form antibodies against both A and B antigens. While individuals with type AB blood are universal recipients, individuals with type O blood are called universal donors, because their blood may be given to anyone without fear of invoking an immune response.

The importance of blood type with respect to organ transplantation is best illustrated by the recent case of Jesica Santillan, a 17-year-old girl who required a heart-lung transplant to correct a congenital lung defect that also damaged her heart. On February 7, 2003, physicians at Duke University Hospital in Durham, North Carolina, replaced Jesica's heart and lungs without checking the blood type of the donor. Jesica was blood type O, but the donor was type A. Jesica's immune system rejected the mismatched organs and she lapsed into a deep coma soon after the operation was completed. In a desperate attempt to correct the mistake, Jesica's surgeons replaced the mismatched heart and lungs with organs obtained from a type O donor, but it was too late. Jesica had already suffered severe and irreparable brain damage, and on February 22, 2003, she died.

The A and B antigens, as critically important as they are to the success of transplant surgery, are only two of many thousands of cell-surface antigens that play a role in the rejection of foreign tissue. A second major group of antigens, called the *human leukocyte antigens* (HLA), may in fact number in the millions. These antigens are glycoproteins that cover the surface of virtually every cell in the body; they are called *leukocyte* antigens simply because leukocytes were the cells from which they were originally identified. When faced with this level of complexity, transplant surgeons have had to content themselves with matching only five or six of the most common HLA antigens between the recipient and donor. This, of course, leaves many mismatched antigens, but it seems that some antigens elicit a much stronger immune response than others, an effect that is likely quantitative in nature. That is, a million copies of antigen X will catch the attention of the immune system much more effectively than will 10 copies of antigen Y. By matching the dominant antigens, surgeons hope to avoid what is called the hyperacute immune response, which leads to the immediate destruction of the transplanted organ and death of the patient. It was a hyperacute response brought on by a mismatch of dominant antigens that killed Jesica Santillan. Matching dominant antigens does not mean the transplanted organ is compatible, but only that the patient has a good chance of surviving the first year. Beyond that, the immune system begins a slow, chronic attack on the remaining mismatched antigens, leading to eventual failure of most transplanted organs. The slow chronic attack is responsible for the poor five- and 10-year survival of transplant patients.

Human Genome Project

Sequencing the entire human genome is an idea that grew over a period of 20 years, beginning in the early 1980s. At that time, the DNA sequencing method invented by the British biochemist Fred Sanger, then at the University of Cambridge, was but a few years old and had only been used to sequence viral or mitochondrial genomes. Indeed, one of the first genomes to be sequenced was that of bacteriophage G4, a virus that infects the bacterium *E. coli*. The G4 genome consists of 5,577 nucleotide pairs (or base pairs, abbreviated bp) and was sequenced in Dr. Sanger's laboratory in 1979. By 1982 the Sanger protocol was used by others to sequence the genome of the animal virus SV40 (5,224 bp), the human mitochondrion (16,569 bp), and bacteriophage lambda (48,502 bp). Besides providing invaluable data, these projects demonstrated the feasibility of sequencing very large genomes.

The possibility of sequencing the entire human genome was first discussed at scientific meetings organized by the U.S. Department of Energy (DOE) between 1984 and 1986. A committee appointed by the U.S. National Research Council endorsed the idea in 1988 but recommended a broader program to include the sequencing of the genes of humans, bacteria, yeast, worms, flies, and mice. They also called for the establishment of research programs devoted to the ethical, legal, and social issues raised by human genome research. The program was formally launched in late 1900 as a consortium consisting of coordinated sequencing projects in the United States, Britain, France, Germany, Japan, and China. At about the same time, the Human Genome Organization (HUGO) was founded to provide a forum for international coordination of genomic research.

By 1995 the consortium had established a strategy called hierarchical shotgun sequencing that they applied to the human genome as well as to the other organisms mentioned. With this strategy, genomic DNA is cut into one-megabase (Mb) fragments (that is, each fragment consists of 1 million bases) that are cloned into bacterial artificial chromosomes (BACs) to form a library of DNA fragments. The BAC fragments are partially characterized, then organized into an overlapping assembly called a *contig*. Clones are selected from the contigs for shotgun sequencing. That is, each shotgun clone is digested into small 1,000 bp fragments, sequenced, and then assembled into the final sequence with the aid of computers. Organizing the initial BAC fragments into contigs greatly simplifies the final assembly stage.

Sequencing of the human genome was divided into two stages. The first stage, completed in 2001, was a rough draft that covered about 80 percent of the genome with an estimated size of more than 3 billion bases (also expressed as 3 gigabases, or 3 Gb). The final draft, completed in April 2003, covers the entire genome and refines the data for areas of the genome that were difficult to sequence. It also filled in many gaps that were present in the rough draft. The final draft of the human genome gives us a great deal of information that may be divided into three categories: gene content, gene origins, and gene organization.

Gene Content

Analysis of the final draft has shown that the human genome consists of 3.2 Gb of DNA, which encodes about 30,000 genes (estimates range between 25,000 and 32,000). The estimated number of genes is surprisingly low; many scientists had believed the human genome contained 100,000 genes. By comparison, the fruit fly, *Drosophila*, has 13,338 genes, and the simple roundworm, *Caenorhabditis elegans*, has 18,266. The genome data suggests that human complexity, as compared to the fruit fly or the worm, is not simply due to the absolute number of genes, but involves the complexity of the proteins that are encoded by those genes. In general, human proteins tend to be much more complex than those of lower organisms. Data from the final draft and other sources provides a detailed overview of the functional profile of human cellular proteins.

Gene Origins

Fully one-half of human genes originated as transposable elements, also known as jumping genes. Equally surprising is the fact that 220 of our genes were obtained by horizontal transfer from bacteria, rather than ancestral, or vertical, inheritance. In other words, we obtained these genes directly from bacteria, probably during episodes of infection, in a kind of natural gene therapy, or gene swapping. We know this to be the case because while these genes occur in bacteria they are not present in yeast, fruit flies, or any other eukaryotes that have been tested.

The function of most of the horizontally transferred genes is unclear, although a few may code for basic metabolic enzymes. A notable exception is a gene that codes for an enzyme called *monoamine oxidase* (MAO). Monoamines are neurotransmitters, such as dopamine, norepinephrine, and serotonin, which are needed for neural signaling in the human central nervous system. Monoamine oxidase plays a crucial role in the turnover of these neurotransmitters. How MAO, obtained from bacteria, could have developed such an important role in human physiology is a great mystery.

Gene Organization

In prokaryotes, genes are simply arranged in tandem along the chromosome, with little, if any, DNA separating one gene from the other. Each gene is transcribed into messenger RNA (mRNA), which is translated into protein. Indeed, in prokaryotes, which have no nucleus, translation often begins even before transcription is complete. In eukaryotes, as we might expect, gene organization is more complex. Data from the genome project shows clearly that eukaryote genes are split into subunits called *exons*, and that each exon is separated by a length of DNA called an *intron*. A gene consisting of introns and exons is separated from other genes by long stretches of noncoding DNA called intervening sequences. Eukaryote genes are transcribed into a primary RNA molecule that includes exon and intron sequences. The primary transcript never leaves the nucleus and is never translated into protein. Nuclear enzymes remove the introns from the primary transcript, after which the exons are joined together to form the mature mRNA. Thus, only the exons carry the necessary code to produce a protein.

13

PANCREATIC CANCER

The pancreas is composed of two major compartments: (i) the exocrine pancreas, which consists of the digestive enzyme-producing acinar cells and ducts that conduct these enzymes to the intestines, and (ii) the endocrine pancreas, composed of the hormone-producing cells in the islets of Langerhans. All of these cells arise developmentally from a common endodermally derived pancreas progenitor cell. Tumors arise in the pancreas with the features of the three major cell types of the pancreas: the acinar cells, endocrine cells, and the pancreatic duct cells.

According to the American Cancer Society, an estimated 1,268,000 new cases of cancer were diagnosed in the year 2001, and an estimated 553,400 Americans died from cancer. Pancreatic cancer now ranks fourth and fifth as a cause of cancer death in men and women, respectively, with an estimated incidence of 31,860 cases in the year 2004, and 31,270 deaths. More than 50,000 Europeans are also estimated to die of the disease annually. Pancreatic cancer is highly aggressive and characterized by extensive local invasion and early formation of metastases, which occur mainly in the regional lymph nodes and liver. The overall prognosis for this cancer remains grim, with a 5-year survival rate of only 4%. The mortality rate is nearly identical to the incidence rate, affirming the poor prognosis of this disease.

Unfortunately, more than 90% of patients with pancreatic cancer present with metastatic disease or advanced local disease and are precluded from a curative surgical resection. However, surgical resection remains the only hope for cure, although only 5% of patients are candidates at the time of presentation because of the biologically aggressive nature of these tumors. Even in this group of patients, only 25% can hope to survive for 5 years. Although adjuvant chemotherapy and radiation may allow for some increases in survival, the effectiveness of these treatments is uncertain. In fact, chemotherapy has not resulted in a significant survival benefit, and the 5-year survival rate with this treatment is <1–3% in the United States, with a median survival of 4.1 months. The risk of pancreatic cancer in certain individuals can approach 50%. Considering these data, it is apparent that new molecular targets are needed for the prevention and treatment of pancreatic cancer.

Although pancreatic tumor is manifested most often in a solid, infiltrating pattern, cystic and solid/cystic variants are not uncommon. Even when confined to the pancreas, adenocarcinoma usually carries an unfavorable prognosis because a diagnosis is usually not established until an advanced tumor stage. In these cases, palliative surgery, often associated with significant morbity, and/or chemotherapy is usually required. Because of the deep retroperitoneal location of the pancreas, a less invasive alternative method for establishing a diagnosis of pancreatic carcinoma is *computed tomography* (CT)-guided core biopsy or *fine-needle aspiration* (FNA) biopsy. Percutaneous image-guided FNA is thought to be the most suitable method for tissue diagnosis of this disease before surgery.

The knowledge of molecular alterations in pancreatic cancer has increased significantly during the last decade. For example, alterations have been identified in the *K-ras, p16, p35, DPC4 (Smad 4), COX-2,* and *KAI1* genes. In addition, increased expression of growth factors, growth factor receptors, and cytokines has been identified in pancreatic cancer specimens; one example is neurokinin-1 receptor that stimulates pancreatic cancer cell growth. This *in situ* hybridization and immunohistochemical study suggests a link between the neural system and pancreatic cancer.

Pancreatic Adenocarcinomas

Adenocarcinomas of ductal origin histologically account for ~85–90% of all pancreatic tumors. The World Health Organization recognizes several histomorphologic variants of ductal adenocarcinomas, including mucinous noncystic carcinoma, signet ring carcinoma, adenosquamous carcinoma, undifferentiated (*anaplastic*) carcinoma, undifferentiated carcinoma with osteoclastlike giant cells, and mixed ductal-endocrine carcinoma. These variants are in addition to the classic tubuloglandular ductal adenocarcinomas. Clear-cell carcinoma of the pancreas is characteristically rich in glycogen and poor in mucin. A unique case of infiltrating ductal adenocarcinomas with predominantly clear cell morphology was reported by Ray *et al.* (2004). They suggest that it should be regarded as a rare variant of pancreatic ductal adenocarcinoma.

Pancreatic adenomacarcinoma presents a particular challenge in clinical management because of very poor response to current therapeutic modalities. An understanding of the genetic regulatory pathways involved in this malignancy may provide the necessary targets for therapy. Special efforts have been made to analyze potential precursor lesions of the ductal adenocarcinoma to gain insights into the development of this malignant tumor. An accumulation of inherited and acquired genetic defects results in the neoplastic transformation and progression of this and other carcinomas.

Pancreatic adenocarcinoma has activating mutations in the *K-ras2* oncogene in >90% of cases, as well as loss of the *INK4A* locus that encodes p16 tumor suppressor protein. In addition, *DPC4, TP53,* and *MADH4* tumor suppressor genes are functionally inactivated in ~50% of the cases. These genes may also be affected in precursor lesions. Crnogorac-Jurcevic *et al.* (2003) have listed 29 genes that were up-regulated fourfold or more in pancreatic adenocarcinoma specimens, using complementary deoxyribonucleic acid (cDNA) arrays method. They have also listed 46 genes that were down-regulated at least fourfold or more in similar specimens, using the same method. These data were confirmed by serial analysis of gene expression database and digital differential display.

The molecular information discussed earlier has been integrated into a tumor progression model that is based on the recently proposed classification of putative ductal adenocarcinoma precursor lesions, i.e., *pancreatic intraepithelial neoplasia* (PanIN) grades 1–3, and even in normal-appearing duct epithelium obtained from carcinoma-associated tissue or from nonneoplastic pancreas. They also report noninvolvement of *K-ras* mutations in apoptotic activity in low-grade PanINs, although such mutations may have an effect on proliferation in PanIN-1 and PanIN-2.

Pancreatic adenosquamous carcinoma (PASC) is a rare variant of ductal adenocracinoma and is characterized histologically by variable proportions of classic, often mucin-producing glandular epithelium and malignant squamous epithelium. Like classic ductal adenocarcinomas, PASC carries a poor prognosis. It usually represents a high-grade tumor and demonstrates features of both glandular and squamous differentiation. A specific diagnosis of PASC is feasible when aspirates show evidence of both squamous and glandular differentiation. The diagnosis of PASC and its distinction from squamous cell carcinoma and ductal adenocarcinomas can be made using FNA biopsy.

Mucinous Tumors of the Pancreas

Pancreatic neoplasms associated with significant amounts of extracellular mucin production include mucin-producing ductal adenocarcinoma, *mucinous cystic neoplasm* (MCN), and *intraductal papillary mucinous tumor* (IPMT). Ductal adenocarcinoma is the most common of these tumor types and often develops in older people. It presents as a firm, ill-defined mass usually involving the head of the pancreatic gland. Ductal adenocarcinoma associated with significant mucin production differs from conventional ductal adenocarcinoma.

The MCNs are classified as mucinous cystadenomas, borderline mucinous tumors, or mucinous cystadenocarcinomas, depending on the degree of atypia of the mucinous epithelium lining the cystic spaces. They are uncommon tumors, representing 2–5% of all pancreatic tumors, and occur predominantly in middle-aged women, with a peak incidence in the fourth and fifth decades. Most often MCNs are found in the body and tail of the pancreatic gland and represent unilocular or multilocular cystic masses filled with thick mucoid material and surrounded by an ovarian type of stroma. The cystic mass does not communicate with the pancreatic duct system.

The IPMTs are characterized by dilation of the main pancreatic duct or its branches, which are filled with mucus and lined by papillary proliferation of the epithelial lining encompassing varying degrees of atypia. Unlike MCNs, IPMTs are more common in men and occur mainly in the sixth and seventh decades of life.

Intraductal Papillary Mucinous Tumors

The IPMTs are classified as adenoma, borderline, or malignant based on the degree of epithelial dysplasia present. Malignant IPMTs are further subclassified into noninvasive and invasive. In the IPMT, dilated pancreatic ducts and ductules are lined by tall columnar mucin-producing neoplastic epithelial cells. Pathologic and clinical features of IPMTs are entirely different from those of the pancreatic duct cell carcinoma. The prognosis is usually good but depends on the presence of invasive carcinoma. Operative strategy should be based on routine frozen sections of the surgical margin and perioperative endoscopic examination of the Wirsung duct with staged intraductal biopsies when technically feasible.

Some information is available regarding the genetic alterations that occur in the IPMTs. A number of examples are presented later. Using polymerase chain reaction (PCR)-based microsatellite analysis, loss of heterozygosity was detected at chromosomal sites 6q, 8p, 9p, 17p, and 18q in IPMT, suggesting that targeted genetic inactivation may occur at these loci. *DPC4* (*MADH4, SMAD4*) is a tumor-suppressor gene on chromosome 18q. This gene is genetically inactivated in ~55% of pancreatic adenocarcinomas. However, immunohistochemical studies demonstrate that *DPC4* inactivation, detected as loss of DPC4 protein expression, is an infrequent event in IPMT. This evidence contrasts with the important role that DPC4 inactivation has been shown to play in the progression of conventional pancreatic ductal adenocarcinoma. The difference in DPC4 protein expression between IPMT and ductal carcinomas suggests a fundamental genetic difference in tumorigenesis of these two types of pancreatic tumors.

Pancreatic Neuroendocrine Tumors

Pancreatic neuroendocrine tumors (PNTs) represent less than 10% of all pancreatic tumors. Routine histologic examination is usually not predictive of their behavior. These tumors are diagnosed at an advanced stage because they usually manifest few symptoms except when there is a hormone syndrome associated with them. Although infrequent, PNTs can cause acute pancreatitis even in patients younger than 50 years.

Capella *et al.* (1995) have classified neuroendocrine tumors of the pancreas, lung, and gut to assess tumor prognosis in terms of the degree of differentiation and the predominant cell type as well as tumor size; the presence or absence of a clinical syndrome; and the degree of local, vascular, and/or metastatic involvement. Histologic and immunohistochemical studies confirm this classification, which is very useful in routine practice for predicting the behavior of PNT.

Acinar Cell Carcinomas

Acinar cell carcinomas (ACCs) are rare neoplasms of the exocrine pancreas, comprising less than 1% of primary pancreatic tumors. The ACCs are distinct from the more common pancreatic ductal adenocarcinomas. The prognosis of ACCs is poor because the majority of patients show evidence of metastatic disease either at or subsequent to diagnosis; the mean survival is ~18 months after diagnosis.

Genetic alterations, such as *K-ras* oncogene and *p53* and *DPC4* tumor-suppressor genes, have been either absent or only rarely present in ACCs, although aneuploidy and ACC allelotype are present. Allelic loss on chromosome 11p is the most common genetic alteration in the ACC. In contrast, activation of *K-ras* oncogene and inactivation of *DPC4* and *p53* are common in conventional pancreatic ductal adenocarcinomas. This difference indicates that ACC is genetically distinct from pancreatic ductal adenocarcinomas. It is interesting to note that morphologic, immunohistochemical, and clinical features of ACC overlap with those of another rare pancreatic neoplasm, pancreatoblastoma.

Biomarkers for Pancreatic Cancer

It is established that gene mutations confer increased risk of cancer. The majority of mutations found in tumor cells occur in signal transduction pathways that ultimately regulate transcription factors involving a large number of genes and their transcription patterns. Therefore, abnormalities in gene expression are characteristic of neoplastic tissues. Adenocarcinomas are correlated with specific sequential genetic mutations. Although the total accumulation of mutations is the principal factor in most cancers, the causative mutations in tumor-suppressor genes and oncogenes occur in a specific order. However, cancer is an exceedingly complex disease that refers to conditions that emerge as a result of the interaction of genes and environment. Genes impart susceptibility or protection, which is neither necessary nor sufficient for disease to develop. Environmental factors are required, and these can promote, delay, or prevent disease. Not only gene–enviroment interactions but also gene–gene interactions (e.g., p53-mdm 2) play a role in complex disease genetics.

Despite improved diagnostic and therapeutic modalities, pancreatic cancer still has a very poor prognosis with a 5-year survival rate of less than 5%. Pancreatic cancer is usually advanced at the time of presentation, but the detection of premalignant pancreatic lesions and earlier detection of malignant pancreatic lesions should improve the clinical outcome of the disease. It is known that pancreatic cancer progression from normal ductal and ductular epithelium to cancer results from a series of lesions (termed PanIN). Recognition of biomarkers in early pancreatic neoplastic ductal lesions can provide effective new diagnostic and treatment approaches. Advances in molecular genetics have resulted in a significant increase in current knowledge regarding the genetic events associated with pancreatic tumorigenesis. Further characterization of the molecular changes associated with tumor initiation and progression will elucidate the essential cellular pathways responsible for maintaining noncancerous states. Such information will identify novel, effective, therapeutic and diagnostic strategies. Molecular characterization of tumors will also provide clinically useful information for guiding further therapy after surgical resections.

Like most other cell types, pancreatic cells experience a constant barrage of mutations. Many of such mutations are irrelevant unless the function of a critical gene is lost or an oncogene is activated. In other words, sequential accumulations of genetic alterations including the activation of oncogene and the inactivation of tumor-suppressor genes play a central role in the development of cancer. Somatic inactivation of a tumor-suppressor gene is usually caused by an intragenic mutation in one allele of the gene with subsequent loss of chromosomal region that spans the second allele. Such an affected cell has growth advantage over normal cells with subsequent clonal expansion. It has been clear that up-regulation and/or down-regulation of certain genes initiates pancreatic cancer. Detailed immunohistochemical and *in situ* hybridization methods for analyzing the following markers for pancreatic cancers are presented: *K-ras* protooncogene, p27 protein, cyclooxygenase-2, synaptic vesicle protein, activated stat3 protein, transcription factor E2F-1, maspin, chromogranins, DUSP6/MKP-3, carbohydrate antigens, mucins, mast cells, and endocrine cells.

The pancreas can contain several different types of tumors with distinct genetic profiles and clinical behavior. Furthermore, genetic alterations are not always the same in different areas of the pancreatic tumor or in the sites with same histologic dysplasia in each tumor. This means that the tumor is hetrogenous, and the pattern of association of histologic features with genetic alterations differs from tumor to tumor.

Table 13.1. Types of pancreatic tumors and their mutations

Tumor types	*Mutations*
Acinar cell carcinoma	APC/β-catenin
Ductal adenocarcinoma	KRAS, SMAD, TP53, CDKN1A
Pancreatic endocrine tumors	MEN1
Serous cystadenoma	VHL

Importance of Biomarkers

Although pancreatic cancer is fairly well-characterized at the histopathologic level, the molecular mechanisms leading to cell transformation are beginning to be elucidated. Identification of key players in the process of cellular transformation is a crucial step toward our understanding of pancreatic cancer progression and toward the development of new, effective cancer therapies. There is an urgent need for determining such players (pancreatic cancer biomarkers). The use of inherited genetic markers to evaluate pancreatic cancer outcome could enhance our ability to identify those persons who are more likely to develop clinically significant pancreatic cancer and to intervene in these persons to reduce morbidity resulting from this disease.

Biomarkers are molecules detectable in the primary tumor, metastatic lesions, blood, or bodily fluids of patients with cancer, providing diagnostic, prognostic, or predictive information. The detection of clinically useful tumor markers whose expression predicts tumor stage or clinical outcome is an important priority in cancer research. The identification of markers is a major advance in the understanding of cancer because their alterations result in a high predisposition to malignancy. The elucidation of the effect of candidate tumor markers can be used to derive biological insight regarding the mechanisms underlying tumor initiation and progression. Furthermore, early detection of a marker can lead to prevention of certain cancers.

Another important advantage of detecting markers is to elucidate their behavior when tumors are exposed to the stress of cytotoxic therapy.

Proportions of cells expressing a particular marker profile in a heterogeneous tumor can change in response to this stress. The question is: Will identifying or targeting altered marker expression in response to cytotoxic therapy be of prognostic or therapeutic value? Such information is available with regard to some markers. For example, the short half-life of the p53 protein is substantially increased following genotoxic stress such as irradiation- and chemically induced DNA damage. It has been shown that radiation-induced DNA damage causes *p53* to arrest the cell cycle in G1 or (depending on cell type and external stimuli) triggers apoptosis.

Ideally, a tumor marker should have clinical utility in the management of cancer. For a marker to be clinically relevant, it must be notably overexpressed or underexpressed in the majority of the tumor samples of a given histology. For a marker to have prognostic significance, it should also show expression alterations concordant with tumor stage or clinical outcome. A number of prognostic biomarkers for pancreatic cancer, with varying degrees of specificity, have been determined. Although most of them have not demonstrated clinical utility as yet, most have proved to be useful for diagnosis, whereas some require further testing. The expression of most of them can be assessed with reliability in formalin-fixed and paraffin-embedded pancreatic tissue specimens, using immunohistochemistry (IHC) or flourescence *in situ* hybridization (FISH). It should be noted that some of these markers (e.g., *p53, BRCA2*, and *HER-2*) are involved not only in pancreatic cancer but also in other cancers such as breast cancer and ovarian cancer. Despite the multitargets of a biomarker, immunohistochemical specificity can be obtained by using monoclonal antibodies.

The identification of tumor markers, however, is not a simple biological problem. Unlike clonal cell cultures, the molecular analysis of human tissue specimens necessarily involves heterogeneous cell populations whose messenger ribonucleic acid (mRNA) composition is proportionally complex. Similarly, the variability in gene expression from one individual tissue sample to another is substantial and may obscure common patterns of gene expression that are predictive of clinical outcome. Furthermore, because a gene may be responsible for a variety of tumor types, its value as an independent prognostic factor is considerably diminished. For example, *p53* amplification is not likely to be an independent marker for pancreatic cancer. Mutations of *p53* occur not only in pancreatic cancer but also in many other cancers including endometrial and ovarian cancers. Genes exert different effects in different populations (genetic heterogeneity). Therefore, identifying the targets, developing target-specific interventions, and validating biological effects of an intervention are daunting tasks. Molecular target expression is certainly a dynamic phenomenon. Nevertheless, the future of oncology undoubtedly involves the detection, validation, and targeting of tumor-specific molecules. In fact, cancer risk assessment has developed into a distinct discipline.

The question is: To what extent it is possible to predict phenotypes from genotypes? This can be accomplished relatively easily for monogenic diseases such as genetic disorders of hemoglobin (e.g., thalassemias), muscular dystrophy (muscle weakness), cystic fibrosis, Gaucher's disease, and familial adenomatous polyposis. In contrast, attempts to identify the genes in the multigenic diseases are fraught with difficulty. These diseases include diabetes and asthma. A wide variety of approaches is being used to dissect the genetic factors in these diseases. Many different classes of genetic markers have been used, including candidate genes, microsatellite DNA, and *single nucleotide polymorphisms* (SNPs). A closely integrated partnership between the clinical and basic biomedical sciences is needed.

The era of molecular medicine for cancer has dawned. Progress in cancer prevention and early cancer detection will be delayed by the failure to adopt a critical and nondogmatic approach to the pathogenesis of cancer. The advent of DNA chip technology will catalyze the development of revised paradigms. Specifically, modern genomics will allow cancers to be grouped within pathogenic pathways on the basis of shared gene expression profiles.

Biomarkers

Most of the well-known genes (biomarkers) and their products involved in pancreatic cancer are discussed next. A large number of up-regulated and down-regulated genes in pancreatic adenocarcinoma specimens is also presented by Crnogorac-Jurcevic *et al.* (2003).

ADAM9

ADAM9 is a member of the large family of proteases that are type I transmembrane proteins with both metalloproteinase and disintegrin–containing extracellular domains. The ADAMs are involved in modulating cell–cell and cell–matrix interactions. ADAM9 is one of the genes that is overexpressed in pancreatic ductal adenocarcinomas, in comparison with normal pancreatic tissues. Overexpression of this gene also occurs in prostate, breast, and liver cell carcinomas. ADAM9 may exert its action via its disintegrin domain, its metalloproteinase domain, or both. Various matrix metalloproteinases (e.g., MMP2 and MMP9) have been described as being overexpressed in pancreatic ductal adenocarcinomas and seem to play an important role in the progression of this carcinoma.

Immunohistochemical studies demonstrate that ADAM9 is overexpressed in pancreatic ductal adenocarcinomas but not in endocrine tumors or ACCs. Pancreatic ductal adenocarcinomas showing cytoplasmic ADAM9 expression correlate with poor tumor differentiation as well as with shorter overall survival than in cases showing only an apical membranous staining pattern. Cytoplasmic ADAM9 overexpression is thought to be a useful diagnostic marker and could be used as a potential target in the treatment of pancreatic ductal adenocarcinomas.

BRAF

BRAF is a member of the RAS-RAF-MEK-ERKMAP kinase growth signal transduction system. The three RAF genes (BRAF is one of them) code for cytoplasmic serine/threonine kinases, which are regulated by binding to RAS. Regarding these three RAF genes, BRAF somatic missense mutations are found in 66% of malignant melanomas and at a lower frequency in a wide range of human cancers. All mutations are found within the kinase domain, with a single substitution (V599E) accounting for 80%. Mutated BRAF proteins also have elevated kinase activity and could transform NIH3T3 cells. Mutated K-ras constitutively activates the RAF-MEK-ERK-MAP kinase system, which is linked to cell growth stimulation. Because up to 90% of pancreatic cancers show active *K-ras* mutation (codon 12), activation of the RAS-RAF-MEK-ERK-MAP kinase pathway may be critically important for pancreatic cells to be transformed to cancer cells. In fact, BRAF V599E mutation is an important mutation in pancreatic cancers, provided *K-ras* codon 12 mutation is also present.

BRCA2

BRCA2 is a tumor-suppressor gene that participates in DNA damage repair. There is an increased risk of pancreatic cancer development in patients with germline BRCA2 mutations. Goggins *et al.* (1996) evaluated 41 pancreatic adenocarcinomas, and 15 demonstrated loss of heterozygosity at BRCA2, and 4 harbored mutations. Germline BRCA2 mutations were responsible for 7.3% of inactivating events, including that both germline (hereditary) and sporadic (nonhereditary) events play a role in pancreatic cancer development.

Extensive studies have been carried out to elucidate the comparative role of BRCA2 germline mutations and sporadic mutations in families with familial pancreatic cancer. The term familial pancreatic cancer is applied to families with at least two first-degree relatives with pancreatic ductal adenocarcinoma but that do not fulfill the criteria for other familial cancer syndromes. The risk for pancreatic carcinoma developing among first-degree relatives of a patient with pancreatic cancer is estimated to be 18-fold in people with two affected family members and as high as 57-fold in people with three or more affected family members.

The majority of pancreatic cancer cases are sporadic. It is estimated that ~10% of patients with pancreatic cancer may have an inherited form of the disease. To study the relationship between BRCA2 germline mutations and familial pancreatic cancer, Hahn *et al.* (2003) identified 26 European families in which at least two first-degree relatives had a histologically confirmed diagnosis of pancreatic ductal adenocarcinoma. They sequenced genomic DNA isolated from peripheral blood lymphocytes obtained from these family members to identify germline mutations in BRCA2. This study supports an important role for BRCA2 germline mutations in a subpopulation of families with familial pancreatic cancer. Based on this and other studies, it is recommended that BRCA2 mutation analysis be included in molecular genetic testing and counseling strategies in families with at least two first-degree relatives affected with ductal adenocarcinoma of the pancreas.

Cartilage Oligomeric Matrix Protein

Cartilage oligomeric matrix protein (COMP) is a member of the thrombospondin family of extracellular glycoproteins. This protein is found in articular nasal cartilage, tracheal cartilage, and tendons. In the growth plate, COMP is primarily observed in the proliferative region, indicating a role in cell growth and matrix development. Immunohistochemical and *in situ* hybridization studies have been carried out for investigating COMP mRNA and protein in normal pancreatic tissues, chronic pancreatic tissues, and cultured pancreatic cancer cells. (Chronic pancreatitis is an inflammatory disease of the pancreas characterized histomorphologically by progressive development of fibrosis and atrophy of the pancreatic parenchyma.) These studies indicate that COMP is preferentially expressed in degenerating acinar cells in chronic pancreatitis and in chronic pancreatitis-like areas in pancreatic cancer, suggesting a potential role of this gene in the course of acinar cell degeneration and dedifferentiation.

Although COMP is not a disease-specific marker for chronic pancreatitis, because it is also present in chronic pancreatitis-like changes in pancreatic cancer tissues, the marker may serve as an important progression marker to monitor the activity of tissue destruction in chronic pancreatitis.

CDKN2A

Loss of CDKNA2 tumor-suppressor gene and its function, as a result of mutation, deletion, or promoter hypermethylation, occurs in 80–90% of sporadic pancreatic adenocarcinomas. Loss of heterozygosity occurs at chromosome 9q21. The inheritance of mutant CDKN2A alleles confer a 13-fold increased risk of pancreatic cancer. Loss of this gene is seen in moderately advanced lesions that show features of dysplasia. The tumor-suppressor locus at 9q21 encodes two tumor suppressors: INK4A and ARF via distinct first exons and alternative reading frames in shared downstream exons. Many pancreatic cancers sustain loss of both the INK4A and ARF transcripts. INK4A is thought to be the more important pancreatic-cancer suppressor at this locus. Loss of INK4A usually occurs only in later stages of pancreatic neoplasia. Because INK4A is implicated in the cellular response to DNA damage *in vivo*, the absence of INK4A might contribute to the chemo-resistance of pancreatic adenocarcinoma.

Cyclooxygenase-2

Most pancreatic neoplasms are adenocarcinomas, which are the most lethal malignancies. Cyclooxygenase-2 (COX-2) is expressed in adenocarcinomas of the human pancreas. Quantitative reverse transcription (RT)-PCR, immunoblotting, and IHC have been used for assessing the expression of COX-2 in this tumor. This study showed an increase of ~60-fold in the level of COX-2 mRNA in the pancreatic cancer compared to that in the adjacent nontumorous tissue. Also, COX-2 protein was commonly present in the adenocarcinoma of the pancreas but was absent in the nontumorous pancreatic tissue. It means that COX-2 is up-regulated in pancreatic cancer. Mutations in the *Ki-ras* oncogene are common in pancreatic cancer. Levels of COX-2 are increased in *Ras*-transformed epithelial cells.

Therefore, activation of the *Ras* pathways contributes to the upregulation of COX-2 in this cancer. These results suggest that COX-2 may be a target for the prevention or treatment of pancreatic cancer. It should be noted that COX-2 expression is also up-regulated in a variety of other human cancers, including colon, lung, gastric, and esophageal cancer. Biological consequences of such up-regulation include inhibition of apoptosis, increase in metastatic potential, and promotion of angiogenesis.

Cysteine-Rich Secretory Protein-3

Human cysteine-rich secretory protein-3 (CRISP-3: SGP28) is the third member of the cysteine-rich secretory protein family. This protein has been detected in several types of human tissues, with predominance in the pancreas, prostate, and salivary gland. The distribution of CRISP-3 in gastrointestinal tissues is predominantly in the pancreas. *In situ* hybridization and immunohistochemical analysis reveal high levels of CRISP-3 in acinar cells differentiating into small proliferating ductal cells in chronic pancreatitis and chronic pancreatitis-like lesions in pancreatic cancer, suggesting a role of this protein in the pathophysiology of chronic pancreatitis. In contrast, CRISP-3 expression is weak to absent in the cytoplasm of cancer cells as well as in acinar cells and ductal cells in pancreatic cancer tissues and normal pancreatic tissues.

In vivo studies have shown that CRISP-3 is under androgen control in the salivary gland. Studies of the androgen profile in patients with chronic pancreatitis and pancreatic cancer have revealed that serum testosterone, dihydrotestosterone, and androstanediol glucuronide levels are significantly lower in patients with pancreatic cancer compared to patients with chronic pancreatitis. This changed androgen profile might contribute to the differential expression of CRISP-3 in chronic pancreatitis and pancreatic cancer.

Cystic Fibrosis Transmembrane Conductance Regulator

Cystic fibrosis transmembrance conductance regulator (CFTR) gene is associated with a wide spectrum of respiratory and pancreatic disorders as well as classically defined cystic fibrosis. Several mutations of CFTR, such as F508del, G542X, and N1303K, are associated with severe cystic fibrosis phenotypes and display high disease penetrance. Many other mutations of CFTR are associated with monosymptomatic diseases of lung, pancreas, or vas deferens, which show partial penetrance. Recent studies indicate that CFTR mutations of M470V-Q1352H, IVS8T5-M470V, and E217G are associated with bronchiectasis and chronic pancreatitis. Defects in CFTR-dependent ion transport are an important aggravating factor in the disease development or progression in addition to other genetic and environmental factors. Mutations of CFTR gene are not independent markers for the diagnosis of chronic pancreatitis.

DPC4

DPC4 (Smad 4) tumor-suppressor gene is deleted in 50% of pancreatic cancers.

Epidermal Growth Factor Receptor

The human epidermal growth factor receptor (EGFR), a 170-kDa transmembrane glycoprotein, is a member of a family of tyrosine kinase receptors that are characterized by an extracellular domain, a transmembrane region, and a cytoplasmic domain. The EGFR was one of the first cellular molecules identified to play a fundamental role in the regulation of cell proliferation, differentiation, and tumorigenesis. It is also involved in tumor angiogenesis, a critical step in the progression of pancreatic tumors as well as other tumors. The activity of angiogenesis depends on the net effects of stimulatory and inhibitory factors secreted by the tumor and its microenvironment. The EGFR is one of these stimulatory factors. The EGFR has the ability of transforming normal cells to a neoplastic phenotype when it is expressed at a high level or when an activation mutation is introduced into it. It is known that overexpression of this receptor accompanied by production of one or more of its ligands is a characteristic feature of a large number of human epithelial tumors, including tumors of the pancreas, brain, urinary bladder, prostate, lung, breast, ovaries, and head and neck. Changes in the expression and activity of the EGFR correlate with continued proliferation of many types of malignant cells. Clinical studies have shown that coexpression of EGFR and epidermal growth factor (EGF) or transforming growth factor (TGF)-α is associated with increased tumor size, advanced clinical stage, and decreased survival of patients. Both EGF and TGF-α are potent inducers of vascular endothelial growth factor (VEGF), the most effective angiogenesis stimulator in human cancer.

Because EGFR is a tumor-associated surface antigen and rarely is expressed on normal tissue cells, it presents an appropriate target for immunotherapy. Blockade of EGFR not only abrogates its effect on cell proliferation but also inhibits angiogenesis. Therefore, such blockade provides a novel strategy for the treatment of cancer, including pancreatic carcinoma. This strategy comprises the application of monoclonal antibodies, immunotoxins, and tyrosine kinase inhibitors. The selectivity of the monoclonal antibodies for the pancreatic tumor does not seem to affect normal cells expressing EGFR. Currently, several phase II and III clinical trials with EGFR inhibitor IMC-C225 are under way, justifying the EGFR as a suitable target for therapy of pancreatic carcinoma. Xiong and Abbruzzese (2002) have also used IMC-C225 in combination with gemcitabine for patients with advanced pancreatic cancer in a phase II clinical trial. This therapy induced apoptosis and suppressed proliferation of tumor cells.

It should be noted that immunohistochemical expression of EGFR and TGF-α, either alone or in concert, does not show any correlation with size, functional status, secretory profile, or biological behavior in the pancreatic endocrine tumors. Hence, expression of these factors cannot be used as a marker of malignancy in this group of pancreatic tumors. Some information is available regarding the use of immunotoxins. It is known that the chimeric (mouse/human) anti-EGFR is very effective in suppressing the growth of pancreatic tumors. Bruell *et al*. (2003) have demonstrated the elimination of the metastatic pancreatic cancer cell line L3.6 pl *in vitro* after incubation with the recombinant anti-EGFR immunotoxin 425(scFv)-ETA. The use of this immunotoxin in *in vivo* studies in a mouse model is awaited.

Hypoxia-Inducible Factor-1 Alpha

Growth of malignant epithelial tumors is limited to only several square millimeters in the absence of neoangiogenesis because of insufficient oxygen and glucose diffusion from blood vessels. Neoangiogenesis and cellular adaptation to hypoxia are therefore essential events for cancer progression. One of the key factors involved in this adaptation is hypoxia-inducible factor-1 alpha (HIF-1α). This is a basic helix–loop–helix–Per–AHR/Arnt–Sim homology sequence transcription factor that plays a major role in cellular oxygen homeostasis. This factor transactivates genes whose protein products function either to increase O_2 availability or to allow metabolic adaptation to O_2 deprivation. These genes include VEGF and insulin-like growth factor 2. Protein products of these genes are implicated in tumor progression, and overexpression of HIF-1α has been demonstrated in a variety of human malignancies. Overexpression of HIF-1α has been reported in pancreatic carcinoma *in vivo* and *in vivo*.

Kitada *et al.* (2003) have investigated the expression of HIF-1α protein in primary and metastatic pancreatic cancer tissues using IHC. This study has demonstrated a significant association between HIF-1α expression and certain clinicopathologic parameters (cell proliferation, microvessel density, tumor size, and advanced TNM stage) known to be prognostic factors in pancreatic carcinoma. It is concluded that HIF-1α can be used as a therapeutic target in pancreatic ductal carcinoma.

Id Protein

Id proteins are members of a family of basic helix–loop–helix (bHLH) transcription factors lacking the DNA-binding domain and are inhibitors of differentiation. Therefore, they act as dominant negative regulators of HLH proteins by forming transcriptionally inactive Id-bHLH protein complexes. Id proteins play important roles in the regulation of cell differentiation during neurogenesis, lymphoiesis, and angiogenesis. Their functions also include promotion of cell growth and cell cycle progression and apoptotic induction. Id proteins, in addition, can induce cell proliferation, increase DNA synthesis, and immortalize mammalian cells in association with other oncogenes.

Id protein overexpression has been found in a number of primary human cancers including cervical, breast, prostate, skin, and pancreatic cancers. Moreover, Id-1 protein is an essential factor in the promotion of G1/S cell-cycle transition in certain cancers by inactivating p16 and increasing cDK4 activity/RB. Several lines of evidence strongly suggest that these proteins have a potential role in the aggressiveness of malignant tumors and formation of tumor angiogenesis. It has been demonstrated that Id-I is significantly overexpressed in pancreatic cancer but not in chronic pancreatitis, suggesting that this protein may be associated with the enhanced proliferative potential of pancreatic cancer cells. Immunohistochemical studies have demonstrated overexpression of Id-1 in human primary pancreatic cancer, which is closely related to tumor angiogenesis. Thus, Id-1 can be used as a target molecule for antiangiogenic drug design in pancreatic cancer treatment.

Integrin

Transmembrane receptors of the integrin family mediate dynamic cell-adhesion processes. Integrins can mediate signaling entering the cell or leaving the cell, these signals play principal roles in various aspects of tumor biology, such as growth, differentiation, invasion, and metastasis formation. Increased expression of laminin-binding integrins or decreased expression of fibronectin-binding integrins is correlated with aggressive growth and metastatic potential in several types of tumors, including human pancreatic carcinoma.

It is also known that human metastatic pancreatic cancer cells express interleukin-1α (IL-1α) mRNA. Immunohistochemical studies have demonstrated that enhanced integrin $\alpha_6\beta_1$ levels by IL-lα signaling is an important determinant of metastasis formation in pancreatic cancer. Expression of both integrin $\alpha_6\beta_1$ and IL-1α is increased in pancreatic cancer, and both play important roles in metastasis formation. Such expression might provide valuable prognostic information for treatment strategies. The role of another component of extracellular matrix, cartilage oligomeric matrix protein, in pancreatic cancer is also discussed in this chapter.

Interleukin-8

Interleukin-8 (IL-8) is a member of the CXC chemokine family and has a wide range of proinflammatory effects. This protein is expressed in normal cells such as monocytes and fibroblasts as well as several types of tumor cells, including pancreas cancer cells. Two receptors for IL-8, CXCR1 and CXCR2, have been identified. Both receptors bind to IL-8 with high affinity. The role of these receptors in pancreatic cancer is presented later.

The protein IL-8 can act multifunctionally to induce angiogenesis and proliferation of pancreatic carcinoma. Immunohistochemical and RT-PCR analysis have shown overexpression of IL-8 and its receptors in pancreatic cancer. This study also suggests that IL-8 regulates matrix metalloproteinase in supernatants of the PANC-1 human pancreatic cancer cell lines. A Vectastain Elite ABC kit was used to perform IHC; antibodies used were a rabbit polyclonal antibody (1:100 dilution) for IL-8 and a rabbit polyclonal antibody (1:200 dilution) for CXCR1 and CXCR2.

KOC

KOC is one of the differentially expressed genes in pancreatic cancer. It encodes a protein with four K-homologous (KH) domains, which are overexpressed in pancreatic cancer. These domain-containing proteins are involved in fundamental biological processes such as development, cell growth, differentiation, and carcinogenesis. KOC is thought to play a role in the regulation of tumor cell proliferation by interfering with transcriptional or post-transcriptional processes. Mueller *et al.* (2002) have used the KOC assay for detecting malignant cells in aspirates of fluids containing ascites, liver fluid, cerebrospinal fluid, and pancreatic and mediastinal cysts. This assay could be useful to facilitate screening for malignant disease and to improve the diagnostic accuracy of fine-needle aspirates.

K-rasGene

One of the most frequent types of protooncogene activation is the *ras* protooncogene activation. The family of these genes has three well-characterized members (H*ras*, K-*ras*, and N-*ras*). The K-*ras* protooncogene located at chromosome 12p codes for a 21-kDa guanosine triphosphate (GTP) binding protein (p21 *ras*) that is involved in the signal transduction of activated tyrosine kinase cell membrane receptors to downstream signal cascades. Activation of this gene usually results from point mutations at codons 12, 13, or 16, causing the oncogenic *ras* protein to be in a permanently active GTP-bound state. In fact, *ras* group of proteins functions as a part of the membrane-associated signal-transduction pathway of GTP-binding proteins. Once activated, these proteins code for key mediators in a number of pathways regulating cell growth and differentiation. In other words, *ras* functions as a molecular switch in a network of intracellular signaling pathways, mainly controlling cell differentiation or proliferation.

Ras-activating mutations result in constitutive signaling, stimulating not only cell proliferation but also apoptosis inhibition. However, according to Lüttges *et al.* (2003), K-*ras* mutations are not involved in apoptotic activity. They suggested that in PanIN there is a relationship between K-*ras* mutations and proliferation but not between mutated K-*ras* and apoptosis or apoptotic markers. Cells carrying K-*ras* mutations therefore may not be eliminated but persist as dormant cells until an additional genetic hit triggers further malignant transformation. Alterations of the apoptotic pathway are thought to be late events in pancreatic cancerogenesis. According to these scientists, molecular pathology and epidemiologic studies suggest that wild-type K-*ras* carcinomas of the pancreas may arise through a genetic pathway distinct from that involved in carcinomas that harbor a K-*ras* mutation only.

Nevertheless, oncogene *ras* mutations are one of the fundamental initiating events in several types of cancers, including pancreatic carcinoma. In fact, K-*ras* is the most commonly altered gene in pancreatic cancers. High frequencies of *K-ras* gene mutation in the adenomas, borderline tumors, and carcinomas of mucin-producing tumors of the pancreas indicate that this mutation is a common and early event in these tumors. At diagnosis, pancreatic tumors show the highest prevalence of K-*ras* mutations of all human cancers, ranging from 75–85%. K-*ras* point mutations are found in ~90–95% of all pancreatic ductal adenocarcinomas and represent the earliest known genetic alterations in premalignant or precursor lesions. K-*ras* mutations are involved in the entire progression of pancreatic carcinogenesis, including early and late stages. Almost all K-*ras* mutations occur in codon 12.

Because up to 90% of pancreatic cancers show active K-*ras* mutation, activation of the RAS-RAF-MEK-ERK-MAP kinase pathway is critically important for pancreatic cells to be transformed to cancer cells. This pathway mediates cellular responses to growth signals. It is concluded that K-*ras* oncogene is strongly associated with the tumorigenesis of pancreatic cancers, because mutations of this gene at codon 12 are detected at a level (up to 90%) higher than in other cancers. Accumulated evidence indicates that K-*ras* mutations play an important role in the development of premalignant stages not only in the pancreas but also in other cancers such as stomach cancer. This information can be translated into effective chemopreventive and therapeutic strategies.

Although K-*ras* mutations are important initiating events, inactivation of the *Rb-1, p16*, and *p53* tumor-suppressor genes, as well as the *Smad* genes, are also important in pancreatic tumor development and progression, which are discussed later in this chapter. Unlike ductal adenocarcinoma, pancreatic acinar carcinomas frequently contain alterations in the *APC* or *CTNNB1* genes, which lead to deregulated Wnt signaling but do not harbor mutations in the K-*ras, p16, p53,* and *Smad* genes. Indeed, it has been suggested that the mutation in K-*ras* may require combination with inactivation of one or more of these genes to induce cancer. Thus, pancreatic adenocarcinomas arise in ductal epithelial cells and undergo a carefully orchestrated program of genetic alterations that arise in premalignant lesions. In other words, multiple oncogene types are involved in this cancer and many other cancer types in a coordinated way. As an example of coordination, the relationship of the *p53* gene with the K-*ras* gene is presented next.

A relationship between alterations in K-*ras* genes and those in *p53* genes has been reported in the pancreatic tumors. Both of these alterations occur, for example, in the intraductal stage of mucin-producing tumors of the pancreas, and the latter is superimposed on the former during the course of tumor progression. With regard to the distribution of K-*ras* mutation and loss of heterozygosity (LOH) of *p53* gene, the former is distributed widely throughout the tumor, whereas the latter appears only in some limited areas of the tumor. The specificity of K-*ras* mutations is relatively easy to detect because they are generally limited to one codon (codon 12), whereas the detection of *p53* is more difficult because of its multiple sites of mutations. A stepwise increase in the frequency of codon 12 mutations correlates with the stage of neoplastic evolution to cancer. With respect to clonal progression, certain clones with K-*ras* gene mutations gain a growth advantage to form a tumor, and then a selected subclone harboring alteration of a different gene (e.g., LOH of *p53* gene) obtains a further growth advantage.

A relationship has also been reported between K-*ras* mutations and serum organochlorine compounds in pancreatic cancer. However, these results require replication before their acceptance as a diagnostic tool for this cancer. Similarly, the measurement of markers, such as carcinoembryonic antigen, cancer-associated carbohydrate antigen, and pancreatic oncofetal antigen, in the pancreatic juice is not useful in the diagnostic modalities of this cancer. Also, the detection of point mutations in the K-*ras* gene at codon 12 even in pure pancreatic juice has little or no specificity for pancreatic neoplasms.

Additional information regarding the functional relevance of Ras proteins in pancreatic cancer has been obtained by studying the effect of these proteins on transforming growth factor beta (TGFβ). Such information is meaningful because overexpression of TGFβ and its receptor (TGFβR) as well as inactivating mutations of TGFβ pathway components (e.g., Smad 4 and TGFβ2) have been described in pancreatic cancer. Expression profiling analyses have been used for studying the relevance of *Ras*-signaling events in the TGFβ1-mediated transcriptional phenotype of the pancreatic cancer cell line PANC-1. These cells have a functional TGFβ pathway with an intact TGFβR system and wild-type *Smad* 4, which react to TGFβ1 treatment by a moderate inhibition of cell growth.

Comparative studies have shown significant differences in the overall frequency of K-*ras* mutations in pancreatic cancer among persons of different ethnicities. In addition, the effect of these mutations in terms of poor prognosis of this cancer differs depending on the ethnicity of the patient. For example, the frequency of K-*ras* point mutations is lower in Chinese patients than in Japanese patients, but is similar to that in White patients. The primary reason for these differences is different lifestyles of individuals of different ethnicities in different countries.

Maspin

Maspin protein is related to the serpin family of protease inhibitors. Protease inhibitors have the ability to prevent tumor invasion and metastasis by inhibiting degradation of extracellular matrix proteinase. Accumulated functional evidence demonstrates that maspin blocks tumor metastasis *in vitro*. It has been shown that maspin expression is lost at the critical transition from noninvasive to invasive breast and prostate carcinomas. Maspin also suppresses tumor progression by enhancing cellular sensitivity to apoptotic stimuli. Cellular, molecular, and biochemical studies demonstrate an essential role of Bax in the proapoptotic effect of maspin. Bax is up-regulated in maspin-transfected prostate and breast tumor cells. The link between maspin and Bax up-regulation explains the loss of maspin-expressing tumor cells in invasive breast and prostate carcinomas.

Maspin is down-regulated but not mutated in cancer cells. Down-regulation of maspin is also involved in carcinomas other than breast and prostate cancers. Oh *et al.* (2002) have investigated the usefulness of maspin as an adjunct diagnostic marker in various pancreatic neoplasms. This immunohistochemical study showed that all of the pancreatic ductal adenocarcinomas were positive for maspin, although a significant correlation between the maspin expression and the clinical stage was not determined. In contrast, nonneoplastic pancreatic parenchyma and chronic pancreatitis lacked maspin expression. This and other studies suggest that maspin may be of importance in the pathobiology of pancreatic neoplasms with epithelial origin, especially pancreatic tumors that are composed of mucin-producing cells. Using

IHC of maspin may be useful in separating ductal adenocarcinoma from ACC, pancreatic endocrine tumor, solid-pseudopapillary tumor, and chronic pancreatitis, particularly in needle biopsy specimens. It is suggested that maspin may be used as a modifier for apoptosis-based cancer therapy.

Metastasis-Associated Gene 1

The metastasis-associated gene (*MTA1*) is mapped to the center of a 1.6 Mb region of human chromosome 14q 31.2 and encodes a protein of 715 amino acids with a calculated molecular mass of 80.8 kDa. Enhanced expression of MTA1 mRNA is found in a variety of human cancerous tissues and carcinoma cell lines, including colorectal, gastric, and esophageal. Comparative analyses reveal differential expression of this mRNA in nonmetastatic and metastatic tumors, pointing toward a role of MTA1 in enhancing the metastatic potential of malignant tumor cells. Immunofluorescence studies also demonstrate enhanced expression of MTA1, which triggers the development of motile, invasive pancreatic carcinoma cells by altering the organization of the cellular cytoskeleton. Thus, enhanced expression of MTA1 is thought to be of considerable importance to understand the malignancy of pancreatic neoplasms.

Microvascular Density

A brief comment on the role of microvascular density, a marker for tumor angiogenesis, in pancreatic cancer is given later. It is known that the process of angiogenesis is essential for tumor growth and is important for the tumor capacity to metastasize. Routinely, IHC is used to measure the angiogenic activity. This technique has shown that high microvascular density is correlated with decreased survival rate in several types of cancers. Microvascular density has also been demonstrated to be a valuable indicator of overall and relapse-free survival in patients with pancreatic adenocarcinoma and may therefore be useful for prognostic evaluation and treatment of patients with pancreatic ductal carcinoma.

The prognostic value of microvascular density in pancreatic neuroendocrine tumors has also been investigated. Tan *et al.* (2004) have evaluated microvascular density in these tumors and correlated it with clinicopathologic features and patient outcome for determining whether this information is a useful prognostic indicator for these patients. In their study, 25 pancreatic neuroendocrine tumors from archival files resected between 1981 and 2000 were studied. According to this study, microvascular density in pancreatic neuroendocrine tumors is not correlated with the patient outcome and is not a useful prognostic indicator in these patients. These results suggest that factors other than the number of microvessels are important in determining pancreatic neuroendocrine tumor behavior. However, most tumors, including these tumors, are highly vascularized.

Mucins

Mucins are a group of genes that transcribe for glycoproteins (MUC1-9) and that are differentially expressed in various tumor types. Epithelial mucins (MUC1, MUC2, and MUC5) are frequently overexpressed in epithelial cancers, particularly those arising in the gastrointestinal tract and pancreas. MUC1 (mammary-type mucin) is a membrane-associated glycoprotein detected in most epithelial tissues and is highly expressed in the pancreas and breast. MUC2 is an intestinal-type secretory mucin, expressed in goblet cells of the intestine. The expression of MUC1 is commonly observed in invasive pancreatic adenocarcinoma at both the transcript and protein levels, whereas MUC2 expression is a marker of the indolent pathway.

The differential expression of mucins described earlier is important in differentiating pancreatic invasive ductal carcinoma (IDC) from pancreatic intraductal papillary mucinous tumor (IPMT) because patients with IDC show poor outcome of radical surgery. However, patients with IPMT can be cured by appropriate surgery and a considerable number can survive without surgery. Patients with IPMT, however, sometimes show invasive proliferation and poor outcome. Thus, it is important to know which subtype of IPMT has a high potential for malignancy and needs surgical treatment. Such subtype can be determined by targeting the type of mucin present.

Immunohistochemical and *in situ* hybridization studies have been carried out for differentiating malignant pancreatic tumors from benign. Invasive ductal carcinoma usually showed positive MUC1 and negative MUC2 expression, whereas IPMT was negative for MUC1 and positive for MUC2. This information is of value in assessing the biological behavior of the IPMTs and their potential for malignancy and improved surgical management. This and other evidence indicates that a dichotomy in carcinogenesis exists in the pancreas in the forms of IDC and IPMT.

A uniform nomenclature and standardized diagnostic criteria for pancreatic precursor lesions have been adopted, and the accepted terminology is now PanIN, the precursors of ductal adenocarcinoma. The PanINs are small incidental duct lesions that progress to invasive ductal adenocarcinomas. Immunohistochemical labeling with MUC1 and

MUC2 antibodies has been performed on PanINs, intraductal papillary mucinous neoplasms, ductal carcinoma, and colloid carcinomas. This study indicates that colloid carcinomas are MUC2 positive, whereas this labeling pattern is reverse for ductal adenocarcinomas that are rich in MUC1 and poor in MUC2. Because these two pathways often lead to different types of invasive carcinomas, they are an invaluable model for the study of pancreatic carcinogenesis.

A high-throughput tissue microarray study demonstrates that molecular abnormalities in pancreatic cancer are not random; they can usually be stratified into early changes (expression of MUC5 and prostate stem antigen, or loss of p16), intermediate changes (expression of D1), and late changes (expression of p53, proliferation antigens, MUC1, mesothelin, or loss of Smad4/ Dpc4). Invasive pancreatic adenocarcinoma, once established, is almost always fatal, and, therefore, the systematic identification and targeting of molecular abnormalities in the precursor lesions of invasive cancer is one of the strongest avenues for combating this lethal disease.

Neurokinin-1 Receptor

Neurokinin-1 receptor (NK-1R) belongs to the class of seven transmembrane domain receptors that interact with intracellular effector systems via guanine nucleotide-binding regulatory proteins (G-proteins). Neurokinin-1 receptor is up-regulated in human pancreatic cancer, and pancreatic cancer cell growth is stimulated by the neurotransmitter substance P (SP). The expression of NK-1R mRNA and protein in human pancreatic cancer specimens has been investigated by quantitative RT-PCR, *in situ* hybridization, IHC, and Western Blot analysis and compared with normal controls. This study indicates that the NK-1R pathway is activated in human pancreatic cancer and has the potential to contribute to cancer cell growth.

Nuclear Factor Kappa B

Nuclear factor kappa B (NF-κB) is a member of the Rel family of transcriptional regulatory proteins, including p50 and p52. The untethered NF-κB translocates to the nucleus and binds to the specific *cis*-elements located in the promoters of various genes, including adhesion molecules, enzymes, cytokines, and chemokines. The activation of NF-κB has been shown to involve multiple immune and inflammatory mechanisms. Many experimental studies have implicated the activation of NF-κB as an important step in the pathogenesis of acute pancreatitis and the development of systemic complications.

Considerable evidence indicating that the expression of NF-κB in peripheral blood mononuclear cells (PBMCs) is increased in pathologic conditions such as sepsis, trauma, inflammation, and diabetes mellitus is available. Such expression level might therefore serve as an indicator of clinical severity. It has been shown the NF-κB is activated in experimental pancreatitis models and that there are quantitative differences in the degree of NF-κB expression between the macrophoges from rats with severe pancreatitis and those from rats with mild pancreatitis. In 2003, it was demonstrated that NF-κB is involved in the clinical course of acute pancreatitis. In this study it was suggested that altered features of NF-κB in PBMCs may predispose patients to a higher risk of serious systemic complications if these altered features are prolonged.

A brief comment on the development of acute pancreatitis is in order. The natural course of severe acute pancreatitis constitutes two phases: The early phase is characterized by multiple organ failure, chiefly during the first 2 to 3 weeks after the onset, and the late phase is dominated by septic complications, mostly later than 3 weeks from the onset. A relationship between an impaired immune reaction and susceptibility to bacterial infection has been suggested. An immune disorder is thought to be present even in the early phase of acute pancreatitis and continues for a long time in the patients who develop sepsis in the later clinical course. Elucidation of immunologic status during acute pancreatitic may contribute to the development of an effective approach for improving the prognosis of the disease.

Osteopontin

Osteopontin (OPN), a glycoprotein normally produced by osteoblasts, arterial smooth muscle cells, various epithelia, activated T cells, and macrophages, is secreted into most body fluids. As a member of the small integrin family, OPN is able to bind to extracellular matrix proteins. It functions as a signaling molecule, either in the soluble form or as an immobilized cell-adhesion protein. The functions most likely related to tumorigenesis include facilitation of anchorage-independent growth in transformed cells, stimulation of migration and invasion, binding and activation of matrix metalloproteinases, protection from apoptosis, enhancement of metastatic ability, and direct stimulation of cancer cell proliferation and progression.

In clinical studies, OPN has been associated with decreased survival in patients with cancer, increased metastatic potential, and advanced disease stage. Using global gene expression technology, OPN was identified as overexpressed (7.9-fold) in pancreatic cancer. Because of the secreted nature of the OPN, it was evaluated as a serum marker of pancreatic adenocarcinomas. This ISH study has shown strong OPN mRNA in tumor-infiltrating macrophages in pancreatic adenocarcinomas, compared with normal pancreatic tissues. This and other studies demonstrate that serum OPN has a diagnostic potential as a marker for pancreatic adenocarcinomas.

p16

The *p16* gene product is a 16-Kd protein that inhibits formation of cyclin D/CDK4 complexes. Loss of p16 function results in the release of activated transcription factors and progression of the cell cycle through the G1/S checkpoint. Frequent alterations of p16 occur in a number of human malignancies, and mechanisms of inactivation include homozygous deletion, mutation, and aberrant methylation of 5' CpG islands. It is known that 5' CpG island methylation of pancreatic cancers exhibits abrogation of the Rb/p16 tumor-suppressive pathway by potentially inactivating *p16* gene alterations. This evidence and immunohistochemical results indicate a significant role for *p16* inactivation in pancreatic cancer.

p21$^{WAF1/CIP1}$

p21 is an inhibitor of cyclin-dependent kinase and acts to prevent protein retinoblastoma (pRb) phosphorylation by inhibiting activation of cyclin E/cdk2 complexes that are required for Rb phosphorylation. Expression of *p21* is regulated by a number of signaling molecules, including *p53* and *K-ras*. However, an agreement on the role of these two genes in the induction of *p21* in pancreatic cancer is lacking. Some studies indicate that *p21* is induced by wild-type *p53* but not mutant *p53*. Other studies report that *p21* expression in pancreatic adenocarcinoma may be induced by a *p53*-independent pathway. Immunohistochemical studies have demonstrated that overexpression of p21 is an early event in the development of PanIN. Overexpression of *p2l* increases progressively from normal ducts through the spectrum of PanIN lesions in resection specimens of chronic pancreatitis and invasive carcinoma.

Activating mutations of *K-ras* are known to increase intracellular levels of *p21* in experimental models. However extensive immunohistochemical and PCR-restriction fragment length polymorphism (PCR-RFLP) studies indicate the absence of activating *K-ras* mutations in specimens containing normal ducts and PanIN lesions that overexpressed *p21*. An alternative pathway to explain the activation of *p21* is the overexpression of HER-2/neu that is detected in a significant proportion of PanIN lesions and pancreatic carcinomas. The role of HER-2/neu biomarker in pancreatic cancer is discussed elsewhere in this chapter.

p27

The p27/Kip 1 protein belongs to the family of proteins called cyclin-dependent kinase inhibitors (CDKIs). It prevents progression of the cell cycle from G1 phase into S phase by binding to and inhibiting the cyclin E/Cdk2 complex. Because p27 also interacts with various other cyclin complexes, it is designated as a universal CDKI. The highest levels of *p27* expression occur during the quiescent G0 and prereplicative G1 phases.

Neoplastic cells progress rapidly through the cell cycle, often ignoring the mechanisms that control cell division. Cyclin-dependent kinases (CDKs) play an important role in cell cycle control. They form cyclin-CDK complexes that facilitate entry into the S phase. The CDKs are bound and inactivated by various proteins, including p27, thus reducing cell proliferation. In this role, p27 is a potential tumor suppressor, and its levels are reduced in many tumor types, including pancreatic ductal adenocarcinomas. In this cancer, a loss of p27 expression is correlated with high tumor grade, advanced clinical stage, and aggressive character of the disease. The prognostic value of p27 is discussed later.

Immunohistochemical expression of p27 and its prognostic value in a series of 147 human pancreatic ductal adenocarcinomas has been investigated. This study demonstrated loss of p27 expression, which was associated with poor prognosis in stages 1 and 2 of pancreatic adenocarcinoma. The 5-year survival for patients negative for p27 was only 3.6% compared with 20% for patients positive for p27. Another immunohistochemical study has analyzed the relationships among p27 expression, pathologic features, and clinical outcome in resected pancreatic ductal adenocarcinomas from 46 European patients and in associated lymph node metastases from 13 patients. The extent of p27 expression (the percentage of cells expressing p27) was lower in carcinomas than in non-neoplastic ductal epithelia. No significant difference was seen between the extent of p27 expression in lymph node metastases and their corresponding primary tumors, and p27 expression did not correlate with patient gender.

p53

The *p53* tumor-suppressor gene is ubiquitous in the discussion of biomarkers for human cancers. It is inactivated in 40–75% of pancreatic cancers. The protein product of the *p53* gene responds to cellular DNA damage. Like *p16,* it tends to block the progression of cells through the G1 phase of the cell cycle. This protein also mediates cell death or apoptosis by detecting irreversible DNA damage within a cell. Interactions of p53 with many regulatory pathways have been identified, which are highly complex. In pancreatic cancer the primary mechanism of p53 inactivation is thought to be mutation because homozygous deletions have not been observed. Mutated p53 protein inhibits wild-type p53, and biallelic inactivation may not be necessary for loss of function. Alterations of p53 are associated with K-ras mutations, suggesting a cooperative effects in tumorigenesis.

Rad51

In the DNA repair pathway, recombinational processes function to maintain genetic stability, but if this process is deregulated or enhanced, genomic instability and malignant transformation can result. Rad51 is one of the key enzymes of homologous recombination and repairs DNA double-strand breaks. Overexpression of wild-type Rad51 is correlated with histologic grading of invasive ductal breast carcinoma as well as with human pancreatic adenocarcinoma. Because overexpression of Rad51 is restricted to tumor cells, it is a tumor-specific antigen. This antigen has been localized in pancreatic adenocarcinoma using monoclonal antibody 1 G8 and IHC.

S100P

S100P belongs to the family of S100 Ca-binding proteins. *S100* genes are small (9–12 kD), displaying 30–50% homology within the group. The *S100P* gene is located on 4p16. The functions of the S100 proteins are multiple, including interaction with cytoskeletal elements leading to dysfunction in microtubule assembly and increased motility and invasion. S100 proteins are of major interest owing to their differential expression in a variety of tumors and their putative involvement in the metastatic process. The IHC (using anti-S100P monoclonal antibody) of S100P protein has been carried out and correlated S100P expression with the level of its transcript detected on cDNA arrays to determine the site of protein expression. This study suggests specific increase of S100P at both RNA and protein levels almost exclusively in pancreatic adenocarcinoma. In addition, this protein is highly elevated in intraductal papillary mucinous tumors, pointing to the involvement of the S100P gene in early stages of pancreatic tumor development. This evidence suggests a potential value of S100P for diagnostic and disease-monitoring purposes.

S100A6

S100A6 is a low molecular mass (10 kDa) Ca^{2+} binding protein. It belongs to a family of S100 proteins, members of which are expressed in a cell- and tissue-specific manner. These proteins are implicated in a variety of diseases, including cancer development and metastasis. Immunohistochemical analysis of a pancreatic cancer tissue array has revealed that the normal ductal cells in 83% of cases were devoid of detectable cytoplasmic S100A6, whereas more than half lacked nuclear S100A6. The level of S100A6 expression was weak or intermediate in the normal ducts that exhibited staining. Well-differentiated tumors showed slightly more cytoplasmic staining but similar nuclear staining.

In contrast, moderately and poorly differentiated pancreatic cancers showed both a greater frequency and a higher intensity of S100A6 expression. This pattern of staining indicates that this protein is potentially involved in pancreatic cancer progression. Microarray technology has also identified Sl00A6 as highly expressed at the RNA level in this cancer. This proteomic approach can uncover changes in protein expression that correlate with the malignant pancreatic phenotype. The exact function of S100A6 and the mechanism(s) underlying its overexpression in pancreatic cancer cells are not known.

Serine Proteinase Inhibitor

SERPINE2 (protease nexin I) is an extracellular serine proteinase inhibitor with activity toward trypsin, thrombin, plasmin, uPA, and other serine proteinases. This inhibitor plays a central role in a physiologic process of invasion—namely, neurite outgrowth during embryogenesis and nerve regeneration. The mechanism by which SERPINE2 exerts its effect on the invasiveness of tumor cells is derived from the observation that SERPINE2-expressing tumors, especially highly invasive specimens, contain significantly higher amounts of extracellular matrix (ECM) components organized in prominent fibrous bundles than their non–SERPINE2-expressing counterparts. It is known that the ECM, depending on its cellular context, can actively regulate growth, death, adhesion, cell migration, invasion, gene expression, and differentiation in neighboring cells. Invasive cancer cells benefit in many ways from inducing specific changes in the ECM composition in and around the tumor. Immunohistochemical studies demonstrate that SERPINE2 overexpression enhances the invasive potential of pancreatic cancer cells in nude mice xenografts by altering ECM production and organization within the tumors. This experimental system provides the opportunity to model the desmoplastic reaction of pancreatic cancer and represents a new tool for studying tumor–stroma interactions.

Smad 4

The Smad signal inhibits the growth of most epithelial cells. Impairment of the Smad pathway causes escape from growth inhibition and leads to the promotion of cell proliferation, thereby contributing to carcinogenesis. Several genetic or epigenetic alterations of the components of the Smad pathway have been identified in several human cancers. Mutations or deletion of the Smad gene have been detected in ~50% of all pancreatic cancers. (Smad gene was originally designated as the tumor-suppressor gene that DPC4 deleted in pancreatic carcinoma, locus 4.) Many pancreatic cancer cell lines also have impaired TGFβ-Smad signaling owing to a functionally inactivated Smad 4.

Stk11 Gene

Stk 11 (LKB11) mediates cell cycle arrest through induction of the cyclin-dependent kinase inhibitor $p21^{WAF1}$, through a p53-dependent process. The Stk11 protein also interacts with brahma-related gene-1 (BRG1) and ATPase that is associated with SW1/SNF chromatin-remodeling complexes. Exogenous expression of BRG1 induces cell cycle arrest and senescence. The tumor-suppressor function of Stk11 is related to its ability to affect the cell cycle proliferation. It is also known that germline mutations of Stk11 gene located on distal chromosome 19p cause Peutz-Jeghers syndrome (PJS). This syndrome is an autosomal-dominant disorder characterized by hamartomatous polyps in the gastrointestinal tract and pigmented macules of the lips and buccal mucosa. The syndrome is also associated with an increased risk of developing cancers, including pancreatic cancer. Somatic mutations of Stk11 are involved in a small proportion of sporadic pancreatic adenocarcinomas, intraductal papillary mucinous neoplasms, and biliary adenocarcinomas.

An antibody specific for the protein product of the Stk11 gene has been used for characterizing its distribution in pancreatobiliary neoplasms. This study included a large series of pancreatic (n = 56) and biliary (n = 38) neoplasms with known Stk11 gene status. The inactivation of Stk11 was observed in 7% of pancreatic adenocarcinomas and 27% of intraductal papillary mucinous neoplasms. This difference suggests genetic disparity in the pathogenesis of these closely related neoplasms. Because IHC has the advantage of detecting genetic abnormalities irrespective of the mechanism of gene inactivation, immunohistochemical analysis of the abrogation of Stk11 expression may be a valid surrogate for genetic analysis of this mutation in cancer.

Telomerase

Telomerase is an enzyme involved in the *de novo* synthesis of telomere at chromosomal ends. Telomerase is activated in various human malignant tumors, including lung, gastric, and colorectal tumours. This enzyme has also been detected in the pancreatic cancer but not in benign tumors or precancerous lesions. It has also been detected in some types of normal cells, especially in proliferative stem cells and activated lymphocytes. To avoid the false-positive results by contaminating lymphocytes, Murakami *et al.* (2002) have detected telomerase activity in the pure pancreatic juice that was obtained preoperatively by endoscopic retrograde pancreatic juice aspiration; the juice was analyzed by telomeric repeat amplification protocol (TRAP) assay. This study was carried out when a 52-year-old man complained of abdominal pain and was diagnosed with malignant IPMT of the pancreas. This malignancy is difficult to diagnose by imaging examination. It is concluded that detection of telomerase activity of the pure pancreatic juice can be useful to distinguish benign from malignant IPMT preoperatively.

Transforming Growth Factor Beta 1

The gene *TGF β1* plays a dual role in pancreatic carcinogenesis. In early phases of carcinogenesis, *TGF β1* is a potent mediator of antiproliferative effects such as cell-cycle arrest and growth inhibition. In later stages, this factor contributes to tumor progression by inducing cell spreading, migration, angiogenesis, and tumor cell invasion. One of the main mechanisms responsible for this dual role is thought to be the introduction of an epithelial-mesenchymal transdifferentiation (EMT) of epithelial tumor cells. During this transdifferentiation, the epithelial phenotype is lost and a mesenchymal phenotype is acquired that is associated with enhanced invasiveness and metastasis.

The *Ras* pathway is implicated in mediating these effects of TGFβ1 on tumor cell morphology. It has been shown that TGFβ1 causes reversible and time-dependent EMT in TGFβ1-responsive pancreatic cancer cell lines that harbor activating mutations of the *Ras2* oncogene. Expression-profiling analyses have been used for studying the functional relevance of Ras proteins to the TGFβ1-mediated transcriptional phenotype of the pancreatic cancer cell line PANG-1. This study indicates that in these cells *Ras*-dependent signal-transduction pathways are intimately involved in the induction of EMT following TGFβ1 stimulation. It is known that TGFβ1 activates several signaling pathways such as the RAS-RAF-MEK-MAPK pathway in addition to Smad-dependent signal transduction.

Vascular Endothelial Growth Factor

The VEGF is a potent angiogenic peptide with specific mitogenic activity on endothelial cells. It is the best characterized of the angiogenic factors and has been associated with increased angiogenesis and poor prognosis in patients with a variety of solid tumors, including pancreatic carcinoma. Members of the VEGF family mediate both vascular permeability and endothelial cell proliferation through three tyrosine kinase receptors: VEGFR receptor-3 (VEGFR-3; Flt-4). The VEGF exists in four isoforms generated by alternative mRNA splicing. The shorter isoforms ($VEGF_{121}$ and $VEGF_{165}$) are secreted peptides that may act as diffusible agents with $VEGF_{165}$ being the predominant soluble isoform, whereas the longer isoforms ($VEGF_{189}$ and $VEGF_{206}$) are bound to the extracellular matrix.

The VEGF affects not only endothelial cells but also tumor cells. Up-regulation of VEGF and its receptors at both mRNA and protein levels has been demonstrated in pancreatic ductal carcinoma cell lines and in human pancreatic cancer tissues. Furthermore, tissue VEGF expression is an independent prognostic marker for early recurrence after curative resection of the pancreatic tumor.

Immunohistochemical and immunofluorescent studies demonstrate that the VEGF receptor neuropilin-1 (NRP-1) is associated with human pancreatic adenocarcinoma but not with nonmalignant pancreatic tissue. Regulation of NRP-1 expression is thought to be involved, at least in part, in VEGF-dependent signaling pathways. This receptor is also involved in the potential mechanism by which EGF affects the growth of pancreatic carcinoma.

Soluble forms of VEGF are also detectable in the serum from patients with various types of adenocarcinomas, often correlating with tumor stage, microvessel density, and tumor VEGF expression. Karayiannakis *et al.* (2003) also report that patients with pancreatic cancer have significantly higher serum VEGF levels compared with healthy controls, with a significant association between serum VEGF levels, disease stage, and the presence of both lymph node and distant metastases. Serum levels of VEGF decrease markedly after radical resection of the tumor. Elevated preoperative serum VEGF level is an important prognostic factor for patient survival, although not independent of tumor stage. These findings suggest that serum VEGF concentrations tend to reflect pancreatic cancer progression, and their determination may be clinically useful.

Validity of Biomarkers in Clinical Practice

Tumor markers are usually proteins associated with a malignancy, which might be clinically usable in patients with cancer. A tumor marker can be detected in a solid tumor; in circulating tumor cells in peripheral blood; in lymph nodes; in bone marrow; or in other body fluids such as urine, stool, and ascites. Screening for early diagnosis via marker detection generally results in lower mortality for diseases such as breast cancer and cervical cancer. Many malignancies, including pancreatic cancer, however, are still diagnosed after the metastatic process has already begun, indicating poor prognosis.

A tumor marker can be used to define a particular disease entity; in this case it can be used for diagnosis, staging, or population screening. In addition, markers can be used to detect the presence of occult metastatic disease, to monitor response to treatment, or to detect a recurrent disease. Markers can also be used as targets for therapeutic intervention in clinical trials. Although biomarkers are being introduced into clinical decision-making at an increasing rate, the basic understanding of the underlying molecular mechanisms and their clinical use is not always clear. Some aspects of such molecular mechanisms, including molecular pathways, are explained in this volume. Caution is warranted in the use of biomarkers because only a few guidelines have been established to standardize a biomarker for a specific type of cancer. The guidelines will help to interpret the data correctly to reach correct clinical decision-making.

Hayes *et al.* (1996) have proposed a tumor marker utility grading system, a framework to evaluate clinical utility of tumor markers. In support of this proposal, the editor of the *International Journal of Biomarkers* has suggested a checklist for designing studies using biomarkers. More recently, Sweep *et al.* (2003) have discussed in detail various factors that may play a role in discordant test results; these factors include method of specimen collection (FNA, core biopsy, or large biopsy obtained during surgery), source of tissue (fresh or frozen), storage (duration, temperature, or freeze-thawing cycles), and processing (e.g., differences in antibody specificity or affinity used in different test kits and reference materials provided with the kits).

The size of the tissue specimen is also important because of the heterogeneity of tumors. Subclonal diversity results in a heterogeneous tumor. Because of this, sampling bias may occur, leading to different test results if different areas of a tumor are examined. The major question that remains is how and when to transfer technologies from the research setting to the clinic (translational research). This question is answered by the type of biomarker, its relevancy to a certain malignancy, and the demand by both the patient and the clinician.

Molecular Detection of Micrometastases in Pancreatic Cancer

Despite advances in surgical oncology, local recurrence and distant metastases are the major problems in treating pancreatic cancer. Only 25% of all pancreatic cancers are resectable, and only patients who have been curatively resected (R0) enjoy a favorable outcome. However, the survival after surgery still remains poor. Most surgeons and oncologists treating pancreatic cancer believe that local recurrence represents the growth of residual tumor. Despite histologically confirmed curative resection (no residual tumor: R0) and tumor-free lymph nodes, most patients will suffer from postoperative local recurrence or distant metastases. Occult dissemination of tumor cells beyond resection margins is of paramount importance for prognosis. This is impressively shown by a 50% recurrence rate within 2 years after surgery for pancreatic cancer.

In recent years, numerous new techniques to detect minimal residual disease (MRD), including immunohistochemical and molecular assays, have been introduced to reveal the accurate resection status (R0 versus R1) and enrich the routine histopathology. These techniques detect micrometastases and disseminated tumor cells not only in lymph nodes that had appeared tumor free in routine histology but also in body compartments such as bone marrow, peritoneal cavity, and blood. From the current data, it has been concluded that routine histopathology often under-estimates the true tumor stage. It is well known that micrometastases of a diameter of 3 cells are diagnosed only in 1% based on serial 5-μm sections. Diagnosing micrometastases with routine histopathology can be accomplished only on extensive serial sections and extensive lymph node dissection, which are not useful in pancreatic cancer. However, occult metastases can be more easily detected by immunohistochemical or molecular methods designed to recognize certain tumor-associated antigens, lineage-specific markers, or distinct tumor-related gene mutations. Immunohistochemical methods use antibodies against a variety of epithelial cell markers such as cytokeratins, CA 19.9, carcinoembryonic antigen (CEA), or Ber-Ep 4. These markers are often not specific because nonmalignant cells are also able to express them and thus might deliver falsepositive results. It has been demonstrated that CA 19.9 antibodies can be detected in 60% of regional lymph nodes dissected as a result of chronic pancreatitis. As in histopathology, the limiting factor is the analysis of tissue in stepwise serial sections and not as a whole specimen.

As shown in other gastrointestinal malignancies, specific genetic disorders, e.g., mutations, can be used in pancreatic cancer to detect micrometastases in different body compartments. According to various analyses, mutated K-*ras* gene has been found in a range from 70% to 95% of pancreatic adenocarcinomas, and the site of mutation is restricted to codon 12 of the K-*ras* gene. Therefore, mutant K-*ras* is one of the most promising genetic alterations in ductal adenocarcinoma to detect malignant cells by molecular techniques. In several studies, micrometastases have been detected at the molecular level by sensitive polymerase chain reaction (PCR) and restriction fragment length polymorphism (RFLP) assays for the detection of mutant codon 12 K-*ras* allele.

Nevertheless, it has been discussed whether micrometastases are of prognostic significance or if these are only "dormant" tumor cells arrested in G0-phase. This chapter attempts to answer these questions and provides detailed information of immunohistochemical and molecular methods to detect lymph node micrometastases in pancreatic cancer.

The following investigations were carried out with 69 specimens of resected ductal pancreatic adenocarcinomas. In all cases, corresponding paraaortic lymph nodes were obtained by *en bloc* dissection from the suprarenal para-aortic region. All cases had tumor-free margins. We used nine surgical specimens of patients diagnosed for adenomas of Vater's papilla (n = 4), chronic pancreatitis (n = 4), and one cystadenoma with corresponding paraaortic lymph nodes as controls. Normal pancreatic tissue served as a negative control for each individual subject. Tumor, normal tissue, and paraaortic lymph nodes were used for histopathology and immunohistochemistry, and extended deoxyribonucleic acid (DNA) investigations were prepared. Each paraaortic lymph node was divided into two portions, one of which was formalinfixed and paraffin-embedded for immunohisto-chemistry, and the other one was stored frozen at -80°C until PCR analysis.

Materials

Immunohistochemistry for Pan-Cytokeratin

1. Buffered formalin (4%): 100 ml phosphate buffer saline (PBS) buffer (PBS-buffer: 200 g Natriumhydrogenphosphat, 325 g Dinatium-

hydrogenphosphat, bring volume to 5 L with distilled water), 100 ml formalin (37%), bring volume to 800 ml with distilled water.

2. Paraffin wax.
3. Microtome.
4. Xylene.
5. Alcohol 100%, 96%, and 80%.
6. Brood-cupboard.
7. 0.1% Trypsine solution: 100 mg trypsine, 100 mg calciumchloride, bring volume to 100 ml with distilled water.
8. Deionized water.
9. Blocking-solution.
10. Primary anti-pan-cytokeratin antibody (Zymed; NCC-pan-ck, dilution 1:50).
11. Tris-buffered saline (TBS) (pH 7.6): 6.055 g Tris buffer, 8.52 g NaCl, 37 ml 1 N HCl, bring volume to 1 L with distilled water, 0.5 ml Tween 20.
12. Secondary biotinylated antibody (Zymed).
13. Streptavidin-labeled immunoalkaline phosphatase.
14. Substrate-chromogen-mixture (SCM): 0.121 g Tris-buffer and 0.5 ml 1 N HCl, bring volume to 10 ml distilled water, 2 mg Naphtol AS-MX Phosphat, 2.4 mg Levamisole hydrochloride, and 10 mg Fast Red TR Salt.
15. Hematoxylin.
16. Kaiser's glycerine gelatin.

Molecular Detection by Mutated K-Ras

1. Human pancreatic adenocarcinoma cell line Pa-Tu-8902 (DSMZ).
2. QIAamp DNA mini Kit.
3. Photometer.
4. Thermocycler.
5. 0.5-ml tubes (for PCR) and 1.5-ml/2-ml tubes (for DNA extraction).
6. Thermocycler.
7. 25 mM $MgCl_2$.
8. 5 mM of each dNTP (deoxyribonucleotide-triphosphate).
9. 0.3 μM 3'-primer (5'-GTC CTG CAC CAG AAA TAT TGC-3') and 5'-primer (5'-ACT GAA TAT AAA CTT GTG GTA GTT GGA CCT-3').
10. Two units of *Taq* polymerase in PCR-buffer containing 500 mM KCl, 15 mM $MgCl_2$, and 100 mM Tris-HCl.

11. Ampermeter.
12. Agarose.
13. Tris-acetat-ethylenediamine tetraacetic acid (TAE)-buffer: dilution 1:10.
14. Ethidium bromide.
15. Electrophoresis-box.
16. Loading buffer.
17. DNA-ladder.
18. Gel documentation system.
19. Endonuclease *Mva* I system containing *Mva* I and incubation-buffer.

METHODS

Immunohistochemistry for Pan-Cytokeratin

1. Fix tissue blocks in 4% buffered formalin for 24 hr and embed in paraffin.
2. Cut serial sections of 5 μm thickness of paraaortal lymph nodes with microtome.
3. Deparaffinizing and rehydration: Rinse the samples for 5 min in xylene, then for 2 mm in 100% alcohol; repeat the procedure with 96% alcohol and 80% alcohol.
4. Dry the samples for 12 hr in brood-cupboard at 37°C.
5. Incubate the samples for 40 min in 0.1% trypsine solution at 37°C for antigen retrieval.
6. Rinse sections in deionized water for 5 min.
7. For immunohistological detection the biotinstreptavidin- amplified indirect immunoalkaline phosphatase method was used.
8. Add 100 μl of blocking solution to each sample and incubate for 15 min at room temperature; rinsing is not necessary.
9. Thereafter, the primary anti-pan-cytokeratin antibody is applied (100 μl) for 1 hr at room temperature.
10. Control sections are incubated with TBS instead of the primary antibody.
11. Rinse all samples for 5 min in TBS.
12. The sections are incubated for 10 min with the secondary biotinylated antibody (100 μl).
13. Rinse the samples for 5 min in TBS.
14. Streptavidin-labeled immunoalkaline phosphatase is added for 10 min (2 drops or 100 μl).

15. Rinse the samples for 5 min in TBS.
16. The SCM-staining is applied for 30 min at room temperature.
17. Sections are washed in tap water.
18. Counterstain the samples with hematoxylin for 1–3 min at room temperature, and mount them in Kaiser's Glycerine Gelatin.

Molecular Detection by Mutated K-Ras

1. The human pancreatic adenocarcinoma cell line Pa-Tu-8902 from DSMZ serves as a positive control.
2. Distilled water without tissue is used as an internal negative control.
3. For DNA extraction, the scheme of the QIAamp DNA mini Kit is used.
4. After DNA extraction, the optical density (OD) at 260 and 280 nm, respectively, is measured.
5. Aliquots corresponding to 200 ng of genomic DNA are submitted to PCR.
6. The PCR is performed using 0.5 ml tubes and a thermocycler.
7. Reactions are carried out in a total volume of 50 μl containing final concentrations of 20 μl aliquot of genomic DNA; 5 μl PCR buffer; 1 μl 25 mM $MgC1_2$; 2 μl with 5 mM of each dNTP; 3 μl 0.3 μM of each 3'- and 5'-primer, respectively; 0.4 μl with 2 units of *Taq* polymerase; and 15.6 μl distilled water.
8. Experiments using the technique of mismatch PCR are carried out starting with an initial step for denaturation at 95°C for 5 min; then, 35 cycles are run including denaturing at 95°C for 45 sec, annealing at 59°C for 45 sec, and DNA synthesis at 72°C for 90 sec, followed by a final step at 72°C for 10 min. The primers used are leading to a PCR product of 147 base pairs (bp) in length.
9. Successful PCR is shown by ethidium bromide agarose gel (2%) electrophoresis.
10. Bring 1 g agarose in 50 ml TAE buffer, and heat the solution until agarose is completely dissolved.
11. Add 2.5 μl ethidium bromide after 2 min cooling of the solution.
12. Pour the solution into the electrophoresis box and bring into the gel-comb.
13. After cooling for 30 min at room temperature, fill TAE buffer until complete coverage of the gel is obtained.
14. After, bring 10 μl DNA aliquot and 2 μl loading buffer into the gel-pouch.

15. Fill reference line with 5 μl DNA ladder and 2 μl loading buffer.
16. To run gel, use ampermeter (70–100 V) for 1 hr. Digital analysis is recommended.
17. After electrophoresis digest, aliquots of genomic DNA with restriction endonuclease *Mva* I according to the manufacturer's instructions.
18. Reactions are carried out in a total volume of 20 μl containing final concentrations of 10 μl DNA aliquot after PCR, 1 μl Mva I, 2 μl incubations buffer, and 7 μl distilled water; incubate the aliquots for 5 hr at 37°C.
19. Analyze PCR again in ethidium bromide agarose gel electrophoresis (2%) as described in Steps 9–12, then fill in 20 μl aliquot with 3 μl loading buffer into the gel-pouch and run gel using ampermeter (70–100 V) for 90 min.
20. Each individual sample is analyzed in triplicate manner.

Results

Immunohistochemical Examination

Using the pan-cytokeratin, antibody-positive immunoreaction of single or grouped carcinoma cells within the lymphoreticular tissue of the nodes was found. Positive immunoreactivity was observed in 5 out of 69 specimens (7.2%). As a consequence, these five cases were diagnosed for micrometastases in paraaortic lymph nodes. No positive staining was found except in cancer cells. In comparison, using routine histology with hematoxylin and eosin staining, one could find occult tumor cells in paraaortic lymph nodes only in 3 of 69 specimens (4%).

Molecular Detection of Micrometastases

The use of the described mismatch primers results in amplification of a 147-bp product. A restriction site for *Mva* I is created in wild-type (wt), but not in mutated K-*ras* using the 5'-primer, whereas 3'-primer inserts a restriction site in both, serving as an internal control for a successful *Mva* I digestion. Thus, a wildtype allele, is detected by the appearance of a 107-bp band, whereas in cells harboring K-*ras* mutations, an additional band of 136 bp can be visualized. Forty-two of 69 (61%) ductal adenocarcinomas harboring the K-*ras* mutation in primary tumor were identified, visualized by appearence of the additional 136-bp band after *Mva* I digestion and subsequent gel electrophorsis. In the control specimen K-*ras* mutation was found in 1 of 4 (25%) adenomas of Vater's papilla but in no other case of the control group. In addition, no mutation was detected in all individual negative controls (normal pancreatic tissue). In pancreatic adenocarcinoma specimen, 12 cases (12/69, 17.4%) showed mutant K-*ras* gene in corresponding paraaortic lymph nodes. Therefore, in subjects with K-*ras*-positive primary tumors, micrometastases could be found in 29% (12/42). Immunohistological staining was able to detect tumor cells in lymph nodes in only five of these subjects. Mutated K-*ras*, an indicator for tumor-cell DNA, that is found in para-aortic lymph nodes, can be set equivalent with micrometastases. There was no mutated K-*ras* found in paraaortic lymph node specimen of the control group.

Discussion

Ductal adenocarcinoma of the pancreas is associated with the worst 5-year survival rate of any form of gastrointestinal cancer, even after curative resection. However, until now, the question of why some patients die within a few months after curative resection because of metastases or local recurrence, whereas others enjoy a more favorable outcome has not been sufficiently answered. We argue that the present histologic sectioning may lack sufficient sensitivity for assessing lymph nodes and surgical resection margins for tumor involvement and minimal residual cancer, respectively.

Therefore, highly sensitive methods have been investigated to assess patients with other types of gastrointestinal cancers for minimal residual disease. In 2001, PCR-based assays were used for detecting MRD in histologically negative lymph nodes from patients with gastric and colorectal cancer. For pancreatic cancer, it has been suggested that immunohistochemical antibodies be used against epithelial- or tumor-associated antigens, such as cytokeratin (CK) or CEA in various body compartments for the detection of occult micrometastases at the time of surgery. One group suggested combining routine histopathology with CK immunohistology for detection of MRD after surgery because the latter method increases the sensitivity for micrometastases.

Because mutant K-*ras* is the most evident genetic alteration in pancreatic adenocarcinoma, several investigators have performed analyses for this gene as a marker for occult tumor cells, e.g., in stool, blood, or tissue specimens. It has been demonstrated that detection of K-*ras* mutation in regional and para-aortic lymph nodes is superior to routine pathologic examination, and it has been suggested that using this for prognostic reevaluation. Tamagawara *et al.* (1997) could reveal that evidence of MRD in regional lymph nodes by detection of mutant K-*ras* was a predictive marker for recurrence in patients with pancreatic adenocarcinoma.

From our investigations the following conclusions can be drawn: (1) patients with positive K-*ras* mutations in para-aortic lymph nodes will have a significantly worse prognosis than those without, (2) K-*ras* positive para-aortic lymph nodes are an independent prognostic marker after curative resection, and (3) patients with K-*ras* mutations in para-aortic lymph nodes will suffer significantly earlier from recurrent cancer.

With the described method one could find K-*ras* mutations in a similar range, as described by other authors. Minimal residual disease in paraaortic lymph nodes after curative resection can be detected in 7% by cytokeratin immunohistochemistry and in 17% by the PCR-based assay to detect mutant K-*ras*, underlining the sensitivity of the presented molecular detection system. In comparison, in routine histology with hematoxylin and eosin staining, occult tumor cells in those lymph nodes can only be diagnosed in 4%. Therefore, we believe, in accordance with other authors, that the identification of K-*ras* mutations for the detection of MRD in lymph nodes is superior to the morphologic approach of the pathologic examination and that cancer cells may have already spread to lymph nodes that were histologically diagnosed as negative.

In conclusion, the routine, stepwise sectioning pathologic examination lacks the detection of micrometastases in many patients, whereas PCR-based assays to screen for mutated K-*ras* analyzes tumor cell DNA of the whole sample reveals a higher sensitivity. This can enrich the routine histopathologic examination in resectable pancreatic cancer and might precisely identify the "real" tumor stage.

Aspiration Biopsy of Pancreatic Adenocarcinoma

Pancreatic malignant tumors are the fifth most common cause of cancer death among both men and women in the United States, and the incidence of these tumors continues to increase. Approximately 2900 Americans are diagnosed with pancreatic malignancies each year, and nearly all of them die of the disease, with an overall 5-year survival rate of less than 5%. Among these pancreatic malignant tumors, ductal adenocarcinoma and its variants account for 90% of the total cases.

Fine-needle aspiration biopsy (FNAB) of the pancreas has become a method of choice to establish a tissue diagnosis in many institutions before chemotherapy or surgery. The primary indication of FNAB of the pancreas is a pancreatic mass suspected as a carcinoma radiographically and clinically, in most instances. Such biopsies generally provide better diagnostic sensitivity and specificity and fewer complications such as pancreatitis and bleeding, than tissue (large core or wedge) biopsies.

An FNAB is most frequently performed with computed tomography (CT) guidance or endoscopic ultrasound (EUS) guidance preoperatively. Both of the procedures provide similar diagnostic specificity and sensitivity. The overall accuracy of FNAB of the pancreas is variable, but it increases with experience. The average sensitivity is about 80–90%, and specificity approaches 100%. In our study series of 291 cases of CT-guided FNAB of the pancreatic lesions, the diagnostic sensitivity increased to 98% if special criteria are used. Similar diagnostic sensitivity was also reported. The main advantages of EUS-guided FNAB over CT-guided FNAB include the ability to detect smaller lesions, to identify a possible local invasion of the tumor, and to simultaneously sample the adjacent lymph node for cancer staging. Intraoperative FNAB can be performed as well, which allows direct visualization or palpation of the lesion during the sampling process. As the result of this, the diagnostic sensitivity of intraoperative FNAB is more than 90%, with at least one reported series of 100%, and the specificity is usually 100%.

Unfortunately, an interpretation of FNAB of the pancreas is not always straightforward. False-positive results, which are rare, and a significant number of false-negative results do occur. The distinction of well-differentiated adenocarcinoma (WDA) from benign/reactive glandular epithelium represents the major diagnostic challenge. Other diagnostic problems may include differential diagnosis of WDA from pancreatic endocrine neoplasms, acinar cell carcinoma, solid pseudopapillary tumor of the pancreas (SPTP), mucinous cystic neoplasms, serous microcystic adenoma, and metastasis.

Materials

1. The specimens in this study, including 291 CTguided FNABs of pancreatic lesions.
2. Carnoy's solution (1:6, glacial acetic acid:70% ethanol).
3. Harris Hematoxylin.
4. Ethanols (70% ethanol, 95% ethanol, 100% ethanol).
5. Eosin alcohol (EA) polychrome-modified dye.
6. Xylene.
7. Eosin.
8. Quik-Dip Solution I (100% methanol).

9. Quik-Dip Solution II.
10. Quik-Dip Solution III.
11. Plus slides.
12. Coverslips.

Methods

Preparation of slides

1. Direct smears are obtained from CT-guided biopsies, endoscopic-ultrasound guided biopsies, or intraoperative FNABs.
2. Two slides are recommended from each pass of the FNAB. It is recommended to have one airdried slide for Diff-Quik stain and one ethanol (Carnoy's solution) fixed slide for Papanicolaou Quick-staining or hematoxylin-eosin stain (for intraoperative FNABs if a Papanicolaou quick-staining is not available).

Staining methods

Papanicolaou quick-staining technique

1. 10 dips in water.
2. 8 sec in Harris Hematoxylin.
3. 10 dips in water.
4. 10 dips in 95% ethanol.
5. 10 dips in 95% ethanol.
6. 2 min in EA polychrome-modified dye.
7. 10 dips in 95% ethanol.
8. 10 dips in 100% ethanol.
9. 10 dips in xylene.

Diff-quik stain

1. 5 sec in Quik-Dip Solution I.
2. 20 sec in Quik-Dip Solution II.
3. 20 sec in Quik-Dip Solution III.
4. Rinse slides with water.
5. Allow to air-dry.
6. Coverslip.

Hematoxylin-eosin stain

1. 5 sec in fixation solution (100% methanol).
2. 10 dips in water.
3. 1 min in Harris Hematoxylin.
4. 10 dips in water.

5. 10 dips in blueing solution (0.5% ammonium hydroxide).
6. 10 dips in water.
7. 10 dips in 70% ethanol.
8. 5 dips in eosin solution.
9. 10 dips in 70% ethanol.
10. 10 dips in 95% ethanol.
11. 10 dips in 100% ethanol.
12. 10 dips in xylene.
13. 10 dips in xylene.
14. Coverslip.

Cytologic criteria for adenocarcinoma

1. Anisonucleosis (variation in nuclear size greater than 4× within a same epithelial group).
2. Nuclear membrane irregularity.
3. Nuclear crowding/overlapping/three-dimensionality.
4. Nuclear enlargement (if more than two red blood cells).
5. Hypercellularity.
6. Gap versus confluent cell spacing.
7. Hyperchromasia.
8. Macronucleoli.
9. Mitosis.
10. Chromatin clearing.
11. Necrosis.
12. Single intact cells.

Evaluation of fine-needle aspiration biopsy smears

Microscopic observations at low magnification (40X and 100X)

1. Cellularity.
2. Epithelial group shape, architecture, and cohesiveness.
3. Background of smears, such as necrosis, inflammation, mucin, and cystic changes.
4. Nuclear enlargement.

Microscopic observations at intermediate magnification (200X)

1. Architectural changes, such as nuclear crowding, loss of nuclear polarity, nuclear overlapping, threedimensional clusters, and papillary groups.
2. Gap versus confluent cell spacing.

3. Single intact cells (pleomorphic cells, columnar cells, mucin-containing cells, plasmacytoid cells).
4. Nuclear enlargement.

Microscopic observations at high magnification (400X and 600X)

1. Anisonucleosis (variation in nuclear size greater than 4× within a same epithelial group).
2. Nuclear membrane irregularity.
3. Macronucleoli.
4. Mitosis.
5. Nuclear chromatin, such as salt and pepper, chromatin clearing, and hyperchromasia.

Results and Discussion

The diagnostic sensitivity and specificity of FNAB of pancreatic lesions have improved greatly as a result of several articles on the cytologic criteria for the diagnosis of pancreatic malignancies. In 1985, Mitchell and Carney published the first comprehensive study on diagnostic criteria. They focused on three-dimensional cellular fragments, nuclear enlargement, and nuclear membrane irregularity.

Following their publication, several modified cytologic criteria based on those of Mitchell and Carney were reported. Cohen *et al.* (1991) identified anisonucleosis (variation in nuclear size of at least three times within a same epithelial group), nuclear molding, and large nuclei as the significant cytologic features for the diagnosis of pancreatic adenocarcinoma.

Robins *et al.* (1995) were the first to propose major criteria (overlapping nuclei/crowded groups, nuclear contour irregularity, and chromatin clearing and/or clumping) and minor criteria (single epithelial cells, necrosis, mitosis, and nuclear enlargement) for pancreatic adenocarcinoma. According to these authors, the sensitivity and specificity for diagnosing pancreatic adenocarcinoma are 100% when two or more major criteria or one major and three minor criteria are identified, although these data have not been validated prospectively. In addition, they proposed that at least six groups of atypical ductal epithelial cells were needed to confirm a diagnosis. Additionally, several authors also considered single epithelial cells, necrosis, mitosis, hyperchromasia, and prominent nuclei as significant cytologic features for a diagnosis.

It is our experience, and that of others as well, that establishing a correct diagnosis of pancreatic adenocarcinoma from FNAB specimens is generally straightforward unless the tumor is a WDA, which could be extremely difficult, and in rare instances impossible, to distinguish from reactive conditions such as chronic pancreatitis. The previous published cytologic criteria generally apply to all grades of adenocarcinomas, but do not specifically focus on WDA. We have tried to add, redefine, and test these cytologic criteria in a large series of WDA in our article. In this retrospective study, 291 cases of CT-guided FNABs of pancreatic lesions were included. Available surgical specimens (84 cases) and cell blocks (131) prepared from a needle rinse solution were also reviewed. The original cytologic diagnoses were nondiagnostic in 24 (8%) cases, benign in 27 (9%), suspicious for malignancy in 15 (5%), and malignant in 225 (77%). The diagnoses among the 225 malignant cases were as follows: WDA, 74 (25%); moderately differentiated adenocarcinoma (MDA), 58 (20%); poorly differentiated adenocarcinoma (PDA), 62 (21%); mucinous adenocarcinoma, 8 (3%); neuroendocrine tumor, 12 (4%); and metastasis, 11 (4%).

We have applied 10 cytologic criteria to evaluate this group of tumors classified as WDA. These criteria included the following: (i) anisonucleosis (variation in nuclear size greater than four times within a same epithelial group), (ii) nuclear membrane irregularity, (iii) nuclear crowding/overlapping/three-dimensionality, (iv) nuclear enlargement (if more than two red blood cells), (v) gap versus confluent cell spacing, (vi) hyperchromasia, (vii) macronucleoli, (viii) mitosis, (ix) chromatin clearing, and (x) necrosis. Our data showed that the most prevalent criteria for diagnosing WDA were anisonucleosis (97% of cases), nuclear membrane irregularity (97% of cases), nuclear crowding/overlapping/three-dimensionality (92% of cases), and nuclear enlargement (99% of cases). In contrast, the criteria of gap versus confluent cell spacing, hyperchromasia, macronucleoli, mitosis, chromatin clearing, and necrosis were seen in 38%, 36%, 14%, 22%, 14%, and 7% of WDA cases, respectively.

Six cases in the suspicious category with a subsequent histologic or clinical confirmation of adenocarcinoma met most of these criteria (67–100%). For example, anisonucleosis, nuclear membrane irregularity, nuclear crowding, and nuclear enlargement were present in 100%, 83%, 67%, and 83% of the six cases, respectively. Additionally, there were four false-negative cases in this study, all of which also exhibited many of these four criteria (50–100%).

It should be emphasized that some of the nonprevalent cytologic features of WDA from this study, such as macronucleoli, mitosis, and necrosis, have been claimed as significant cytologic features for a diagnosis by some of the previous articles. Our findings suggest that these criteria are important in diagnosing adenocarcinoma in general, but there is limited value in diagnosing WDA. We do observe these cytologic features (marked nuclear pleomorphism, single malignant cells, tumor necrosis, prominent nucleoli, and many mitoses) in less differentiated adenocarcinoma, especially in a PDA.

Fraig *et al.* (2002) applied 10 cytologic criteria to evaluate the 33 cases of pancreatic adenocarcinoma with false-negative diagnoses. The cytologic criteria used in their study were very similar to our criteria, including the following: (i) loss of polarity, (ii) nuclear enlargement, (iii) nuclear membrane irregularity, (iv) pleomorphism, (v) pale or granular chromatin, (vi) gaps between cells versus confluence, (vii) increased cellularity, (viii) hyperchromasia, (ix) macronucleoli, and (x) necrosis. Their results demonstrated that loss of polarity, nuclear enlargement, and nuclear membrane irregularity were the most prevalent cytologic criteria, followed by nuclear pleomorphism, chromatin pattern (pale or granular), gap versus confluence, and hypercellularity. Also, similar to our findings, hyperchromasia, macronucleoli, and necrosis were only observed in 22–27% cases.

As mentioned in the section on methods, our general approach to an FNAB smear is as follows. Scan the entire slide at low-power field, getting an overall impression of the cellularity and the background of the smear. The majority of adenocarcinomas exhibit moderate to high cellularity of ductal epithelial cells.

Hypercellularity is also frequently seen from normal pancreatic tissue. However, the cellular components are groups of acinar cells and few ductal cells. Pancreatic endocrine neoplasms, solid and pseudopapillary tumor of the pancreas, and acinar cell carcinoma usually demonstrate high cellularity as well. It is important to pay attention to background of the smear, such as any necrosis (tumor or pancreatitis) inflammation (acute and chronic pancreatitis), granular debris with pigmented histiocytes (pancreatic pseudocyst), mucin (mucinous cystic neoplasms or mucinous adenocarcinoma), or clear fluid (microcystic serous adenoma).

Nuclear enlargement can be easily observed at low power. As a general rule, benign ductal cells are the same size or slightly larger than red blood cells. The cytologic details of benign ductal cells would not be easily appreciated at low power. Therefore, it is almost certain that there is nuclear enlargement if you can see some of the nuclear features of these ductal epithelial groups at low magnification (4X). A hypercellular smear containing many groups of ductal cells with nuclear crowding and nuclear enlargement is suspicious for adenocarcinoma.

At intermediate magnification, pay attention to the architectural features of these epithelial groups. Loss of nuclear polarity, nuclear crowding, nuclear overlapping, and three-dimensionality are the common findings in pancreatic adenocarcinoma. The finding of papillary groups lined by one to two layers of cytologically bland epithelial cells should raise a concern of SPTP and pancreatic endocrine neoplasms. Loss of cohesion at the edge of an epithelial group can be seen in adenocarcinoma. However, the cohesive groups of ductal cells are the most consistent finding in a case of WDA. Gap cell spacing (as opposed to confluent cell spacing) means there is a distinct open space formation within a confluent sheet of epithelial cells. This feature has been observed in 38% of WDAs.

Nuclear enlargement and single intact cells should be easily identified at this magnification. Following a diligent search, a few intact malignant cells are frequently seen, even in a WDA. A few very large, well-formed columnar malignant cells, referred to as "tombstone cells", may be present in a less-differentiated adenocarcinoma. If many single intact cells with bland cytomorphology are present, pancreatic endocrine neoplasms and SPTP should be included in the diagnostic considerations. Bland single columnar cells are commonly present in a mucinous tumor.

At high magnification, attention should be shifted to observe the detailed features of nuclei. Anisonucleosis is one of the most significant cytology criteria and was observed in the vast majority of WDAs in our study. Anisonucleosis was probably first introduced by Cohen *et al.* (1991) in the cytology literature for diagnosis of pancreatic adenocarcinoma, but it also served as one of the three major criteria for identifying pancreatic adenocarcinoma on frozen sections. We strongly suggest that anisonucleosis, variation in nuclear size greater than four times in the same epithelial group instead of three times as proposed by Cohen *et al.*, should be observed because this is somehow subjective among interobservers from our limited experience. It is our experience that small-sized nuclei tend to present in the peripheral portion of the epithelial group if anisonucleosis is seen focally.

Nuclear membrane irregularity is one of the most significant cytologic features for diagnosing WDA, and it is present in nearly all of cases of WDA in our study series, although the finding could be very focal. The degree of the nuclear membrane irregularity can range from small notch and groove to popcorn and resinoid. A combination of anisonucleosis and nuclear membrane irregularity is highly suggestive of adenocarcinoma because such combinations are nearly absent in a reactive condition. Extensive nuclear clearing or pale chromatin is a relatively unique feature for WDA if it is present. Hyperchromasia, granular chromatin, macronucleoli, and mitosis may be seen. Unfortunately, a WDA usually lacks these features.

As mentioned earlier, 90% of pancreatic malignancies are ductal carcinoma and its variants. We have discussed the cytologic features for a diagnosis of pancreatic adenocarcinoma, especially for a WDA. However, before a final diagnosis of adenocarcinoma is rendered, one should be certain to exclude the possibility of other neoplasms, such as pancreatic endocrine neoplasms, acinar cell carcinoma, SPTP, microcystic serous adenoma, mucinous cystic neoplasms, and metastasis. More importantly, a reactive condition, such as chronic pancreatitis, should be excluded as well.

Chronic pancreatitis

Chronic pancreatitis is probably the most important nonneoplastic disease, which needs to be distinguished from adenocarcinorna of the pancreas. It may mimic pancreatic adenocarcinoma both clinically and cytologically. Clinically, obstructive jaundice, pain, and weight loss may present. A mass lesion or diffuse involvement of the pancreas may be seen radiographically. The main cytologic features include chronic inflammation, acinar atrophy, fibrosis, ductal hyperplasia, and relatively increased numbers of islet cells. The cytologic findings largely depend on the stage of chronic pancreatitis. In the early stage, evidence of acute and chronic inflammation, fat necrosis, and granulation tissue may be the dominant features. In the late stage, as a result of an extensive acinar atrophy, the smear may be composed predominately of ductal epithelial cells, fibrosis, chronic inflammatory cells, and islet cells. Squamous metaplasia has been described. Ductal epithelial proliferation associated with significant cytologic atypia may present. The nuclear atypia more frequently show a combination of nuclear enlargement and prominent nucleoli. Marked anisonucleosis and/or nuclear membrane irregularity are rare findings. However, in some instances, the differential diagnosis from well-differentiated adenocarcinoma is virtually impossible.

If a cell block is available, some immunohistochemical markers, including clusterin, mesothelin, and prostate stem-cell antigen (PSCA), may provide some valuable information. Clusterin is a heat shock protein and has been shown to play a role in cell proliferation. A 2002 study of 8 cases of adenocarcinoma of the pancreas and 7 cases of chronic pancreatitis demonstrated a strong expression of clusterin in pancreatic duct and chronic pancreatitis and nearly absent expression in pancreatic adenocarcinoma. The study by McCarthy *et al.* (2003) showed that PSCA was present in 16 of the 19 pancreatic adenocarcinomas and was absent in 10 of the 11 benign lesions, with the sensitivity of 84% and specificity of 91%. They also demonstrated that mesothelin was present in 11 of the 19 cases of adenocarcinoma of the pancreas and absent in 10 of the 11 benign lesions, with a sensitivity of 68% and specificity of 91%.

Pancreatic endocrine neoplasms

Pancreatic endocrine neoplasms are relatively rare tumors, accounting for less than 5% of all pancreatic neoplasms. The neoplasms frequently occur in adults; they rarely occur in children. The majority of pancreatic endocrine neoplasms are functional. Nonfunctional tumors account for 15–30% of the reported cases. It is important to distinguish pancreatic endocrine neoplasms from adenocarcinoma because some of the pancreatic endocrine neoplasms are benign or borderline tumors. In fact, pancreatic endocrine neoplasms encompass a spectrum of lesions, including adenoma, borderline tumor, well-to moderately differentiated carcinomas, and poorly differentiated/ undifferentiated carcinomas.

There are no reliable histologic criteria to predict the malignant potential of these tumors, risk of recurrence, or metastasis. However, tumors exceeding 2 cm in size, 0–3 mitoses/10 high-power field (HPF), and 1–5% of Ki-67 proliferation index are indicative of borderline malignant potential. Most low-grade (differentiated) pancreatic endocrine carcinomas are larger than 3 cm, with 1–10 mitoses/10 HPF and 1–10% of Ki-67 proliferation index. In contrast, poorly differentiated (undifferentiated) pancreatic endocrine carcinomas generally have more than 10 mitoses/10 HPF and greater than 10% of Ki-67 proliferation index. Tumors exceeding 6 cm in size usually are regarded as malignant, as documented in a large series in which 93% of malignant pancreatic endocrine tumors were of this size. Tumor necrosis is a good indicator for malignancy. However, it occurs only rarely in a differentiated pancreatic endocrine carcinoma. The unequivocal indicators for malignancy are metastasis and invasion of adjacent organs.

The FNAB specimen is usually hypercellular. It frequently consists of a 50–50 mixture of loosely cohesive clusters and single cells. Acinar-like formation, perivascular tumor growth, or trabecular pattern can be seen. The neoplastic cells are typically monotonous, with focal nuclear pleomorphism. Individual cells with well-defined cytoplasm or even a plasmacytoid appearance are the common findings. The nuclei tend to be round to oval with smooth nuclear membranes and a salt-and-pepper nuclear chromatin pattern. Binucleated and multinucleated neoplastic cells are usually seen. In less-differentiated tumors, predominated single cells with high nuclear/cytoplasmic ratio, prominent nucleoli, and mitoses are characteristic features. Immunohistochemical stains for chromogranin, neuron specific enolase (NSE), and synaptophysin may confirm the nature of neuroendocrine differentiation. As stated earlier, reliable histologic criteria, as well as cytologic criteria, to predict the malignant potential are not available.

Solid-pseudopapillary tumor of the pancreas

SPTP is an unusual low-grade malignant epithelial tumor, predominately occurring in adolescent girls and young women. The cell origin of these neoplasms is uncertain. However, the neoplasm has been shown to express epithelial, mesenchymal, and neuroendocrine markers. The long-term prognosis following an adequate local surgery is generally excellent, although local recurrence or even metastasis has been reported. An accurate preoperative diagnosis on FBAB specimen is crucial because it should lead to a more conservative surgery.

The FNAB specimen is highly characteristic. It is a highly cellular smear with clusters of papillary fronds and dissociated single cells. The papillary fronds are composed of delicate fibrovascular core covered by one to two layers of bland neoplastic cells. The tumor cells are monomorphic, bland nuclei with evenly distributed nuclear chromatin and frequent nuclear grooves. Nuclear pleomorphism, mitosis, and prominent nucleoli are consistently absent. Cytoplasmic process and hyalin globules may present. Foamy histiocytes, multinucleated giant cells, and cystic background are the common features. Immunoreactivity for vimentin and alpha-1 antitrypsin in all of the reported cases, and for progesterone receptor in some cases, is helpful in confirming the diagnosis. Focal pancytokeratin positivity can be seen from our experience and others.

Acinar cell carcinoma

Acinar cell carcinoma is a rare tumor, accounting for less than 1% of all pancreatic malignancies. This tumor has been reported in a wide age distribution, from 3–90 years, with higher frequency in males. Approximately 15% of the patients may be associated with a clinical syndrome, which is characterized by extrapancreatic fat necrosis, polyarthralgia, and eosinophilia. The FNAB specimen is usually highly cellular. It is composed of a mixture of cohesive groups and single acinar cells. The neoplastic cells tend to have high nuclear/cytoplasmic ratio, irregular nuclear contour, and prominent nuclei. Many naked nuclei may present in the background. A well-differentiated tumor may resemble benign acinar tissue. Ductal epithelial cells are usually absent. The overall cytologic features are similar to acinar cell carcinoma of the parotid gland.

Serous microcystic adenoma

Serous microcystic adenoma or serous cystadenoma is an uncommon, but benign, cystic tumor, with a striking predilection for elderly women. The tumors frequently occur in the head of the pancreas, with an average size of 10 cm. The tumors are sharply demarcated, multilocular cysts and may have a central stellate scar and a sunburst type calcification on a CT scan. The FNAB specimen is usually hypocellular and characterized by the presence of few groups of ductal-like cells in a background of clear, watery fluid. The epithelial cell groups are usually tightly cohesive, with mild nuclear pleomorphism. Focal nuclear crowding and nuclear membrane irregularity may present. Single atypical cells, marked nuclear pleomorphism, prominent nucleoli, and mitosis are not the cytologic features. Periodic acid-Schiff stain should demonstrate positive reactivity for the cytoplasmic glycogen. Mucicarmine stain for intracytoplasmic mucin is uniformly negative.

Mucinous cystic neoplasms

Mucinous cystic neoplasms are uncommon tumors of the pancreas, accounting for approximately 1% of total pancreatic tumors. It usually occurs in middle-age patients and is more common in females than males. The average size of tumors is 10 cm (ranging from 2–20 cm), and they are frequently located in the body or tail of the pancreas. All mucinous cystic neoplasms are currently regarded as having at least borderline malignant potential. However, it has been proposed that mucinous cystic tumors of the pancreas can be classified into mucinous cystadenoma, mucinous cystic tumor of borderline malignant potential, and mucinous cystadenocarcinoma, according to their grade of dysplasia. An important diagnostic clue for mucinous cystic neoplasms can be appreciated grossly, when an FNAB specimen of pancreatic lesion contains watery or viscid mucoid material. Mucoid material tends to be metachromatic on Diff-Quick stain, but it may not be very visible on the Papanicolaou stain. An additional unstained slide for mucicarmine stain is recommended. The cellularity of FNAB specimen is variable depending on the amount of mucin obtained or if the solid area is aspirated. The degree of architectural and nuclear atypia may be variable depending on the nature of the lesion. Papillary clusters may present. Unequivocal cytologic features of malignancy are diagnostic for mucinous cystadenocarcinoma. However, mucinous cystadeno-carcinoma may be noninvasive or invasive. Unfortunately, no reliable cytologic criteria are available to differentiate invasive versus non-invasive mucinous cystadeno-carcinoma.

Dpc4 protein is a nuclear transcription factor and has been demonstrated in the inactivation of more than half of the infiltrating ductal adenocarcinomas of the pancreas. The study of Dpc4 expression in 36 mucinous cystic neoplasms showed that only 1 of the 7 mucinous carcinomas was positive for Dpc4, whereas 29 noninvasive mucinous cystic neoplasms were positive.

Metastasis

Distinction of primary ductal adenocarcinoma of the pancreas from metastatic carcinoma may be impossible. As reported in the literature, the most common sources of metastatic malignant tumors of the pancreas are lung, kidney, breast, liver, and gastrointestinal tract; sarcoma; and melanoma. In our study, 11 cases of metastatic malignant tumors were identified, including renal (4 cases), stomach (3 cases), prostate (1 case), squamous cell carcinoma (1 case), liver (1 case), and sarcoma (1 case).

If a cell block is available, a panel of immunohistochemical markers may provide some useful information, including cytokeratin 7 (CK-7), cytokeratin 20 (CK-20), cytokeratin 17 (CK-17), thyroid transcription factor-1 (TTF-1), and estrogen receptor (ER). The most common staining profiles for these tumors are as follows: adenocarcinoma of the pancreas –CK7+, CK20-, CK17+, TTF-1-, ER-; adenocarcinoma of the lung –CK7+, CK20-, CK17-, TTF-1+; renal cell carcinoma –CK7-, CK20-, TTF-1-; and ductal carcinoma of the breast –CK7+, CK20-, ER+, TTF-1-. Metastatic renal cell carcinoma is frequently positive for RCC marker, CD-10, and P504S.

In summary, the majority of pancreatic lesions can be accurately diagnosed on FNAB specimens. The high diagnostic sensitivity and specificity in diagnosing adenocarcinoma of the pancreas, including WDA, can be achieved by observance of nuclear crowding/three-dimensionality, anisonucleosis, nuclear membrane irregularity, and nuclear enlargement. Other cytologic criteria, such as mitosis, necrosis, prominent nucleoli, and hyperchromasia, which are frequently present in less-differentiated adenocarcinomas of the pancreas, are of little value in diagnosing WDA. Some immunohistochemical markers, including CK-17, clusterin, Dpc4, mesothelin, and PSCA, may provide useful information in diagnosis and differential diagnosis of pancreatic adenocarcinomas on FNAB specimens. Exploration of global gene expression of pancreatic carcinomas by complementary deoxyribonucleic acid (cDNA) microarray analysis will identify more specific genes as potentially important in diagnosis and treatment of pancreatic carcinomas.

Adenocarcinoma

Endocrine cells are frequently observed in a wide variety of ordinary adenocarcinomas. In pancreatic ductal adenocarcinomas, scattered endocrine cells have been reported to be either lined up along the base of the neoplastic glands or to lie between the neoplastic columnar cells. They should be separated from endocrine cells in mixed ductal-endocrine carcinomas in which ductal and endocrine cells, which compose at least one third to one half of tumor tissue, are intimately admixed in the primary tumors as well as in their metastasis. Endocrine cells in ductal adenocarcinomas might be neoplastic considering their close association with neoplastic glands. However, metastases from ductal adenocarcinomas usually lack the endocrine cell population seen in the primary sites, and thus these endocrine cells may represent nonneoplastic rather than true neoplastic cells. Therefore, it has not been clearly concluded whether these endocrine cells are neoplastic.

To clarify whether endocrine cells are neoplastic, we studied the localization of the endocrine cells in the primary, invasive, and metastatic sites of pancreatic invasive ductal adenocarcinomas by immunohistochemistry (IHC) for chromogranin A (CgA), islet hormone (insulin, glucagon, and pancreatic polypeptide [PP]), serotonin, and gastrin.

Materials

Twenty-nine invasive ductal adenocarcinomas of the pancreas, which had been surgically resected, were collected from the University of Tokushima, Tokushima Prefecture Central, and Tokushima Municipal Civic Hospitals. The age of the 29 patients, 17 men and 12 women, ranged from 36 to 82 years, with a mean of 64.3 years. Primary sites in the pancreas were the head in 20 cases, the body in 6, and the tail in 3. Seventeen cases had metastatic lesions: lymph nodes in 15 cases, liver in 1 case, and both lymph nodes and liver in 1 case.

Methods

For immunohistochemical study, formalin-fixed and paraffin-embedded tissues were used. The labeled streptavidin biotin (LSAB) method was adopted for all reactions except for a double staining of CgA and Ki-67. Monoclonal CgA antibody (clone DAK-A3, 1:100, Dako, Glostrup, Denmark) was used to detect endocrine cells in adenocarcinoma and nonneoplastic pancreatic tissue around adenocarcinomas. Cases with CgA-immunoreactive (IR) cells in adenocarcinomas were further stained with antibodies to insulin (polyclonal, 1:100, Dako), glucagon (polyclonal, 1:75, Dako), PP (polyclonal, 1:600, Dako), serotonin (clone 5HT-H209, 1:50, Dako) and gastrin (polyclonal, 1:500, Dako). All CgA-IR adenocarcinomas were double stained with CgA and laminin (polyclonal, 1:200, Dako) to see whether endocrine cells in neoplastic glands are located within the basal membrane of the neoplastic glands. Ten CgA-positive adenocarcinomas were also double stained with CgA and Ki-67 (clone MIB-1, 1:50, Dako). The incubation time for all primary antibodies was 30 min at room temperature. Antigen retrieval was performed by autoclave (15 min) in 10 mM/L citrate buffer, pH 6.0 for CgA, and by microwave (2× at 600 W for 6 min) for serotonin. For the double staining of CgA and laminin, CgA was applied first and cobalt-3,3′-diaminobenzidine (Co-DAB) was used as a first chromogen. For a second staining sequence, antigen retrieval was performed by proteinase K (40 μ 1/3 ml 0.05 M Tris-HCl pH 7.7, Dako) before the application of laminin, and DAB served as a second chromogen. For the double staining of CgA and Ki-67, antigen retrieval was performed by autoclave (15 min) before the application of Ki-67, and Co-DAB was used as a first chromogen. CgA was detected in a second staining sequence using the Envision method (Dako) and DAB as a second chromogen.

Results

Incidence and location of CgA-IR cells

Of 29 cases, 24 (82.3%) had CgA-IR cells in the adenocarcinomas. Regarding the site of the tumor in the pancreas, there was no significant difference between cases with and without CgA-IR cells. However, most of the cases of well- (93.3%) or moderately (88.9%) differentiated adenocarcinomas had CgA-IR cells, whereas only 40% of cases of poorly differentiated adenocarcinomas did. Poorly differentiated adenocarcinomas were, thus, less likely to have endocrine cells ($P < 0.05$). About 70% (12/17) of cases with metastases and all cases (12/12) without metastases had CgA-IR cells in the primary tumors. There was no significant difference in incidence of CgA-IR cells between tumors with and without metastases.

CgA-IR cells in adenocarcinomas occupied a very small proportion of the adenocarcinoma cells, being less than 1% in all 24 cases. The CgA-IR cells lined up along the base of the neoplastic glands, showing a periglandular arrangement, or a single CgA-IR cell was at the base of the neoplastic gland. When tumor cells formed multilayered or papillary architecture, some CgA-IR cells lay between the tumor cells. In one case in which tumor cells predominantly presented papillary architecture, most of the CgA-IR cells lay between tumor cells and a few were on the luminal side. As tumor cells invaded, acini were destroyed, leaving islets. Islet cells were often broken up into small nests, cords, or single cells in the fibrous stroma and often were in contact with neoplastic glands and bordered on part of the neoplastic glands.

The double immunostaining for CgA and laminin revealed that CgA-IR cells along the base of the neoplastic glands were located within the basement membrane. Whether CgA-IR cells were located at the base of the neoplastic glands or between carcinoma cells, CgA-IR cells in neoplastic glands were at least visibly in contact with adjacent nontumorous islets or closely located to them in all 24 cases. In two cases, nests of CgA-IR cells were in the lumen of some neoplastic glands and part of the walls of the neoplastic glands were destroyed. In one of the two cases, nests were connected to the stroma and protruded into the lumen, whereas in the other case they floated in the lumen without connection to the stroma.

Tumor cells sometimes invaded the preexisting interlobular ducts and formed a front with nonneoplastic cells in the same ducts, presenting an intraductal extension in three cases. The CgA-IR cells were located at the base, lay between tumor cells, or were on the luminal side. In one of the three cases, tumor cells within the duct proliferated in cribriform or papillary architecture where CgA-IR cells on the luminal side were also seen. In another case, CgA-IR cells were found in both nonneoplastic and neoplastic epithelia of the same ducts. The CgA-IR cells in the intraductal extensions showed no contact with the surrounding islets. In the remaining 21 of 24 cases, CgA-IR cells were found only in neoplastic glands.

The CgA-IR cells were recognized in nontumorous interlobular ducts near adenocarcinomas in 21 of 24 CgA-IR adenocarcinomas and in 4 out of 5 CgA-IR tumors. They were sparsely present, ranging from 1 to 10 in a duct. There were more CgA-IR cells in hyperplastic than in nonhyperplastic epithelium. Ductuloinsular-complex-like structures, which indicated that the interlobular duct was incorporated in an islet, were found in 3 CgA-IR adenocarcinomas. In 2 CgA-IR tumors of the head, a few nonneoplastic pancreatic lobules around adenocarcinomas contained more than 20% CgA-IR cells of all cells in the lobule.

Among 24 CgA-IR tumors, there were 12 cases in which adenocarcinomas invaded the adjacent tissue beyond the pancreas. In 10 cases of the head, 6 adenocarcinomas invaded to the muscularis or further into the duodenum, 1 invaded the adjacent lymph node, and 3 cases invaded both. In the 2 cases of the body or tail, 1 tumor invaded the muscularis of the stomach and the connective tissue around the spleen, whereas the other went into the subserosa of the stomach and the adjacent lymph node. When an adenocarcinoma invaded these surrounding tissues beyond the pancreas where islets were not present, there were no CgA-IR cells in the invaded site. No pancreatic tissue was recognized in the duodenum in the present cases. Three of five cases without CgA-IR cells in the adenocarcinoma had invaded sites beyond the pancreas, but no CgA-IR cells were found there.

Of 24 CgA-IR tumors, 12 had metastatic sites. Only one case showed several CgA-IR cells in a metastatic site, one regional lymph node. This was a case of poorly differentiated adenocarcinoma of the head, where the tumor cells proliferated in nests or organoid patterns and had several regional lymph nodes as metastatic sites.

Hormonal reactivity of CgA-IR cells

Tests of IHC for insulin, glucagon, and PP were positive in 12 of 16 cases of the head; insulin and glucagon were positive in 2 cases, and insulin and PP were positive in 2 cases. No case showed serotonin positivity. In 6 of the 8 cases of the body or tail, CgA-IR cells showed glucagon and insulin positivity. Insulin, glucagons, and PP were positive in one case and insulin, glucagons, and serotonin were positive in another case, which was the only case that showed serotonin positivity in neoplastic glands. All 24 cases showed two or three islet hormones (insulin, glucagons, and PP). Different types of hormones were recognized in the same neoplastic glands or the same cluster of neoplastic glands in 22 (91.7%) of the 24 cases. Similar to immunoreactive cells for CgA in neoplastic glands, immunoreactive cells for each of the three islet hormones were closely located-to cords or nests of nontumorous islet cells, which showed the same hormonal immunoreactivity as in the neoplastic glands. Among 13 PP-IR adenocarcinomas, 12 were in the head, but only 1 was in the body. In the body case, PP cells were recognized in nontumorous islets near PP-IR cells in the neoplastic glands. The numbers of PP-IR cells were much fewer in both islets and neoplastic glands in the body than in the head. In 1 case presenting serotonin-positive cells, there were no serotonin-IR cells in nontumorous tissue around the neoplastic glands. None of the 24 cases showed gastrin positivity in neoplastic glands. In 2 cases, nests of CgA-IR cells were in the lumen of a few neoplastic glands. The nests were comprised of insulin-IR and glucagon-IR cells.

Two of three adenocarcinomas with CgA-IR cells in the intraductal extensions showed hormonal reactivity. These two were located in the head. In one case, PP-IR cells and serotonin-IR cells were in neoplastic epithelium in the duct, whereas PP-IR cells were in nonneoplastic epithelium of the same duct. The other case had serotonin-IR cells in neoplastic epithelium of the duct. In the last case in the body, CgA-IR cells were seen, but because the carcinomatous component in the duct was observed only in a specimen for HE and CgA, their hormonal activity was unknown. However, in nonneoplastic epithelia of this case, hormonal reactivity was present, which was gastrin and serotonin positivity.

CgA-IR cells were also recognized in nontumorous interlobular ducts near or at the site of invasion in 21 of 24 CgA-IR adenocarcinomas. In 19 of the 21 cases, hormonal reactivity was identified. In 14 cases, only one hormone was positive, but in the other 5 cases, two types of hormones within the same duct were identified: insulin and PP in 3 and insulin and glucagon in 2. Of the 5 CgA-negative adenocarcinomas, 4 had CgA-IR cells in nontumorous interlobular ducts. Of those 4 cases, 3 showed hormonal reactivity, but in 1 of the 3 cases only PP-IR cells were identified. In 2 CgA-IR adenocarcinomas with numerous CgA-IR cells in nontumorous lobules, these cells were PP positive. Numerous PP-IR cells in nontumorous lobules were found in another CgA-IR adenocarcinoma, but they lacked CgA positivity. In the metastatic lymph node with several CgA-IR cells in one case, a few of them showed serotonin reactivity. The other metastatic lymph nodes in this case showed no immunoreactivity for CgA or other hormones.

Ki-67 positivity of CgA-IR cells in adenocarcinoma

Ten CgA-IR adenocarcinomas were double-stained with CgA and Ki-67. None of the CgA-IR cells at the base of neoplastic glands or between tumor cells in neoplastic glands stained with Ki-67 in all 10 cases. In 1 case, tumor cells in the intraductal extension proliferated in cribriform or papillary architecture. CgA-IR cells were at the base or on the luminal side of the duct, but they were negative for Ki-67.

Discussion

Endocrine cells have been recognized in 40–80% of ductal adenocarcinomas of the pancreas and reported to be most common in well-differentiated adenocarcinoma. In our study, 24 (82.8%) of 29 cases had CgA-IR endocrine cells in the primary sites. These cells were located along the base of the neoplastic glands. When carcinoma cells formed multilayer or papillary architectures, some CgA-IR cells lay between tumor cells. Regardless of their arrangement, at least visually they always seem to be in contact with or near to the surrounding CgA-IR islet cells, which sometimes seemed to adhere to the neoplastic glands. Endocrine cells in neoplastic glands and those of the surrounding islets are often located together within the same basement membrane, as revealed by a double immunostaining of CgA and laminin. Interactions between islet and pancreatic adenocarcinoma have been reported. Kodama and Mori (1983) suggested interactions between carcinomatous ductal cells and islet cells in pancreatic carcinogenesis. In hamsters, normal pancreatic islets were necessary for the induction of pancreatic adenocarcinoma by a chemical carcinogen and ductal adenocarcinoma arose from progenitor cells in islets. Cancer cell growth has been shown to be regulated by islet hormones such as insulin and somatostatin *in vitro*. Conversely, an abnormality in islet composition and secretion is common in pancreatic cancer. For example, beta cells of the islets adjacent to the pancreatic cancer secrete increased amounts of islet amyloid polypeptide (IAPP) *in vivo* and *in vitro*. Ding *et al.* (1998) thought that a soluble factor from pancreatic cancer cells selectively stimulated amylin secretion from islet cells. It is understandable that tumor cells and surrounding islets were close in terms of location and that endocrine cells persisted within a basement membrane of neoplastic glands, if some interactions between neoplastic ductal and nonneoplastic adjacent islet cells existed.

Exocrine and endocrine components have the same origin in the developmental stage of human pancreas, the primitive gut endoderm, and originate from branching "protodifferentiated" epithelial cells with the features of duct cells.

In the first phase, i.e., 13–16th gestation week (gw), small aggregates of endocrine cells grow out from pancreatic ducts, losing their contact with ducts from gw 17–20. Because carcinomas can show features comparable to the embryonic pancreas, neoplastic glands in well-differentiated carcinomas could most likely show a close relation to islets, mimicking the developmental stage of pancreas. This may be one reason why endocrine cells are frequently seen in well-differentiated adenocarcinomas. In addition, because even in well-differentiated adenocarcinoma endocrine cells were only focally seen in neoplastic glands, the close relation of endocrine cells to neoplastic glands may only be present during the limited period of neogenesis and growth of carcinomas. Rapidly growing carcinomas such as some poorly differentiated adenocarcinomas might have no chance to present endocrine cells within them. In our study, the presence of endocrine cells in carcinoma was most unlikely in the poorly differentiated carcinoma.

We found that when carcinoma invaded adjacent organs or tissues, such as the duodenum (muscularis or further), stomach, and connective tissue around the spleen where islets of pancreas were not present, endocrine cells in carcinoma were completely absent. Therefore, the existence of islet cells near cancer seems to be a key to the existence of endocrine cells in neoplastic glands. This finding, in addition to the close location of neoplastic glands and nonneoplastic islets, leads us to believe that endocrine cells in neoplastic glands may come from the surrounding nonneoplastic islet cells.

Endocrine cells have been reported to be located in the invasive edge of cancers and to occur in the base of the neoplastic glands, at different distances from the lumen and within the lumen. In those reports it was thought that these endocrine cells were shed and renewed, as were tumor cells and constituents of tumors, and that these findings indicated the neoplastic nature of the endocrine cells. However, the occurrence of endocrine cells on the edge of the invasion may be the result of the presence of the numerous intact or broken islets because compared to acini, islets tend to survive in carcinomatous tissue. None of the endocrine cells, including those in neoplastic glands and those on the luminal side of the intraductal extension, showed Ki-67 positivity with double staining of Ki-67 and CgA. Even in normal pancreatic ducts, endocrine cells sometimes border the lumen and are joined to the neighboring ductal cells by tight junctions. Therefore, being on the luminal side does not mean that they are of a neoplastic nature. The endocrine cells on the luminal side might occur because of intricate folds of lining epithelium protruding into the lumen. In two cases here, there were nests of endocrine cells composed of insulin-positive and glucagon-positive cells, which were thought to be islets in the lumen of some neoplastic glands. It seemed that an artifact had been caused by the destruction of part of the neoplastic glands during the process of invasion to the islets. Thus, an artifact can cause nontumorous endocrine cells to be present in the lumen. Pour *et al.* (1993) reported a lack of colocation of CgA in some somatostatin or glucagon cells in tumor-associated endocrine cells and stated that this abnormality may indicate the neoplastic nature of tumor-associated endocrine cells. In one case in the present study, however, it was recognized that lack of colocation of CgA and PP positivity might indicate some effect by a carcinoma on the islets, as reported in previous articles. We believe that the findings of Pour *et al.* are insufficient to conclude that endocrine cells in pancreatic adenocarcinoma have a neoplastic nature.

As for hormonal reactivity, all four islet hormones and amylin (IAPP), serotonin, and occasionally gastrin have been identified in endocrine cells in pancreatic carcinomas. More than one type of hormonal reactivity has been identified in some cases. Colocation of two types of hormones within an endocrine cell has also been reported. In our study, all 24 cases with endocrine cells in neoplastic glands showed more than one hormonal reactivity of the three islet hormones (insulin, glucagon, and PP), and in 22 (91.7%) of the 24 cases, immunoreactive cells for different types of hormones were seen within the same gland or cluster of neoplastic glands. PP-IR cells were mostly found in neoplastic glands of the head, which is consistent with previous reports. PP-IR cells in the body were seen in one case (8.1%), which has not been reported before. PP-IR cells in nontumorous islets both in the head and body were recognized near neoplastic glands. However, the number of PP-IR cells was much fewer in both islets and neoplastic glands in the body than in the head, which reflected the differences in the numbers of PP cells seen in normal pancreas in the head and body or tail. Therefore, this finding, as well as the heterogeneity in hormonal localization within the same neoplastic glands, seems to support our hypothesis that endocrine cells in neoplastic glands may originate from the surrounding islets.

In the present study, 3 cases had endocrine cells in the intraductal extensions. These endocrine cells showed no contact with adjacent islet cells, suggesting that they could be neoplastic. They could be nonneoplastic, however, because nonneoplastic endocrine cells may be left over after neoplastic cells replaced the preexisting epithelium in the ducts. In the present study, endocrine cells in nontumorous ducts near or at the site of invasion were seen in 25 of 29 cases and most of them showed hormonal reactivity. In 1 case with intraductal extensions, endocrine cells were present in both nonneoplastic and neoplastic epithelium in the same duct. Of the 3 cases with intraductal extensions, 2 showed serotonin positivity, which is not uncommon for endocrine cells in the pancreatic duct, but is not common for those in pancreatic adenocarcinoma. We are inclined to think that endocrine cells in the intraductal extension were present before the carcinomatous invasion and that they are nonneoplastic rather than neoplastic.

There has been a report stating that endocrine cells existed in the metastatic sites of pancreatic exocrine carcinomas. However, the cases were actually mixed ductal-endocrine carcinomas, a different category from ductal adenocarcinoma with endocrine cells. In the present study, only one case showed several CgA-IR cells in one metastatic lymph node. Endocrine cells in the metastatic lymph node showed immunoreactivity for serotonin, whereas the endocrine cells in the primary site showed focal contact with the surrounding islets and immunoreactivity for insulin, glucagon, and PP. We think that these endocrine cells in the metastatic site are neoplastic. Other than this case, there were a few serotonin-positive cells in neoplastic glands of the body in only one case. Because islets usually do not have serotonin cells and there were no serotonin-IR cells in nontumorous tissue near the neoplastic glands and thus there was no source of nonneoplastic endocrine cells nearby, they could be neoplastic. However, the absence of endocrine cells in metastatic sites seen in the other cases strongly supports their nonneoplastic nature. We concluded that most endocrine cells in pancreatic ductal adenocarcinoma are nonneoplastic and are derived from the surrounding islets and that there is a possibility that endocrine cells in the intraductal extensions are preexisting nonneoplastic cells. Neoplastic endocrine cells may exist, although their frequency is low.

Ductal Adenocarcinomas

Cyclooxygenase (COX) is a rate-limiting enzyme involved in the conversion of arachidonic acid to prostaglandin H_2, which is the precursor of several molecules, including prostaglandins, prostacyclin, and thromboxanes. It consists of at least two related but unique isoforms, COX-1 and COX-2. The *COX-1* gene is located on chromosome regions 9q32-q33.3, and *COX-2* maps to 1q25.2-q25.3. The two proteins show structural and enzymatic similarities, both having a molecular weight of approximately 70 kDa and sharing more than 60% identity at the amino acid level. Nevertheless, they serve distinct functions. *COX-1* is constitutively expressed in a large number of human tissues to mediate house keeping, physiological functions such as vascular homeostasis, gastroprotection, and absorption of sodium and water in the kidney. *COX-2* is an immediate, early-response gene whose expression is induced by growth factors, tumor promoters, cytokines, and other inflammatory mediators. Its overexpression, in fact, has been demonstrated in several human inflammatory diseases e.g., *Helicobacter pylori*–infectious gastritis, inflammatory bowel disease, chronic hepatitis, Hashimoto's thyroiditis, and rheumatoid arthritis.

Recent studies have highlighted the potential role of *COX-2* in tumorigenesis. Epidemiologic studies indicate that administration of nonsteroidal anti-inflammatory drugs (NSAIDs) that inhibit both *COX-1* and *COX-2* expression reduces the risk for developing many types of human tumors. Oshima *et al.* (1996) showed that the formation of intestinal polyps in $Apc^{\Delta 716}$ knockout mice was dramatically suppressed by crossing these animals with COX-2 knockout mice. COX-2 overexpression has been found in a variety of carcinomas and several effects of COX-2 have been proposed, including inhibition of apoptosis, stimulation of invasiveness and proliferative activity, and facilitation of neovascularization. Epidermal growth factor (EGF), transforming growth factor beta (TGF-β), and their receptors as well as inducible nitric oxide synthase (iNOS) emerge as significant COX-2–inducers, not only in inflammation but also in carcinogenesis.

Overexpression of *COX-2* is also observed in premalignant lesions such as adenoma of the colon and stomach, Barrett's esophagus, dysplasia of the head and neck and esophagus, prostatic intraepithelial neoplasia, endometrial hyperplasia, and pulmonary atypical alveolar epithelium. This suggests that *COX-2* may be involved in early cellular changes leading to the development of several types of carcinoma. Inhibitors of *COX-2* could therefore play a role in chemoprevention of such cancers in a broad range.

Pancreatic ductal adenocarcinoma (PDAC) accounts for 85–90%of all pancreatic neoplasms and is currently the fifth leading cause of cancer death in Western countries. Because there are no suitable markers for early diagnosis, in the majority of patients PDAC is diagnosed at a stage that is not curable by cancer-directed surgery. Unfortunately, it is also barely affected by any other form of cancer-directed therapy, i.e., chemotherapy, radiation therapy, or immunotherapy. To achieve better insight into the disease mechanism, it is important to understand the molecular characteristics of PDAC. It has repeatedly been shown that distinct genes such as the K-*ras* gene and the tumor-suppressor genes *p53, p16,* and *DPC4/SMAD4* are frequently altered in PDAC, and may therefore be essential for its tumorigenesis. Further genetic studies have demonstrated that some cancer-related genes such as vascular endothelial growth factor (VEGF), *Her-2/neu, c-Myc, Rad51, maspin,* and *COX-2* are overexpressed in pancreatic cancer cells. The identification and characterization of these genes will lead to a better understanding of PDAC pathogenesis and provide therapeutic strategies. Especially notable is *COX-2,* because the *COX-2* inhibitors have been demonstrated to inhibit proliferation and induce apoptosis in human pancreatic carcinoma cells and in PDAC in Syrian golden hamsters. Interestingly, pancreatic islets are among the few tissues that constitutively express *COX-2*. However, only a few studies have been done on *COX-2* expression in pancreatic endocrine tumors (PETs).

Here, we reconfirmed *COX-2* expression in 28 PDACs and 20 PETs immunohistochemically using the EnVision ChemMate method. EnVision is a very sensitive detection method for routine immunohistochemistry (IHC) and is a two-step staining technique in which the primary antibody is followed by a polymeric conjugate in sequential steps. The polymeric conjugate consists of a large number of peroxidase and secondary antibody molecules bound directly to an activated dextran backbone.

Materials

1. Tissue sections: Tumor tissues were fixed in 10% formalin and embedded in paraffin, and the paraffin block sections were cut at into 3-μm thick sections and placed on silane-coated glass slides for immunohistochemical staining.
2. 10 mM citrate buffer: 0.36 g citrate acid•1 H_2O and 2.44 g trisodium citrate•2 H_2O were dissolved in distilled water and made up to 1 L solution.
3. TBS (Tris-buffered saline: 6.06 g trisaminomethane and 3.40 ml HCl) was added to distilled water and the volume was brought up to 1 L with distilled water.
4. TBS containing 0.1% Tween-20 (TBS-T) and 5 ml Tween-20 were added to 5 L of TBS.
5. Primary antibody: Anti-human *COX-2* rabbit polyclonal antibody diluted at 1:200 with antibody diluent.
6. Blocking reagent (DakoCytomation).

7. Visualization system: HRP conjugated dextran polymer reagent (DakoCytomation).
8. Chromogen: 3,3-diaminobenzidine tetrahydrochloride (DAB) (DakoCytomation).

Methods

(ChemMate EnVision working procedure)

1. Bake tumor tissue sections for 30 min at 65°C in incubater, deparaffinize in xylene, and rehydrate through ethanol.
2. Rinse the sections in water.
3. For antigen retrieval, pretreat the sections by microwaving (960 W) for 10 min in 10 mM citrate buffer that has been microwaved for 10 min.
4. Quench the endogeneous peroxidase activity by adding a few drops of 0.3% H_2O_2 onto the sections, and incubate in moisture chamber for 6 min.
5. Rinse the sections with TBS-T, and immerse the sections in TBS-T for 5 min.
6. Add a drop of the blocking reagent onto the sections in order to prevent nonspecific background staining, and place in moisture chamber for 5 min.
7. Tap off the excess blocking reagent and wipe slide; incubate with primary antibody in moisture chamber for 30 min at room temperature.
8. Rinse the sections with TBS-T, and immerse in TBS-T for 5 min.
9. Incubate the sections with dextran polymer reagent (ChemMate, EnVision) in moisture chamber for 30 min at room temperature.
10. Rinse the sections with TBS-T, and immerse in TBS-T for 5 min.
11. Develop the sections with Liquid DAB chromogen in moisture chamber for 10 min at room temperature.
12. Rinse with water.
13. Counterstain lightly with hematoxylin, and rinse in water for 5 min.
14. Dehydrate through ethanol and clear through xylene.
15. Coverslip the sections and mount.

The *COX-2* immunostaining was evaluated as negative, weakly positive, moderately positive, or strongly positive. The cases were then divided into high expressers (i.e., when at least 10% of tumor cells were moderately to strongly positive) and low expressers. We evaluated the *COX-2* expression in relationship to a number of clinicopathological features. Additional immunohistochemical studies used antibodies to Ki-67 (Dako), p53 (Oncogene Research Products, Boston, MA), and DPC4 (Santa Cruz Biotechnology, Santa Cruz, CA). All statistical evaluations were carried out using Student's t-test and χ^2 test for independence (2×2 contingency table). Statistical significance was tested at a probability level of 0.05.

Results and Discussion

All PDACs showed cytoplasmic staining for COX-2 of variable extent. Of PDACs, 19/28 (67.9%) were classified as high expressers and 9 were low expressers. So far, several authors have reported *COX-2* overexpression in PDACs by Western Blot, reverse transcription polymerase chain reaction (RT-PCR), and IHC, and the frequency of *COX-2* immunohistochemical overexpression ranges from 53% to 90%. Tucker *et al.* (1999) showed a more than 60-fold increase in COX-2 messenger ribonucleic acid (mRNA) expression in PDAC tissues in parallel with up-regulation of the COX-2 protein. These findings indicate that COX-2 up-regulation is a frequent event in PDACs.

Okami *et al.* (1999) did not find any significant differences between high expressers and low expressers among clinicopathological parameters, including age, sex, location, histological grade, nodal involvement, metastasis, and stage. We also found no correlation between COX-2 expression and sex, size, location, histological grade, and Ki-67-labeling index except patients' age (high and low expressers; average ages 66.5 and 59.3 years, $p = 0.046$). Therefore COX-2 expression does not seem to be affected by clinicopathological features. Merati *et al.* (2001), however, showed that COX-2 over-expression was significantly related to perineural invasion and was more common in the glandular component than in the solid component.

Our investigation revealed a close relationship between COX-2 expression and abnormalities in *p53* (high and low expressers; 17/19 and 5/9, $p = 0.04$) and DPC4 (15/19 and 4/9, $p = 0.07$). Recent genetic analyses have indicated that the tumorigenesis of PDAC is a complex, multistep process involving the progressive accumulation of alterations in oncogenes such as K-*ras* and tumor-suppressor genes such as *p16, p53,* and *DPC4.* Moreover, the accumulation of genetic changes correlates with increasing grade of dysplasia of pancreatic intraepithelial neoplasias (PanINs), which are considered precursor lesions of PDAC. Since significant COX-2 expression is observed in PanINs, it is possible that COX-2 contributes to the carcinogenesis of PDAC via PanINs and may be interrelated with the previously mentioned cancer-associated genes. Overexpression of COX-2 in premalignant lesions is also observed in intraductal papillary-mucinous neoplasms, where the hypothesis of the adenoma-carcinoma developmental sequence is widely accepted.

PETs, particularly insulinomas, usually show benign behavior, but some can metastasize widely. The diagnosis of malignancy and the prognostic assessment are difficult, because the histological appearance of PETs does not correlate with their biological behavior. A new World Health Organization classification provides three categories: (i) tumors with benign behavior; (ii) tumors with uncertain behavior (borderline lesions); and (iii) carcinomas (low-grade or high-grade malignancy) based on tumor size, angioinvasion, metastasis, mitotic index, Ki-67-LI, and the hormone produced. Like PDACs, PETs showed heterogeneous and cytoplasmic staining for COX-2 in almost all cases, and 13/20 (65%) were high expressers. Further, based on the WHO classification, the 13 high expressers included 3 of 4 borderline lesions and all malignant tumors (10 cases), while the low expressers consisted of 1 borderline lesion and all benign tumors (6 cases). Moreover, the 13 high expressers showed significantly large tumor size, frequent angioinvasion and metastasis, and a high Ki-67 labeling index compared to the low expressers. Therefore, COX-2 may be a potential marker that indicates the malignant behavior of PET. A corresponding result in neuroendocrine tumors has been found in pheochromocytomas. Okami *et al.* (2002), however, showed that COX-2 might well play a role in the endocrine function of PETs, but that its expression is unrelated to its biological behavior. They proposed that, to elucidate whether *COX-2* expression is associated with tumor development and malignant potential, further examinations on more cases focusing on *COX-2* expression in stromal cells as well as tumor cells are required.

The surrounding islet cells, acinar cells, duct cells, or stromal cells showed weak or negative COX-2 expression in most cases of PDAC and PET, and only occasionally exhibited strong expression. However, the significance of intense *COX-2* expression in tumor-surrounding stromal cells remains unclear. *COX-2* was also found to be involved in nonneoplastic diseases such as chronic pancreatitis and diabetes mellitus. Thus, tumor-associated pancreatitis may also have an influence on *COX-2* expression in PDAC-associated stromal cells. In conclusion, this study showed that *COX-2* overexpression is a frequent event in PDACs and PETs, when studied with the EnVision ChemMate method, which is a very sensitive, easy detection system for routine

IHC. For both tumors, *COX-2* seems to be somehow related to their progression from premalignant lesions to definite carcinomas and *COX-2* inhibitors might therefore be effective chemopreventive agents.

Mast Cells in Cancer

Mast cells play a key role in immediate hypersensitivity (type I) immune reactions. Binding of a specific antigen to two adjacent immunoglobulin E (IgE) molecules expressed on mast cell plasma membrane ("cross-linking") initiates the process of degranulation, which is the release of preformed mediators of the inflammatory reaction contained in mast cell granules (e.g., histamine, adenosine, heparin, various proteases). At the same time, the synthesis of new mediators (e.g., prostaglandins, leukotrienes, cytokines, and growth factors) is initiated. Through this and other IgE-independent mechanisms (e.g., under the stimulation of the anaphylotoxins C3a and C5a, dextran, basic peptides and physical agents), mast cells exert their function as major cell mediators of the allergic reactions. At the same time, they are also involved in acute and, at a higher level, chronic fibrogenic inflammatory processes in which they directly induce fibrosis through the production of fibroblast growth factor (FGF), platelet-derived growth factor (PDGF), and transforming growth factor-β. The differentiation of mast cells from bone marrow precursors and their proliferation is promoted by stem cell factor (SCF), which binds to c-kit, a type-3 tyrosine–kinase receptor. Mast cell precursors complete their maturation at peripheral sites, under the influence of the specific local microenvironment. There are many cellular sources of SCF: fibroblasts, endothelial cells, the basal cells of the epidermis, and various tumor cells. Mast cells can also produce SCF and stimulate their own growth in an autocrine way.

Role of Mast Cells in Nonpancreatic Tumors

Studies have provided evidence that mast cells play an important yet controversial role in the pathogenesis of human neoplasms. The accumulation of mast cells at the tumor infiltrative borders was first described by Westphal in 1891. More recently it has been demonstrated that mast cells can produce and release growth factors, proangiogenetic factors, and lytic enzymes, which might influence local tumor growth and invasion. The number of infiltrating mast cells has been found to be associated with the intratumoral microvessel density and to be directly correlated with the presence of lymph node metastases in lung adenocarcinoma. It also correlates with a worse prognosis in non-Hodgkin's lymphoma.

Furthermore, metastatic melanomas show a higher number of vascular endothelial growth factor (VEGF)-positive mast cells at the tumor periphery when compared with nonmetastatic tumors. The expression of VEGF and other proangiogenic factors (tryptase, basic fibroblast growth factor [bFGF]) by peritumoral mast cells has been also described in squamocellular larynx cancer and esophageal cancer. In breast cancer the production of the serin-proteases tryptase and chymase by mast cells has been related to the tumor's invasive ability. In contrast, the number of mast cells has been found to be correlated with a shallower penetration of gastric cancer cells into the gastric walls and with a lower number of lymph node metastases in patients with gastric cancer.

Role of mast cells in pancreatic cancer

Pancreatic cancer is an aggressive disease with a dismal prognosis. In its classic ductal histotype pancreatic cancer appears as a "scirrhous" tumor, characterized by well-to-moderately differentiated neoplastic glands embedded in a dense stroma. The onset of pancreatic adenocarcinoma can be preceded by a chronic inflammatory condition, chronic pancreatitis, which has been recognized as a definite risk factor for the development of pancreatic cancer. This risk increases with the duration of the disease and is particularly high in patients affected by hereditary pancreatitis, who develop the disease at a young age. In 2001, using deoxyribonucleic acid (DNA)-array technology, the expression patterns of 5600 genes in pancreatic tissues were analyzed, comparing chronic pancreatitis with the normal pancreas and pancreatic cancer. The results of this study showed that the mast cell serine-protease tryptase is overexpressed in chronic pancreatitis (11.1-fold), and to a lesser extent in pancreatic cancer (7.3-fold), when compared to the normal pancreas. Tryptase is contained in mast cell granules and is released as a preformed mediator on mast cell degranulation. It is considered a specific marker for mast cells; moreover, tryptase immunostaining can reveal the presence of mast cells with a higher sensitivity than histochemical stainings such as toluidine blue or Giemsa. Therefore, the increased expression of tryptase messenger ribonucleic acid (mRNA) in chronic pancreatitis and pancreatic cancer in comparison with the normal pancreas might correspond to an increased number of mast cells in these disorders.

Tryptase is a proteolytic enzyme that exerts a proinflammatory activity by cleaving multiple substrates, such as prothrombin, fibrinogen, prourokinase, and neuropeptides. In addition, tryptase acts as a signaling molecule by binding to a protein G–coupled receptor named PAR-2 (protease activated receptor-2), thus inducing different cell responses, such as vasodilation, leukocyte adhesion and extravasation, and cytokine synthesis. Moreover, tryptase exerts a fibroproliferative action by binding PAR-2 and then stimulating the synthesis of cyclooxygenase 2 (COX2) and prostaglandins, which ultimately leads to fibroblast proliferation. The induction of angiogenesis is another important function of tryptase, which can specifically induce endothelial cell proliferation and capillary formation. Mast cells, as the cellular source of tryptase, are therefore likely to play an active role in fundamental pathogenic aspects of chronic pancreatitis and pancreatic cancer, such as the induction of stromal cell proliferation and angiogenesis.

A further step in our analysis was the evaluation of mast cell expression (through tryptase immunostaining) in chronic pancreatitis of varying etiology. We demonstrated an increase in total mast cell number in comparison with the normal pancreas and a correlation between mast cell number and the degree of inflammation and fibrosis. However, the etiology of chronic pancreatitis was not related to the number of infiltrating mast cells.

In this chapter we summarize an analysis of mast cell infiltration in pancreatic cancer and of its relation to the SCF-c-kit system, which provides novel information about the biology of this disease. These data have been published in detail elsewhere.

Materials

1. 10% formalin: 37% formalin diluted 1:10 in water.
2. Carnoy's solution: 6 parts of ethanol (absolute or 95%), 3 parts chloroform, 1 part glacial acetic acid.
3. Xylene.
4. Ethanol solutions: 99%, 95%, 70%, 50%, and 30% diluted in deionized water.
5. Tris-buffered saline (TBS) + 0.1% bovine serum albumin (BSA): combine 3.03 g Tris HCl and 8.18 g NaCl, bring volume to 1 L with distilled water, adjust pH to 7.4; add 1 g BSA.
6. Methanol.
7. Methanol/0.6% hydrogen peroxide (H_2O_2): 4 μl of 30% H_2O_2 in 200 μL methanol.
8. Primary antibodies: mouse anti-tryptase (Chemicon International, Temecula, CA) diluted 1:1000 in normal goat serum (NGS) (Kirkegaard and Perry Laboratories, Gaithersburg, MD); mouse

anti-chymase (Chemicon International) diluted 1:4000 in NGS (Kirkegaard and Perry Laboratories); goat anti-SCF (Santa Cruz Biotechnology, Santa Cruz, CA) diluted 1:100 in normal rabbit serum (NRS) (Kirkegaard and Perry Laboratories); rabbit anti-c-kit (Santa Cruz Biotechnology) diluted 1:200 in NGS (Kirkegaard and Perry Laboratories).

9. Pronase (1 mg/ml in TBS, pH 7.5).
10. Biotinylated secondary antibodies (rabbit antigoat, goat anti-rabbit, goat anti-mouse) (Kirkegaard and Perry Laboratories).
11. Streptavidin-peroxidase complex.
12. Diaminobenzidine (DAB): 10 μg/ml in distilled water.
13. Tris-HCl buffer: dissolve 121.1 g of Tris base in 800 ml distilled water. Adjust pH to 7.6 by adding HCl. Bring volume to 1 L.
14. DAB tetrahydrochloride solution (DAB + Tris- HCl + 0.03% H_2O_2): 200 μL DAB + 3 ml Tris-HCl buffer + 3 μl H_2O_2 30%.
15. Mayer's hematoxylin.
16. Mounting medium.

Methods

Immunostaining procedure

1. Fix the tissue samples immediately after surgical removal in 10% buffered formalin or in Carnoy's solution (for chymase detection because formalin fixation destroys chymase immunoreactivity) for 12–24 hr at room temperature; then embed them in paraffin and cut into 4 μm thick sections.
2. Deparaffinize in xylene (3×, 10 min each).
3. Rehydrate in descending ethanol solutions: ethanol 99% (3×, 5 min each), 95% (1×, 5 min), 70% (1×, 5 min), 50% (1×, 5 min), 30% (1×, 3 min), deionized water (1×, 3 min).
4. Rinse the sections in TBS-0.1% BSA (2×, 5 min).
5. Pretreatment: in the case of SCF immunostaining a pretreatment of the tissue sections is necessary to improve antigen retrieval. Incubate the sections with 100 μl of pronase solution for 6 min at 37°C on a warming plate.
6. Rinse the sections in TBS-0.1% BSA (1×, 5 min).
7. Quench the endogenous peroxidase activity: incubate the sections for 1 min in methanol, then for 20 min in methanol/0.6% hydrogen peroxide, then again for 1 min in methanol, and finally for 3 min in deionized water.

8. Rinse the sections in TBS-0.1% BSA (2×, 5 min).
9. Block nonspecific binding by incubating the sections in normal serum (2–3 drops) at room temperature for 30 min in a humid chamber to prevent evaporation.
10. Primary antibody: After removal of the serum, incubate the slides with the appropriate primary antibody (100 μl per section) overnight at 4°C in a humid chamber.
11. Rinse the sections in TBS-0.1% BSA (2×, 5 min).
12. Incubate with the appropriate secondary antibody (2–3 drops) at room temperature for 45 min in a humid chamber.
13. Rinse the sections in TBS-0.1% BSA (2×, 5 min).
14. Incubate with the streptavidin-peroxidase complex (2–3 drops) at room temperature for 30 min in a humid chamber.
15. Rinse the sections in TBS-0.1% BSA (2×, 5 min).
16. Color reaction: Add 100 μl of DAB solution to each section, and incubate in the dark at room temperature for a maximum of 15 min (usually 2–5 min are enough, check under the light microscope); stop the reaction in deionized water.
17. Counterstain the slides in hematoxylin (30 sec– 1 min), then rinse in tap water.
18. Dehydrate the sections in ascending ethanol solutions: ethanol 50% (1×, 5 min), 70% (1×, 5 min), 95% (1×, 5 min), 99% (2×, 5 min).
19. Clear the tissue sections in xylene (3×, 5 min).
20. Mount.

To ensure antibody specificity, consecutive sections can be incubated in the absence of primary antibody or in the presence of a nonimmune serum.

Evaluation of immunohistochemical findings

The number of tryptase/chymase-positive mast cells is assessed by counting the stained cells in each specimen at a 200X magnification after determination of the area of the whole tissue section using a computer-assisted image analysis system. The results are expressed as number of cells/mm^2. The number of SCF and c-kit–positive mast cells is expressed as a percentage of total mast cells present in each section, by comparing two consecutive sections stained with antitryptase and anti-SCF or anti-tryptase and anti-c-kit, respectively. Other methods of mast cell counting have been described. For example, the tissue section can be examined at low magnification (100X) to find the areas with higher mast cell density. Then, the single cells are counted at 200X magnification in the five fields with the highest cell density and the mean value is taken as the mast cell count for that case. Expression of SCF and c-kit by cancer cells is quantified by counting at least 1000 cells in each tumor sample. The immunohistochemical results are scored positive when 5% of the tumor cells are immunoreactive.

Results and Discussion

Demographic and pathologic characteristics of the patient population

The patient population comprised 10 males and 16 females (median age: 69 years; range: 35–83 years) suffering from pancreatic cancer. Normal pancreas tissues were obtained through an organ donor program (n = 17; 11 male, 6 female; median age: 46 years; range: 18–77 years).

The specimens were subjected to histologic analysis; the staging and grading of the cancer specimens were assessed according to the TNM classification of the International Union Against Cancer (1997). All the tumor samples were ductal adenocarcinomas; 7 (27%) were well differentiated (G1), 14 (54%) were moderately differentiated (G2), and 5 (19%) were poorly differentiated (G3). Four tumors (15%) were in stage I, 5 (19%) were in stage II, 15 (58%) were in stage III, and 2 (8%) were in stage IV.

Mast cell count and characterization in the normal pancreas and pancreatic cancer

The presence of inflammatory cells in the neoplastic tissues is considered a mechanism of host defense against cancer. However, it has been demonstrated that the production and release of lytic enzymes and growth factors by the inflammatory infiltrate can promote the growth and invasive capacity of the cancer cells. It is well known that chronic inflammatory conditions favor the development of neoplastic processes in many tissues and organs. Although different mechanisms can be involved in different anatomic sites, it seems that the presence of the inflammatory cells might alter the tissue environment, thus making the normal cells more susceptible to malignant transformation. Free radicals, produced by neutrophils and activated macrophages, are among the factors that can generate this anomalous microenvironment; they induce DNA damage and can be directly mutagenic.

The tissue damage in the context of a chronic inflammatory condition leads to the production and release of cytokines and growth factors that stimulate the regeneration of the damaged cells but at the same time induce the proliferation of genomically altered cells. Mast cell infiltration of the tumor tissues can enhance the invasive capacity of the cancer cells essentially by promoting the angiogenic process. In human and animal tissues two main populations of mast cells have been identified: tryptase-positive mast cells (MCT), also known as mucosal-type mast cells, and tryptase/chymase double-positive mast cells (MCTC), also named connective-tissue–type mast cells.

In this study we used a monoclonal antibody directed against the enzyme tryptase to detect the presence and the number of mast cells in the normal pancreas and in pancreatic cancer tissues. Immunohistochemistry revealed that mast cells are found around blood vessels and nerves, in the interstitial space between acinar lobules, around the neoplastic glands, and at the infiltrative borders of the tumor. The mean number of tryptase-positive cells in cancer tissues was 1.7-fold higher than in the normal pancreas ($p = 0.03$), thus confirming at a morphologic level the increased gene expression levels that resulted from the DNA-array analysis.

After chymase immunostaining of Carnoy-fixed tissue samples, the mean number of positive cells was 2.8-fold higher in pancreatic cancer than in the normal pancreas, thus indicating the presence of connective-tissue-type mast cells in pancreatic tissues as well as their accumulation in pancreatic cancer.

We further characterized the pancreatic cancer–associated mast cells by staining consecutive sections with tryptase and SCF or tryptase and c-kit. Only a small percentage of the mast cells present in the normal samples or in the cancer specimens stained positive for SCF. Cytoplasmic or membrane staining for c-kit was detected in up to 18.5% of total mast cells in the normal pancreas and in up to 16% of total mast cells in pancreatic cancer.

SCF and c-kit expression in the normal pancreas and pancreatic cancer

The acquisition of the mature phenotype by mast cells is tissue-specific and mostly regulated by the SCF–c-kit system. These two factors are produced by different kinds of tumor cells, but their role in the promotion of tumor growth is still under discussion. In some human neoplasms (e.g., lung cancers) the co-expression of SCF and c-kit by tumor cells has been interpreted as an autocrine growth-stimulating loop. In other tissues, the development of malignancy is accompanied by a decrease of SCF–c-kit expression (e.g., thyreocytes, melanocytes). It was therefore interesting to determine the expression of these factors in the human pancreas and to explore their possible relation to the accumulation of mast cells in pancreatic cancer.

In the normal pancreas, SCF immunostaining was limited to mast cell cytoplasm. In contrast, 20% of the cancer specimens exhibited SCF-immunoreactivity in 5–10% of the cancer cells. c-kit was detected in the cytoplasm or on the cell membrane of mast cells. Additionally, moderate to strong c-kit immunoreactivity was present in the cytoplasm of ductal cells of normal and hyperplastic ducts. The c-kit–positive pancreatic ducts were often surrounded by c-kit–positive and, less frequently, SCF-positive mast cells. In addition, pancreatic cancer cells frequently showed c-kit immunoreactivity (73% of the cases). No correlation was found between mast cell number, c-kit or SCF expression, and the histopathologic characteristics (grading, TNM status, stage) of the tumors.

In summary, we have shown an accumulation of mast cells in pancreatic cancer. Pancreatic mast cells belong to the connective-tissue type, they express c-kit and SCF, and they tend to accumulate around c-kit–expressing ducts. Moreover, pancreatic cancer cells frequently express c-kit, whereas SCF expression is restricted to about one-fifth of the tumor cases. Based on these results, it seems that the SCF–c-kit system does not significantly contribute to the growth of pancreatic cancer, although it is possible that SCF-positive cancer cells can recruit mast cells to the tumor mass. The reason for mast cell accumulation in pancreatic cancer is not known. It. is possible that the cells represent a nonspecific inflammatory response to the tissue damage provoked by the growth of the cancer cells. However, examining larger series of pancreatic adenocarcinomas, we have found high expression of proangiogenic growth factors (VEGF, bFGF) by pancreatic mast cells and an association between the number of pancreatic cancer–associated mast cells and the angiogenetic process, measured by the assessment of the intratumoral microvessel density after CD34-immunostaining of endothelial cells.

In conclusion, tryptase and chymase immunostaining reveals with high specificity the presence of mast cells in pancreatic tissues, where they accumulate possibly in response to the chemotactic capacity of tumor-derived SCF. Mast cells produce and release proangiogenic growth factors (tryptase, VEGF, bFGF) that ultimately lead to tumor angiogenesis and invasion and thereby influence the prognosis of pancreatic cancer.

Stat3 Protein in Cancer

Pancreatic cancer is the fifth most common cause of cancer death in the Western World and is a leading cause of cancer death worldwide. The American Cancer Society estimated that there would be 30,700 new cases of pancreatic cancer and 30,000 deaths from pancreatic cancer in the year 2003 in the United States alone. The current 5-year survival rate is approximately 1–2%, and the median survival time after diagnosis is 4–6 months. The prominent cause of death in patients with pancreatic adenocarcinoma is metastatic disease. Unfortunately, patients usually have metastatic disease that is locally advanced or involving the lymph nodes, liver, lungs, or peritoneum at the time of diagnosis. The aggressive nature of metastatic pancreatic adenocarcinoma is caused by the activation of various oncogenes and inactivation of various tumor-suppressor genes, as well as abnormalities in growth factors and their receptors, which together affect the downstream signal transduction pathways involved in the control of cell growth and differentiation. These perturbations confer a tremendous growth advantage on pancreatic cancer cells. One of these transduction pathways is the Stat3 (signal transducer and activator of transcription 3) signal transduction pathway, which is the focus of this chapter.

Stat3 is one of seven Stat proteins that have been identified, which represent a unique group of proteins that are key mediators of various cytokine signaling pathways that control cellular growth, differentiation, development, and survival. The Stat proteins are inactive as transcription factors in the absence of specific receptor stimulation and are located in the cytoplasm of unstimulated target cells. They are activated rapidly in response to receptor-ligand coupling and are recruited to the intracellular domain of the receptor through specific binding of the Stat Src-homology 2 (SH2) domains to receptor phosphotyrosine residues. Stat proteins are then phosphorylated in tyrosine and serine residues. The phosphorylation is mediated most often by the cytokine receptor Janus-associated kinases (JAKs) or growth factor receptor tyrosine kinases. Once phosphorylated, the Stats form homodimers or heterodimers, enter the nucleus, and lead to increased transcriptional initiation, thereby altering the expression of specific target genes and affecting the downstream production of those genes.

Stat3, a member of the JAK-Stat signaling pathway, is ubiquitously expressed in most tissues as a latent transcription factor. Stat3 was first identified as a deoxyribonucleic acid (DNA)-binding factor that selectively interacts with an enhancer element in the promoter of acute-phase genes from interleukin (IL)-6–stimulated hepatocytes. The gene that encodes *Stat3* is located on chromosome 17q21, and it encodes a 92-kD protein. Structurally, Stat3 is similar to other Stat proteins, in that it has a conserved amino-terminus involved in tetramerization, a DNA-binding domain with a sequence specific for a palindromic interferon-gamma (IFN-γ)–activated sequence (GAS) element very similar to that of Stat1, an SH2 domain involved in receptor recruitment and Stat dimerization, and a carboxy-terminal transactivation domain.

Stat3 is activated by many cytokines and growth factors, including epidermal growth factor, plateletderived growth factor, and IL-6; it also is activated by oncogenic proteins such as Src and Ras. On activation, Stat3 is phosphorylated on tyrosine residues (Tyr705) by activated JAK kinases in receptor complexes; this leads to the formation of homodimers and heterodimers and their translocation to the nucleus, where they regulate transcription. Tyrosine phosphorylation is required for Stat3 dimerization, nuclear translocation, and DNA binding. Stat3 can also be phosphorylated in the serine residue in the C-terminal transcriptional domain, which has been found to enhance the transcriptional activity of Stat3. There is also evidence that serine phosphorylation serves a negative function, but the mechanism involved is unclear.

The biological functions of Stat3 are very broad. For example, Stat3 plays a crucial role in the regulation of cell proliferation, survival, apoptosis, and differentiation. In normal cells and in animals, ligand-dependent activation of the Stat3 is a transient process, lasting for several minutes to several hours. In contrast, in many cancer cell lines and tumors, the Stat3 protein is persistently activated. In particular, constitutively activated Stat3 protein has been found in various types of tumors, including leukemia and cancers of the breast, head and neck, melanoma, prostate, and pancreas.

Studies have revealed that altered Stat3 could contribute to oncogenesis. For example, Stat3 activation has not only been observed in cells transformed *in vitro* with v-*src* and v-*abl* oncogenes, but this activation also is demonstrated to be required for v-*src* to mediate cellular transformation. Further, Stat3 activation has been demonstrated to be sufficient to mediate cellular transformation. Overexpression of the constitutively activated Stat3 mutant (Stat3-C) into immortalized NIH 3T3 fibroblasts induced cellular transformation and tumor formation in nude mice, providing genetic evidence that Stat3 has oncogenic potential. Moreover, it has been observed that the level of Stat3 activation correlates with the stages of human malignancies.

In terms of its effects in tumor cells, Stat3 activation has been found to prevent apoptosis and enhance cell proliferation in many human tumor cells by regulating genes that encode proteins involved in cell growth and apoptosis, including cyclin Dl, C-Myc, Bcl-x_L, and Mcl-1. Conversely, the blocking of constitutive Stat3 signaling results in the growth inhibition and apoptosis of Stat3-positive tumor cells *in vitro* and *in vivo*. These results therefore further suggest that Stat3 functions as an oncogene and plays a critical role in transformation and tumor progression.

Several lines of evidence indicate that the constitutive activation of Stat3 contributes to malignant transformation and the progression of human pancreatic cancer. Specifically, the prevalence of activated Stat3 in nontransformed pancreatic tissue, chronic pancreatitis, and pancreatic adenocarcinoma has been analyzed. All carcinoma samples analyzed expressed activated Stat3, whereas ductal epithelium from nontransformed pancreatic tissue obtained from the resection margins of pancreatic tumors or tissue obtained from patients with chronic pancreatitis showed negligible or no activated Stat3 expression. Moreover, most pancreatic cancer cell lines examined have shown constitutively activated Stat3. Further incriminating Stat3 in the oncogenesis of pancreatic cancer was the finding that the blockade of the activated Stat3 inhibited pancreatic cancer cell growth *in vitro* and *in vivo*.

The mechanisms for this inhibition could be the result in part of the down-regulation of Bc1-x_L expression caused by the inhibition of Stat3 activation in pancreatic cancer cells. Furthermore, the finding that activated Stat3 directly regulates the promoter of the angiogenic molecule vascular endothelial growth factor (VEGF) gene is another clue to Stat3's role in the development of pancreatic cancer. This was shown by the fact that the blockade of activated Stat3 by ectopically expressed dominant-negative Stat3 significantly inhibited VEGF expression, and hence angiogenesis and the growth and metastasis of human pancreatic cancer cells. These results therefore collectively show that the activation of the Stat3 signaling pathway is critical for pancreatic tumor progression and that Stat3 activation may constitute both a diagnostic and prognostic marker as well as a molecular target for therapeutic interventions.

In the current study, we examined the expression of activated Stat3 in human pancreatic cancers using a phosphotyrosine-specific Stat3 antibody (p-Stat3 [Tyr-705]). As noted earlier, the tyrosine phosphorylation of Stat3 constitutes an early event in the activation of this transcription factor and is required for its dimerization and DNA-binding activity. Of particular importance, the constitutive tyrosine phosphorylation of Stat3 is necessary for this transcription factor to exert its oncogenic effect. Therefore, this phosphotyrosine-specific Stat3 antibody exclusively detects activated Stat3 and, for this reason, has been used in numerous studies.

Materials

1. Formalin-fixed and paraffin-embedded primary pancreatic adenocarcinoma specimens and normal pancreatic tissue specimens.
2. Xylene.
3. Ethanol.
4. Distilled H_2O (dH_2O).
5. Phosphate buffer saline (PBS): 100 mg of anhydrous calcium chloride, 200 mg of potassium chloride, 200 mg of monobasic potassium phosphate, 100 mg of magnesium chloride 6 H_2O· 8 g of sodium chloride, and 2.16 g of dibasic sodium phosphate 7 H_2O; bring volume to 1 L with dH_2O, and adjust pH to 7.5.
6. 50 mM Tris buffer: 0.6 g of Tris(hydroxymethyl) amino-methane in 100 mL of dH_2O; adjust pH to 7.6 using HCl.
7. 10 mM Sodium citrate buffer: add 2.94 g of sodium citrate to 1 L of dH_2O, and adjust pH to 6.0.
8. Trypsin (Invitrogen Corporation, Carlsbad, CA).
9. 3% H_2O_2 in methanol: add 9 ml of 30% H_2O_2 to 92 ml of methanol.
10. Blocking solution: 5% bovine serum albumin (BSA) and 5% normal horse serum (Jackson Immunoresearch Laboratories, Inc., West Grove, PA) in PBS.
11. Primary antibody: a polyclonal rabbit antibody against activated Stat3 (Phospho-Stat3 [Tyr-705]; Cell Signaling Technology, Inc., Beverly, MA). Phospho-Stat3 (Tyr705) antibody detects endogenous levels of Stat3 only when phosphorylated at tyrosine 705. This antibody does not appreciably cross-react with the corresponding phosphotyrosines of other Stat proteins. Polyclonal antibodies are produced by immunizing rabbits with a synthetic phosphopeptide corresponding to residues around Tyr705 of Stat3. Antibodies are purified by protein A and peptideaffinity chromatography.
12. Secondary antibody: peroxidase-conjugated antirabbit immunoglobulin (IgG).

13. Diaminobenzidine (DAB) solution: dissolve 50 mg of DAB (3,3-diaminobenzidine tetrahydrochloride; Sigma) in 99.5 ml of PBS and add 0.5 ml of 30% H_2O_2; use immediately because solution is good for only 20 min.
14. Hematoxylin.
15. Universal mount.

Methods

Tissue slide preparation

1. Standard tissue sections (5 μm thick) of specimens were cut and mounted on glass slides.
2. Air-dry the slides overnight at room temperature.

Deparaffinization

1. Heat the section slides at 60°C for 30 min.
2. Incubate the section slides in xylene for 6 min at room temperature. Repeat the step 1×.

Rehydration

1. Rinse the slides with 100%ethyl alcohol (ETOH) 2× for 2 min each.
2. Rinse the slides with 95%ETOH 2× for 1 min each.
3. Rinse the slides with 80% ETOH for 1 min
4. Rinse the slides with 50% ETOH for 1 min.
5. Rinse the slides with PBS 2× for 2 min each.

Antigen retrieval

1. Immerse the slides in 10 mM sodium citrate buffer (pH 6.0).
2. Heat the slides in a microwave oven for 1 min at high power, followed by 19 min at medium power.
3. Cool the slides for 20 min after antigen unmasking.

Tissue digestion

1. Incubate sections with 0.025% trypsin in 50 mM Tris buffer (pH 7.6) for 5 min at 37°C.
2. Rinse slides with PBS 3× for 2 min each and continue the immunostaining.

Immunostaining procedure

1. Use paper towel to wipe around the tissue on each slide.
2. Draw a circle with a Pap pen around tissue on each slide.
3. Place all slides in a humidified chamber (care must be taken to prevent tissue from drying out).

4. Quench endogenous peroxidase by placing slides in 3% H_2O_2 / methanol for 15 min.
5. Rinse the slides with PBS 3× for 5 min each.
6. Incubate each slide with 300 μl of blocking solution for 1 hr at room temperature.
7. Remove blocking solution and add 200 μl of diluted primary antibody (diluted 1:50 in blocking solution) to each slide. Incubate the slides overnight at 4°C.
8. Rinse as in Step 2.
9. Incubate each slide with 300 μl of blocking solution for 1 hr at room temperature.
10. Remove blocking solution and add diluted secondary antibody (anti-rabbit IgG, 1:500 diluted in blocking solution). Incubate the slides with the antibody for 2 hr.
11. Rinse as in Step 2.
12. Add 150 μl of DAB solution to each slide. At this point, the slides may be examined under a brightfield microscope to monitor the staining quality. Positive staining is shown by the finding of a reddish-brown precipitate in the nucleus.
13. As soon as the section turns brown, immerse slides into dH_2O.
14. Rinse the slides with dH_2O 3× for 5 min each.
15. Counterstain slides with hematoxylin for 10 sec.
16. Rinse the slides briefly with dH_2O.
17. Rinse the slides with PBS for 1 min.
18. Rinse the slides with dH_2O 2× for 5 min each.
19. Mount the slides with universal mount and place on hot plate (65°C) for 30 min to dry the slides.
20. The slides are now ready for final examination under a bright-field microscope.

Specimen analysis

1. The sections were examined by a pathologist who was blinded to the clinical characteristics of the patients.
2. The intensity of staining of activated Stat3 was evaluated by a digital image analysis system and personal computer equipped with the Optimas Image Analysis software program.
3. The intranuclear staining of tumor cells was considered to indicate the presence of constitutively activated Stat3.

4. Immunohistochemistry (IHC) staining results were classified into three groups depending on the percentage of cells with positively stained nuclei, as follows: negative (<10%), weakly positive (10%–24%), and strongly positive (≥25%). Specifically, if less than 10% of tumor cells showed a nuclear staining pattern, the slide was classified as negative. When the percentage of positive tumor cells was between 10–25%, the slide was classified as weak positive. When the percentage of positive tumor cells was equal or more than 25%, the slide was classified as strong positive.

Results and Discussion

We determined the degree of expression of activated Stat3 in a panel of human pancreatic adenocarcinoma specimens (20 cases) and in normal pancreatic tissue specimens (10 cases) obtained from subjects who did not have cancer, as shown by IHC analyses using an anti-phospho-Stat3 (Tyr705) antibody. This antibody exclusively detects activated Stat3 and does not cross-react with latent Stat3. Fifteen of the 20 (75%) pancreatic adenocarcinomas strongly expressed phosphorylated Stat3 in the foci of pancreatic adenocarcinoma. The Stat3 staining was mainly localized in the nuclei of the pancreatic cancer epithelial cells. In contrast, among 10 normal pancreatic tissues, analysis of the immunohistochemical staining showed either negligible or negative expression of activated Stat3. These results therefore showed that Stat3 is highly activated in pancreatic tumor tissue but not in normal pancreatic tissue. Consistent with the data, several studies have shown that majority of human pancreatic cancer cell lines highly express constitutive activated Stat3.

The mechanisms responsible for the overexpression of activated Stat3 in pancreatic tumors are largely unknown. It is known that Stat3 is activated by various cytokines and growth factors, including epidermal growth factor and fibroblast growth factor, and by oncogenic proteins such as Src and Ras. Significantly, these molecules are also often overexpressed in pancreatic cancers. For example, the epidermal growth factor receptor (EGFR) is overexpressed in approximately 90%of human pancreatic cancers. Further, either an EGFR-specific antagonist or a neutralizing antibody were observed to suppress constitutive Stat3 DNA-binding activity in human pancreatic cancer cells. Because these experiments were performed without exogenous growth factors and cytokines, they clearly identified autocrine or paracrine EGFR signaling as a major upstream stimulus of Stat3 activation in human pancreatic cancer cells. Several groups have additionally observed the overexpression and activation of tyrosine kinase Src in most human pancreatic ductal adenocarcinoma, raising the possibility that the activation of Src contributes to the constitutive activation of Stat3 in pancreatic cancers. The activation of the K-*ras* oncogene is also a common genetic alteration in pancreatic cancers. It therefore seems that the constitutive activation of Stat3 in pancreatic cancers is a result of the previously mentioned aberrant epigenetic and genetic alterations that occur during malignant transformation.

Because of its central position downstream in the signaling pathways from growth factors, cytokines, and oncogenic protein tyrosine kinases, aberrant Stat3 activity is a key mediator in the development and progression of tumors. Stat3 executes its roles in the processes through transcriptional regulation of several important target genes. For example, activated Stat3 has been shown to regulate the expression of the anti-apoptotic regulatory proteins Bcl-x_L and Mcl-1, thereby preventing the apoptosis of tumor cells. It is interesting that, both Bcl-x_L and Mcl-l proteins have been detected in pancreatic cancer tissue. Specifically, Bcl-x_L is up-regulated early in tumor development, and this persists throughout pancreatic carcinogenesis. Moreover, Stat3 activation induces increased Bcl-x_L expression in pancreatic cancer cells. Conversely, the inhibition of Stat3 transcription factor leads to Bcl-x_L down-regulation and induces apoptosis in pancreatic cancer cells. Of further note, in a clinical study, the enhanced expression of Bcl-x_L in pancreatic cancer was found to be associated with shorter patient survival. Stat3 also contributes to cancer cell proliferation by regulating the cyclin Dl, C-*Myc*, and *p21*^{WAF1} genes. In particular, constitutively activated Stat3 has been found to transcriptionally up-regulate cyclin Dl expression; indeed, this gene is overexpressed in 85% of invasive pancreatic carcinomas. The C-*Myc* gene that is also regulated by *Stat3* is commonly deregulated in pancreatic cancer and may be involved in early neoplastic development and progression. Furthermore, activated Stat3 regulation of p21^{WAF1} expression in pancreatic cancer cells could be a cell-type–specific regulatory event. Inhibition of activated Stat3 led to a delay in the G1/S-phase progression of pancreatic cancer cells, which was caused by selective inhibition of p21^{WAF1} expression.

More recently, we have demonstrated that Stat3 may contribute to the angiogenesis of pancreatic tumors by regulating the expression of VEGF, a key mediator of tumor angiogenesis. Like other solid tumors, the growth and metastasis of pancreatic adenocarcinoma is dependent on angiogenesis, the formation of new blood vessels from a preexisting network of capillaries. Of the numerous angiogenic factors discovered so far, VEGF, also known as vascular permeability factor, has been identified as a key mediator of tumor angiogenesis. Indeed, the level of VEGF was noted to be significantly elevated in biopsy specimens of human pancreatic adenocarcinoma, as it has in human tumor biopsy specimens of various other cancers. Physiologically, the pancreas is a highly vascularized organ, and the VEGF level is quite high in the islets of normal pancreas but relatively low in the pancreatic ductal epithelial cells. However, significantly elevated expression of VEGF is found in biopsy specimens of human pancreatic adenocarcinoma.

The mechanism of VEGF expression and its regulation in human pancreatic cancer are mostly unknown. We have shown that the overexpression of VEGF in human pancreatic cancer cells is the result of elevated Stat3 activity. This was shown by several findings. First, we found that both human pancreatic cancer cells and human pancreatic cancer specimens have constitutively activated Stat3 and that its activation directly correlated with the level of VEGF expression. In addition, the overactivation of Stat3 correlated directly with increased blood vessel density.

Further experiments of ours indicated that Stat3 regulates VEGF expression by directly interacting with the VEGF promoter via a Stat3 response element or elements on the VEGF promoter. Our data also indicated that VEGF can be excessively up-regulated as a result of the constitutive overactivation of Stat3. Conversely, the blockade of activated Stat3 by ectopically expressed dominant-negative Stat3 in human pancreatic cancer cells significantly down-regulated the constitutive expression of VEGF.

Furthermore, the inhibition of activated Stat3 suppressed tumor angiogenesis, tumor growth, and metastasis *in vivo*. Taken together, these studies therefore provide evidence that activated Stat3 in human pancreatic cancer cells regulates the expression of genes related to cell survival, cell proliferation, and tumor angiogenesis. Tumor cell proliferation, survival, angiogenesis, and invasion are essential for tumor growth and metastasis; to that end, activated Stat3 is a critical transcription factor in human pancreatic cancer tumor development and progression.

In summary, activated Stat3 is overexpressed in human pancreatic cancers as compared with normal pancreatic tissues. Stat3 has also been found to be constitutively activated in the human pancreatic cancer cell lines examined. Stat3 may contribute to human pancreatic cancer development and progression by collectively affecting the expression of genes related to cell survival, cell cycle control, and angiogenesis, such as the genes that encode Bcl-x_L, p21^{WAF1}, and VEGF. In turn, these results suggest that activated Stat3 might serve as both a molecular marker for the early detection of human pancreatic cancer and a prognostic indicator for use in determining the aggressiveness of the disease. It might also serve as a target for therapy, as indicated by the fact that the blockade of activated Stat3 significantly inhibited VEGF expression, angiogenesis, and the metastasis of human pancreatic cancer cells. Thus, targeting of Stat3 signaling may represent a novel approach to controlling the angiogenesis, growth, and metastasis of human pancreatic cancer.

Maspin in Cancer

Maspin is a recently identified protein related to the serpin family of protease inhibitors. The *maspin* gene is part of a serpin locus cluster at chromosome 18q21.3-q23 closely linked to plasminogen activator inhibitor type 2, Bcl2, the tumor-suppressor gene *DCC*, and squamous cell carcinoma antigen 1 and 2. Maspin was originally isolated from normal mammary epithelium by subtractive hybridization. In cultured human mammary myoepithelial cells, maspin is a predominantly cytoplasmic protein that associates with secretory vesicles and is present at the cell surface.

Maspin is down-regulated but not mutated in cancer cells. It is also known to be a tumor suppressor that inhibits the motility, invasion, and metastasis of the breast and prostatic cancer cell lines. Maspin is also known to be part of the p53 tumor-suppressor pathway and acts as an inhibitor of angiogenesis. However, its functional mechanisms are considered to be unresolved and its role as a protease inhibitor is not clearly established.

Only a few reports of maspin expression in pancreatic neoplasm have been published. In our study, we investigated the expression of maspin in 107 resected pancreatic neoplasms and nontumorous pancreatic lesions. The pancreatic tumors included were 38 ductal adenocarcinomas, 13 intraductal papillary mucinous tumors (IPMTs), 13 mucinous cystic tumors (MCTs), 16 pancreatic endocrine tumors (PETs), 10 solid-pseudopapillary tumors (SPTs), 5 serous cystadenomas, 4 pancreatoblastomas, 2 acinar cell carcinomas, 4 adenosquamous carcinomas, and 2 undifferentiated carcinomas available for assessment. The tumors were classified according to the histologic criteria outlined by the World Health Organization using hematoxylin and eosin stains of formalin-fixed and paraffin-embedded tissue. The stage was classified according to the staging manual of the American Joint Committee on Cancer.

Materials

1. Xylene.
2. Ethanol.
3. Phosphate buffer saline (PBS) (pH 7.4).
4. Tris-buffered saline (TBS) (pH 7.4).
5. 0.01 M sodium citrate buffer (pH 6.0).
6. 30% hydrogen peroxide.
7. Absolute methanol.
8. Primary antibody (Maspin, Pharmingen, San Diego, CA; 1:3,000).
9. Antibody diluent (Dako Glostrup, Denmark).
10. Antibody/peroxidase-conjugated polymer (EnVision+, Peroxidase, Mouse, Dako).
11. Diaminobenzidene (DAB)+ chromogen (Dako).
12. Hematoxylin.
13. Distilled or deionized water.
14. Mounting media.

Methods

1. Paraffin sections (4 μm thick) are mounted onto poly-L-lysine–coated glass slides.
2. Dry slides in an oven for 1 hr at 60°C.
3. Deparaffinize the slides in three changes of xylene.
4. Rehydrate the slides in a graded series of ethanol.
5. Wash the slides 2× in PBS.
6. Microwave 0.01 M citrate buffer of pH 6.0 for 3 min.
7. Place the slides in the citrate buffer and microwave at 97°C for 5 min.
8. Cool the slides in citrate buffer solution at room temperature for 10 min.
9. Rinse slides and place them in the TBS.
10. Incubate slides with 3% hydrogen peroxide in absolute methanol for 10 min.
11. Wash with TBS 3× for 2 min each.
12. Remove excess liquid from around specimen.

13. Apply primary antibody against Maspin (Pharmingen; 1:3,000) to slides and incubate in moist chamber at room temperature for 1 hr.
14. Rinse with TBS 3× for 2 min each.
15. Apply EnVision+, Peroxidase, Mouse (Dako) for 30 min.
16. Rinse with TBS 3× for 2 min each.
17. Apply substrate-chromogen solution (DAB) for 3–5 min.
18. Rinse well with distilled water.
19. Counterstain with hematoxylin.
20. Dehydrate and mount.

Results and Discussion

The cells were considered positive if granular cytoplasmic/nuclear or cytoplasmic staining was observed. The staining was evaluated using the "quick score," where estimation was made of both the proportion and intensity of the cells stained. The proportions were scored as 0 (0), 1 (less than 1/100 of tumor cells), 2 (1/100–1/10 of tumor cells), 3 (1/10–1/3 of tumor cells), 4 (1/3–2/3 of tumor cells), and 5 (more than 2/3 of tumor cells), whereas the intensity was assigned as 0, no staining; 1, weak; 2, moderate; and 3, strong staining. For statistical analysis, the tumors were divided into no (total score of 0), low (total score of 5 or less), and high (total score of 6 or more) expressers.

All cases of ductal adenocarcinomas expressed maspin, of which 30 (78.9%) were classified as high expressers and 8 (21.1%) were low expressers. The majority of tumor cells showed strong cytoplasmic expressions that occasionally accompany nuclear staining. There was no statistical difference between the maspin expression (low versus high) and clinicopathologic parameters including histologic grade, lymph node metastasis, or stage. However, the staining score for maspin was positively correlated with the tumor size ($p = 0.004$). Four cases of adenosquamous carcinoma exhibited high expressions for maspin in both areas of the adenocarcinoma and squamous carcinoma. In two cases of undifferentiated carcinoma, there was low expression in the glandular area but not in the sarcomatous area.

All 13 IPMTs were stained with maspin, as were 11 of the 13 MCTs. Staining patterns were variable and heterogeneous. All six cases of intraductal papillary mucinous carcinoma and two of the three IPMTs of borderline malignant potential expressed high levels of maspin, whereas all four cases of intraductal papillary mucinous adenoma showed a low level of maspin expression. All three cases of mucinous cystic carcinoma, three out of four MCTs of borderline malignant potential, and one out of six mucinous cystadenoma were high maspin expressers. Maspin was expressed more frequently in the dysplastic epithelium. The invasive component of intraductal papillary mucinous carcinoma and mucinous cystic carcinoma showed strong immunoreactivity for maspin. It is interesting that, with increasing degree of dysplasia the localization of maspin seemed to shift from nuclear/cytoplasmic staining to cytoplasmic staining that was prominently seen in ductal adenocarcinoma.

Of the four cases of pancreatoblastoma, one case displayed a high expression for maspin in the glandular and solid portion with squamoid nests, whereas three cases showed focal immunoreactivity for maspin in the solid squamoid cell nests. In the case with a high expression, tumor cells were more pleomorphic with frequent mitosis than those with low expression.

None of the PETs were positive for maspin. One case, which was originally diagnosed as ductal adenocarcinoma and negative for maspin, showed a strong immunoreaction for chromogranin and was reclassified as PET. Some cases of PET that showed vascular invasion, adjacent organ involvement, or metastasis, however, were still negative for maspin. In addition, two cases of acinar cell carcinoma were also negative. These data are not surprising in view of the report by Pemberton *et al.* (1997), which showed that maspin expression was associated almost exclusively with epithelia in many of the human tissues. Our data confirmed the observation that maspin expression may be involved in the tumor of epithelial differentiation but not in endocrine and acinar cell differentiation.

Another interesting observation in our study was the absence of immunoreactivity for maspin in serous cystadenoma and SPT. There are two possible explanations for the lack of maspin expression in these neoplasms. In our experience maspin was focally expressed in the main and interlobular duct epithelium with mucinous cytoplasm but not in the intralobular, intercalated, or centroacinar cells of normal pancreatic tissue. The ductal epithelium of the pancreas is divided into two compartments: the mucinous cells lining the main and interlobular ducts and the ductulocentroacinar (intralobular) compartments. Ductal adenocarcinoma, MCT, and IPMT are closely related to the former, whereas serous cystadenoma and SPT are related to the latter compartment. It is therefore possible that maspin expression may be up-regulated in the neoplasms of the main and interlobular duct origin. However, the absence of maspin expression might be caused by their minimal malignant potential.

In normal pancreatic parenchyma and chronic pancreatitis adjacent to the tumor, maspin expression was rarely seen in the interlobular and the main duct epithelium but not in the intralobular, intercalated or centroacinar cells. Acinar and islet cells were negative for maspin in all cases.

In our study, all of the pancreatic ductal adenocarcinomas were positive for maspin, and the carcinomatous portion of IPMT and MCT showed high expression for maspin in contrast to the reduced or no maspin expression in the advanced breast and prostate cancers. Maass *et al.* (2001) also demonstrated this conflicting expression of maspin in pancreatic cancer. They observed a strong cytoplasmic reaction in 23 of 24 pancreatic ductal adenocarcinomas, but they saw negative staining in normal pancreas by immunohistochemistry using a monoclonal antimaspin antibody (Pharmingen). In their study, there was no correlation between the staining intensity and the histologic grade or stage of the tumors. They also reported that more than half of the pancreatic cancer cell lines expressed maspin messenger ribonucleic acid (mRNA) and suggested that up-regulated maspin mRNA expression is translated into protein in pancreatic cancer cells.

Pemberton *et al.* (1997) also could not detect maspin mRNA expression in intralobular duct epithelia of the pancreas by Northern Blot. However, they observed maspin staining in intralobular duct epithelia of the pancreas using affinity-purified polyclonal antimaspin immunoglobulin G. We thought that this discrepancy of maspin staining in normal pancreas might be caused by different characteristics of the antimaspin antibody.

Of note, Pemberton *et al.* (1997) observed that proliferating epithelial cells at the base of the crypts in the stomach stained strongly with maspin in comparison with surface epithelium. In their study on breast and prostate, myoepithelial cells and basal cells exhibited much stronger staining than adjacent luminal epithelium. Based on these observations, they suggested that maspin down-regulation may be a normal event in cell differentiation and that maspin contributes to the maintenance of normal architecture. However, to date the function and significance of maspin expression in pancreatic cancer is unknown and further investigation is needed.

The up-regulated cytoplasmic maspin expression in pancreatic tumors can be interpreted in several aspects. Maass *et al.* (2001) suggested that the maspin gene could be one of possible genes involved in pancreatic carcinogenesis because the *maspin* gene is mapped on chromosome 18q21.3 in close proximity to the *DCC* and *DPC4/SMAD4* genes and losses of chromosome 18q including *DCC* and *DPC4/SMAD4* are the most frequently identified genetic alterations in pancreatic cancer. However, the cytoplasmic expression of maspin can be speculated as an inactive or nonfunctional form in pancreatic cancers. In summary, maspin may play an important role in the carcinogenesis of pancreatic neoplasm with epithelial origin, especially for pancreatic tumor composed of mucin-producing cells. Maspin immunostaining may also be a useful adjunctive marker for differentiating ductal adenocarcinoma from SPT, PET, acinar cell carcinoma, and chronic pancreatitis.

Pancreatic Endocrine Tumors

Pancreatic endocrine tumors produce and secrete various peptide hormones that induce hormone-related syndromes. For instance, excessive production of gastrin mediates the Zollinger-Ellison syndrome; insulin causes hypoglycemia; and glucagon induces the "glucagonoma syndrome," which is characterized by necrolytic migratory erythema, diabetes, and diarrhea. The Verner-Morrison syndrome, which is brought about by high circulating levels of vasoactive intestinal peptide (VIP), produces severe secretory diarrhea. The "somatostatinoma syndrome" is associated with gallbladder dysfunction and gallstones, diarrhea with or without steatorrhea, and impaired glucose tolerance. Cushing's syndrome, which results from an ectopic adrenocorticotropic hormone (ACTH)-producing tumor of the pancreas, is also noteworthy. The diagnosis of functioning tumors is established by the measurement of the specific tumor marker in the plasma. Specific markers for pancreatic endocrine tumors include insulin, gastrin, glucagon, VIP, somatostatin, serotonin, and ACTH. The immunohistochemical study of peptide hormones is important for the pathologic diagnosis of pancreatic endocrine tumors. Le Bodic *et al.* (1996) have reported an immunohistochemical study of the 100 pancreatic endocrine tumors: 7 were unclassified, 10 were plurihormonal, and 83 produced a predominant hormonal secretion (with 50–90% of the same cell type). Those included 37 glucagonomas, 27 insulinomas, 11 pancreatic polypeptide (PP)-cell tumors, one gastrinoma, and one VIP-cell tumor.

In addition to the peptide hormones, general markers for the diagnosis of pancreatic endocrine tumors are available. Among these, plasma chromogranin A (CGA) has proved to be of great value for diagnosing functioning and nonfunctioning tumors and is considered the most sensitive general marker. Chromogranins are a family of water-soluble, acidic glycoproteins that are present in almost all endocrine, neuroendocrine, and neuronal tissue. This family comprises five members: chromogranin A (CGA), chromogranin B (CGB)/secretogranin I, secretogranin II/chromogranin C, 7B2, and NESP55. The molecules of human CGA and CGB are 48,000 and 76,000 Daltons, respectively. The role of chromogranins has been assumed to be the formation of neuroendocrine granules by aggregating with amines, nucleotides, calcium, and other peptides.

Antisera against CGA and CGB and secretogranin II are used for analyzing the bovine pancreas by immunoblotting and immunohistochemistry (IHC). In IHC, CGA is found in all pancreatic endocrine cell types with the exception of most PP-producing cells. For chromogranin B, only a faint immunostaining is obtained. For secretogranin II, A and B cells are faintly positive, whereas the majority of PP cells exhibit a strong immunostaining for this antigen. For pathologic diagnosis of the pancreatic endocrine tumors, CGA is the most effective general tumor marker independent of the previously mentioned peptide hormones; however, CGB is expressed less. Unlike pancreatic endocrine tumors, CGB is a useful marker for some rectal, ovarian, or testicular carcinoids. When tumors with endocrine tumor-like histology show no immunoreactivity for CGA, immunohistochemical study of CGB is highly recommended.

Materials and Methods

For immunostaining of CGA, pancreatic endocrine tumor tissues are fixed in 10% buffered formalin and embedded in paraffin. Chromogranins in neuroendocrine granules are usually well-preserved, and it is worthwhile to examine the immunohistochemical staining for pathologic diagnosis even in poorly fixed tissues.

For hormone or chromogranin immunostaining, antigen-retrieval pretreatments should be avoided. The antibodies for CGA and CGB are commercially available. Thin sections of 3 μm are suitable for immunostaining. Immunohistochemical procedures using various kits such as the avidin-biotin method, streptavidin-biotin method, amino acid polymer method, or dextran polymer method, are available.

The procedures should be followed according to the manufacturer's manual. For example, CGA staining is given here. After dewaxing, the sections are immersed in ethanol. Endogenous peroxidase activity is blocked with 0.03% hydrogen peroxide in methanol for 10 min. After washing with phosphate buffer saline (PBS), the sections are incubated with normal goat serum for 10 min to decrease nonspecific staining. The sections are incubated for 18 hr at 4°C with rabbit polyclonal antibody for human CGA. After washing, the sections are incubated with biotinylated anti-rabbit goat immunoglobulin (IgG) for 30 min. After washing with PBS, the sections are incubated with streptavidin-biotin peroxidase complex for 30 min. After washing with PBS, the sections are incubated in 0.33% 3,3´-diaminobenzidine tetrahydrochloride in 0.1 M Tris buffer and 0.02% hydrogen peroxide mixture for 10 min. Counterstaining is performed with hematoxylin or methylgreen. A normal pancreas section is simultaneously stained as positive control. For negative control, normal rabbit serum is incubated instead of CGA antibody. The streptavidin-biotin peroxide complex method is applied using a Histofine SAB-PO kit.

Results and Discussion

All pancreatic endocrine tumors examined are positive for CGA. The marker CGA is diffusely stained in cytoplasm. Immunoreactive intensity of CGA is usually weaker in endocine tumors than that of normal pancreatic islets. CGA is used as the tumor marker of first choice for pancreatic endocrine tumors both for IHC and as a serum marker. Then, any peptide hormones should be examined depending on the symptom or syndromes of patients with tumors.

The amino acid sequences of chromogranins have many dibasic sites that, in theory, can still be processed. Actually, sequence homology between the middle portion of chromogranin A and pancreastatin was revealed, and it formulated prohormone concept for the chromogranins. Since then, numerous novel peptides have been described, some of them with biological activity. Human pancreastatin (PST) is deduced to be a 52-residue peptide amide that is present as residues 250–301 of human chromogranin A as a sequence homologous of porcine pancreastatin.

Human PST is reported to suppress insulin release, and a significant increase of plasma PST has been observed in some patients with pancreatic islet tumors. Double immunostaining of PST and pancreatic hormones in human pancreas showed PST immuno-reactivity in all pancreatic endocrine cells, including insulin, glucagon, somatostatin, and PP cells. PST is also detected in pancreatic endocrine tumors. Other chromogranin-derived peptide hormones detected in the pancreatic endocrine tumors are chromacin (the midportion fragment CGA 176-195) in insulinomas and WE-14. Neuroendocrine secretory protein 55 (NESP55) is another novel member of the chromogranin family. Jakobsen *et al.* (2003) showed that 14 out of 25 pancreatic endocrine tumors expressed NESP55. Advances in the study of novel peptides, especially of region-specific antibodies to fragments of chromogranins, could lead to further characterization of pancreatic endocrine tumors.

For the treatment of pancreatic endocrine tumors, especially metastatic endocrine tumors, a somatostatin analog is effective. The presence of somatostatin receptor, especially types 2 and 5, should be confirmed before treatment. The immunohistochemical study of somatostatin receptor combined with chromogranins can contribute greatly to the diagnosis and treatment of patients with pancreatic endocrine tumors.

INDEX